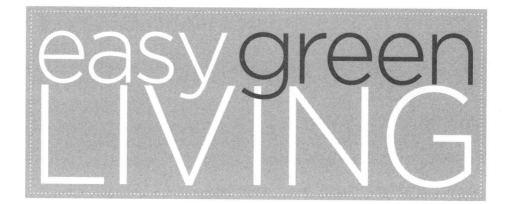

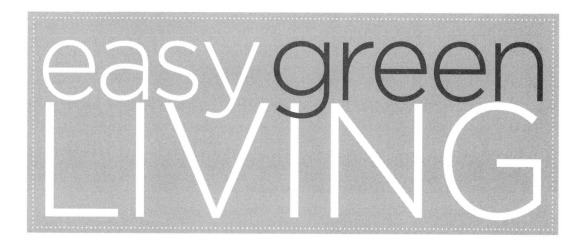

# easy green LIVING

the ultimate guide to simple, eco-friendly choices for you and your home

# Renée Loux

HOST OF FINE LIVING'S *It's Easy Being Green*

RODALE

Rodale books may be purchased for business or promotional use or for special sales. For information, please write to: Special Markets Department, Rodale Inc., 733 Third Avenue, New York, NY 10017

Printed in the United States of America

Rodale Inc. makes every effort to use acid-free ∞, recycled paper ♻.

Book design by Judy Stagnitto Abbate/Abbate Design

Illustrations by Connie Stern, except for the illustrations of the flower and the earth @ImageClub/Fotosearch

**Library of Congress Cataloging-in-Publication Data**

Loux, Renée.
    Easy green living : the ultimate guide to simple, eco-friendly choices for you and your home / Renée Loux.
       p.    cm.
    Includes bibliographical references and index.
    ISBN-10 1–59486–792–5  hardcover
    ISBN-13 978–1–59486–792–7  hardcover
    1. House cleaning—Environmental aspects.   2. Natural products.   I. Title.
  TX324.L68  2008
  640—dc22
                                                       2008005406

Distributed to the trade by Macmillan

2  4  6  8  10  9  7  5  3  1  hardcover

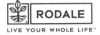

LIVE YOUR WHOLE LIFE™

We inspire and enable people to improve their lives and the world around them

For more of our products visit **rodalestore.com** or call 800-848-4735

TO A GRACEFUL, SUSTAINABLE RELATIONSHIP
BETWEEN ECOLOGY AND ECONOMY

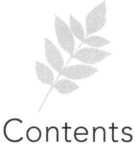

# Contents

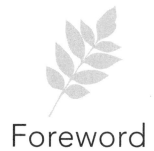

# Foreword

Hawaii is one of those places on Earth that reminds you that you live on a planet. The first time I met Renée, I was walking along the beach in Maui. Renée had been surfing, and she emerged from the ocean like a mythical sea goddess. A beautiful emissary from Atlantis or some other magical place, sent to our world to remind us of our higher selves. I even seem to recall seaweed clinging to her as if she were "of the sea." (This may be an embellishment; however, my artistic license is paid in full.) She was fit, clear-eyed, and energetic and exuded positivity and well-being. She embodied Health.

"Hi, I'm Renée. I'm Shep's friend," she said. She was referring to her husband, Shep Gordon. I had met Shep in 1991 while filming *Wayne's World* with Alice Cooper. Shep is Alice's manager. The type of manager who takes care of his clients diligently while at the same time maintaining his humanity and grace. He is a good friend and a great teacher. Hearing Renée say "I'm Shep's friend" made me realize that she would soon become a good friend as well. She impacts the life of everyone she meets. Just ask Shep. He's never looked better or lived better.

Renée is the type of spiritual seeker who not only speaks of her ideals, but lives them out as well. She believes that spirituality requires a soldier's discipline and not just a bumper sticker's bromide. This book expresses her passion for living green, and my hope is that after you read this book, Renée will have convinced you how easy green living really is.

She will teach you how to create an eco-friendly kitchen, she will explain the environmental hazards in a nongreen household, and, more important, she will offer real and easy green solutions. From this book I learned that cleaning products do not have to list their ingredients even though many aerosol room sprays are publicly registered as "aspiration haz-ards," and that microwave popcorn bags are lined with nonstick chemicals.

I now eat air-popped popcorn and use green cleaning products in my house. I have installed water filters (eliminating plastic water bottles and the fossil fuels used for their delivery). I have switched to energy-efficient lightbulbs that produce the same amount of light while using 25 percent of the energy. I use recycled paper products. Every year, more than 900 million trees are cut down for paper and pulp mills. More than 40 percent of landfill area is paper. I purify my indoor air with houseplants, avoiding aerosols and the electricity wasted on mechanical air purifiers. In my laundry room I use biodegradable detergent, oxygen bleach, and an energy-efficient washer and dryer. I started buying organic foods to avoid the chemicals used in the cultivation of conventional foods and to save the fossil fuels used for their delivery. I continue to buy organic foods because they taste better. If I can't buy organic, which I'm happy to say is less and less common, I now know a great recipe for veggie washing so I can reduce pesticide residue.

Because of this book, *Easy Green Living*, and its author, Renée Loux, I live more greenly. And it is easy.

*Mike Myers*

# Acknowledgments

First, last, and every morsel between, to my beloved Shep, with love that no words can fulfill, you are my everything, more than anything.

To my Mama and Daddio, for always believing in me and instilling in me that the greatest treasure in life is happiness. I always hope to make you proud.

To Lyle and Erika, and my precious niece, Ella.

To Jim and Elizabeth Wiatt and Isabel and Caroline, for love and support like family, I adore you to no end.

To Mike Myers, for wit and intellect that melt and inspire, and for the dear friendship that Shep and I absolutely treasure.

To Tom Kartsosis, my closet earth-muffin pal, I promise to make you cookies no matter what.

To Margaret Hecht, who opens me to where there is no beginning and no end, and for love, friendship, and laughter not bound by this lifetime.

To Lavinia Currier, my dear friend, for always welcoming me as family and for introducing me to my husband, my love knows no bounds.

To Liz Penta, my dearest friend, for reminding me of what's right and good and for walking the talk with passion and poise.

To Marty Kriegel, for a depth of intelligence, compassion, and friendship that I am eternally grateful for.

To Michel Nischan, my hero and friend, for the vision, gifted talent, and contagious passion you share with everyone you touch. And Lori Nischan, you are something! I love you both tremendously.

To Helen Hunt, for beauty through and through, treasured friendship, and grace.

To Owen Wilson, for being an all-time good guy and true friend, *mi casa es su casa*, always.

To Ed McCall, for the way you walk in the world. You are the real deal and I adore you unabashedly.

To Eddie and Nicki, who infuse my body and soul with the breath of life and are with me no matter the time or miles.

To Karen Bouris, my brilliant confidant and savvy sounding board, for embodying dexterous balance with love and goddess intellect.

To Dominique Pandolfi, the lens through which you see the world is one I am honored to be in, thank you for capturing these moments and for treasured, enduring kinship.

To Kelly Tisdale, for smiles that make my toes curl with delight, my adoration runs deep.

To Alicia Silverstone, with dear affection for my best lady, you are like a sister and touch my heart always.

To Alice and Sheryl Cooper, for love like family and kindness like kin, may the good times keep coming.

To Amber Williams, for being exactly who you are and for giving me effervescent hope for the world and the next generation, I love you lots.

To Dick and Lauren Schuler Donner, we love you more on Maui.

To Jerry and Annie Moss, *me ke aloha*, for sharing the joyful dream.

To Paul Newman, Joanne Woodward, and Nell Newman, you have stolen my heart and inspire us all on unparalleled levels, thank you.

To Willie and Annie Nelson, always generous, kind, and insisting that the world keep turning our way.

To Annbeth Eschbach and Julia Sutton, for vision and commitment to Exhale for the future.

To Lora Krulak, for being fabulous, daring to dream big, and celebrating success with genuine friendship.

To Noel Newbolt, for making everything happen with ease, you are the best and I appreciate you so much.

To Steve Murphy, for enveloping me in the Rodale family, there's no place like home.

To Joel Gotler, my keen literary agent, thank you for making it all happen.

To Pat Kingsly for taking me under the wing of PMK; Annie Jeeves, my superwoman publicist; and lovely Lauren Auslander, for mighty media support and green gusto.

To Adam Sher, my savvy and dashing agent, from the moment we met, I knew I was in good hands with a bright horizon, you rock.

To Scott Myers and everyone at Distillery Pictures, for sharing the passion, producing *It's Easy Being Green*, and making dreams come true.

To Karen Bolesta, editing conductor extraordinaire, for taking on this project with dedication and distinction.

To Anne Halpin White, my fearless, brilliant editor, for the insight, passion, and patience to make this book a reality line by line, thank you, thank you.

To Nancy Bailey, project manager superstar, who gracefully and supportively kept all the systems moving forward on point under a fierce schedule.

To Judy Stagnitto Abbate, book designer extraordinaire, and Joanna Williams, senior book design master, for their brilliant fresh design to frame this piece of work with elegant finesse.

To Nancy Elgin, sagely copy editor, for incredible, assiduous accuracy and consistency of presentation.

To Staci Sander, genius fact checker, for verifying each and every of the 1,143 footnotes with superhuman skill; you are my hero.

To Keith Biery, expert layout design specialist, for diplomatically fitting every element with skill and polish.

In memory of Don Ho and Joel Siegel, you are both deeply and dearly missed, *a hui hou*.

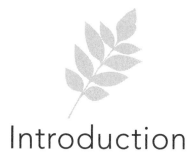

# Introduction

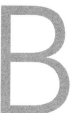eing green is contagious. It starts with one thing, then blossoms and grows into a life-changing, sense-opening natural reflex.

This book is the distillation of years of work, passion, inquiry, and experiential practice in my own life.

I've been green for longer than I've known the word for it. My memories of my childhood are pictures of stretches of meadow, the blazing glory of autumnal foliage, the muffled quiet of fallen snow, smooth stones in meandering creeks, and blue jeans that were stiff as a board because my mom *never* used the energy-hogging dryer. Although I was slightly resentful, I got it: Why waste anything if you don't have to? As an adolescent, I sought autonomy and found a cause to dig my heels into—the environment, stiff jeans and all. In high school, I helped to found an environmental club, which started a recycling program on campus and lobbied the administration to stop using pesticides, even on the sports fields. It was big stuff and we felt empowered to make changes that would make a mark.

When I was in school in Vermont, with my headstrong commitment to walking and biking everywhere, even in the single-digit weather of the long, dark winter, I came to admit that I was a fair-weather bird and wanted to live someplace where fresh food could be grown year-round. In a major leap of faith I moved to Maui, sight unseen, to try my hand at being a chef.

At the ripe age of 21, I opened a raw food restaurant, which was a little ahead of the curve. It was great and it was crazy. I worked my fingers to the bone. About 85 percent of the produce came from local organic farmers, which meant juggling dozens of small accounts to stay stocked, but it was the right thing to do—for the quality of the food, the restaurant patrons, the island, and the local economy. When I sold the restaurant (whew!), I started working privately as an organic chef for a few friends I had met in the Hollywood world and naturally started "greening" their homes, starting with simple things like biodegradable dish soap. Great organic food deserves to be served on dishes that don't have chemical residues from petroleum-derived synthetic soap, right?

And though I try to be as green as can be, I am human. I love creature comforts and convenience. I talk with friends about hand-harvested sea salt in the same sentence as biodegradable plastic and miraculous under-eye cream. It's all part of the same philosophy and it inspires me.

Living on Maui has changed me deeply. The balance of nature is unmistakable. For me, it cracked open the concept of the "life cycle" of things—basically, where things come from and what happens when we are done with them—and this has helped me define a cornerstone of what "green living" is. Everything on an island is closer to home and your backyard. When soap or cleaning products go down the drain on an island, it's pretty obvious where they end up: in the ocean. If it isn't biodegradable, it's a mess in your own beloved backyard.

My husband tells the story of how we fell in love, and it actually involves soap. As he tells it, the first time I visited him at home, I came out of the bathroom and said with a penetrating smile, "Is there any reason you don't use biodegradable soap? You live right on the ocean, after all." Right then, he says, he fell in love. He called the next day and said that in all the years of outrageous guests and traffic through the house (he was in rock 'n' roll and the film industry), no one had ever said such a thing to him. He went right out and bought some biodegradable soap, smart man. I was smitten. Now, when I walk in the bathroom, I smile at the soap, the recycled toilet paper, the fluffy organic towels, and the smell of natural cleaning products. I am smitten with the solar panels on the roof that provide us with more than enough energy to run the household, even with the ongoing outrageous traffic. Though the solar installation was a significant initial investment, I've done the math on how much money we will save over the lifetime of the system, and it's so impressive that our neighbor Tom put some panels up on his roof. Like I said, being green is contagious.

Minding the planet, the environment, and our homes is as essential as life gets. Given our modern amenities and conveniences, it's easy to consider the environment to be something outside of us. A separate entity that we are entitled to, that stages the backdrop of the seasons, that we plead with for good weather on long weekends when we're planning recreation or retreat. But the environment is an integral part of us, and we, a part of it: the air we breathe, the water we drink, the food we eat, and literally every material that we have come to depend on in our daily lives. Without a healthy natural environment, we humans cannot thrive. Yet as adults, in this culture, we have relegated the time we spend in nature to a childhood memory or 1 or 2 weeks on an annual vacation. Interestingly, our best childhood memories—and perhaps the most meaningful adult memories—are often experiences in nature. The precious emergence of spring. A breathtaking vista. The salty air of the sea. Somehow, we have lost the importance of this connection. As a result, the planet is suffering deeply as well.

There have been tipping points and blaring wake-up calls in the past few years.

As a result, being green and eco-friendly has never been hipper. But environmentalism and conservationism have been around for a very long time. Looking at the very prefix *eco-* (which comes from a Greek root meaning *home*) and two words with significant punch in our world—*economy* and *ecology*—it's possible to see how intertwined and enveloping the idea really is. Yet something is amiss. By nature, ecology is meant to govern economy and yet today, it is quite the opposite. Economic gain is all too frequently the impetus for plundering our natural resources, riding Mother Nature's back and bullying her into giving up her treasures. Our treasures. That's neither fair nor sustainable. Having a sustainable relationship with the planet is fundamental for ecology and economy to thrive. Being "eco" embraces everything that supports us. Period.

While recalibrating that relationship will take vision, influence, a little tough love, and developing greener habits, it's well under way. Small choices, like using biodegradable soap and detergent, recycled paper, organic cotton towels and sheets, and energy-efficient lightbulbs; bigger choices, like hybrid cars, solar panels, organic mattresses, and green materials for home renovation; and simple practices, like using cold water to wash clothes, setting the thermostat a few degrees lower, and bringing a cloth bag to the grocery store—all add up to major change.

Every time we decide to do something to be more green, we can use our power to make the world a better place. The tides have been shifting and our options as consumers are being met by a new green frontier in the marketplace, where it's no longer necessary to sacrifice comfort or convenience in the name of eco-friendly living. Let every dollar you spend (or don't spend!) be a vote for green living.

Writing *Easy Green Living* has been an unparalleled education about things I thought I knew a lot about already. It was an intense journey through an extensive field of research and information that sometimes led me into quagmires of confusion. I also found an unprecedented number of promising developments, products, and practices happening everywhere. For instance, while there are few to no regulations on disclosing ingredients in conventional cleaning and personal care products or cosmetics, a bevy of companies are leading the way to make it easy to choose effective, eco-friendly products that are safe for humans and the environment. Also, recycled paper products that are whitened without chlorine are becoming the industry standard and easy to find. Never have I felt more deeply passionate and inspired (though, mind you, all the endnotes in this book nearly drove me insane) that so much is possible and at our fingertips and that even the smallest efforts really add up to great change. We have a voice and a say in what happens under our own roof in the products we buy and use to care for, maintain, and primp the rooms we call home and the skin we live in. And that voice and these choices have dramatic effects on the environment—the water, the air, the land, and the quality of life that embraces all of it, including our very own homes.

Here are a few things to keep in mind for easy green living.

- **Being green is not black and white.** It's about making the best choices whenever we can. Like most things, there is a learning curve, and learning to weigh and balance the pros and cons of a product (and even what to look for on a label) gets easier with practice. For example, weighing the choice of paper versus plastic bags is not black and white. While producing one plastic bag requires less energy and creates less waste than producing one paper bag, plastic is a nonrenewable, petroleum-derived product that will take a *very* long time to break down and photodegrade into toxic microscopic particles, which will eventually contaminate the water and soil and subsequently can enter the food chain. In addition, one paper bag usually holds a lot more stuff than a plastic bag, can be reused or made into wrapping paper, and can be recycled easily, and, ultimately, it will break down and go back to the Earth without leaving harmful toxins in its wake. Of course, the best choice is to bring your own bag to the store!
- **Consider the life cycle of a product.** First, what is it made with (renewable or nonrenewable materials)? Second, how is it made (the impact of its manufacture and transport)? Third, how does it

affect us when it's used (safe or harmful)? And fourth, what happens to it when we're done with it (biodegradable or not)? These four questions will help you make greener choices for your home and lifestyle. The greenest products are made with renewable materials, are produced with little impact on the ecosystem, are nontoxic to humans to use, and do not contaminate the environment when they're disposed of.

- **Start small.** Small changes add up to great change. Try changing one thing a month. Start with one product, like dish soap. Then, change another soap, like the soap you use in the shower, and then your laundry detergent. Next, think about using recycled paper products like toilet paper and facial tissue. Soon, you might think about one whole room at a time. It's contagious and will improve the quality of your life tremendously.

- **Green living is a process.** It's not an all-or-nothing game. If you can't do everything to be green all at once, it's okay—nobody can. Some stuff takes time. Our house is a great example of a work in progress toward green living. Like a lot of American homes, it was built before *eco* or *green* was in the vernacular. So, figuring out how to make it greener without tearing it down has been a practical, exciting, and very real experience. It doesn't happen overnight, but it will happen if you want it to. Be vigilant and uncompromising when compelled, but don't let what you can't change today keep you from making the best choices for being green and balancing out what you can.

While it seems that many of the issues we face as a country and a world are out of our control, there are things each and every one of us can do every day of our lives to be part of the change to make this world a better, cleaner, safer place to live. Being green and eco-friendly is a nonpartisan issue. It's nondenominational and doesn't have to do with your zip code. It's something that we all need to have an interest in because fundamentally, it's part of the fabric of everything. Clean air and water are not luxury items. They're our birthright and precious treasures to pass on with dignity, pride, and compassion. For, unlike petroleum-based soap, we will eventually go back to the earth. And what we leave behind really does matter.

If you crack open this book to any page, you will see that it's easy to be green. I invite you to dog-ear these pages and make them yours. This book is a lens into my heart and soul, growing from a deep passion that we can share a sustainable relationship without sacrificing pleasure, convenience, or our planet. As an adult, I now know to toss my jeans (which are made of organic denim) in the dryer for a few minutes to fluff them up for the best of both worlds—being green and comfortable. Start small. Start anywhere. It feels good because it's the right thing to do—and that's contagious.

# CHAPTER 1

# Green Living Is Easy

**Green** *adjective*

**etymology:** akin to Old English *growan*, to grow;
**3.** pleasantly alluring; 10c. tending to preserve environmental
quality (*Merriam-Webster's Collegiate Dictionary*)

**3.** concerned with or supporting protection of the
environment (*Oxford English Dictionary*)

**Living** *noun*

**1.** the action of leading one's life; alive (*Oxford English Dictionary*)

Green living is easy once you know what to do. Just about every corner of your life and home offers ample opportunities to be green, without requiring you to sacrifice comfort or convenience. This chapter is an opening volley on how to be green by making simple choices that will improve the quality of your life and have a gentler impact the environment. It's an overview of topics that are delved into more deeply in the rest of this book and a look at some basic information that will help you reflexively make smart choices to be a green consumer, such as taking inventory of what labels really mean and identifying the part we can play in the waste stream of trash and recycling. It's a great place to get your bearings and step up to ride the green wave that's happening everywhere.

It seems that one of the great modern conundrums is that we have been convinced, largely by the media, that the environmental, political, and social issues we are facing are so great that they are out of our control. But the truth is that we as individuals and consumers have potent power to influence the laws of supply and demand, of ecology and economy, and of give-and-take that shape our world. The power to do what's good and right is in our hands every day.

Green living is as fundamentally essential as life gets and, frankly, it's our duty. Being green isn't a privilege or a luxury, it's a responsibility we all need to accept, because a healthy, safe environment is the backbone of everything we rely on to live, thrive, and survive. Choosing to be green is not just about the far-flung corners of the planet or generations that have yet to be born, it's about immediately improving our lives and the quality of living every day. The brilliant beauty of being green is that it not only serves the planet, it also serves us. Choosing to clean kindly with nontoxic and biodegradable products not only protects our precious freshwater supplies and aquatic ecosystems from contamination, it also prevents the buildup of chemical residues in our homes and improves indoor air quality. Curbing the use of plastic for food containers, shower curtains, and water bottles not only prevents mass pollution from the petroleum extraction, manufacturing, and disposal of those products, it also reduces our exposure to health-endangering plastic additives as well. Conserving energy with smart, efficient practices and products not only decreases the emissions of overburdened power plants, it also saves us money on our utility bills. Opting for natural personal care products and cosmetics instead of those made with synthetic, petroleum-based ingredients not only curbs the manufacturing of chemicals, which ultimately end up in the water, air, and soil, it will also make your skin and hair healthier and more beautiful. It's a win–win relationship.

Being responsible stewards of our beautiful, complex world and governing our actions with accountable etiquette is both selfless and selfish—it helps the planet and helps us. It's said that "many hands make light work," and if each of us does our own small part in making this world a better, cleaner, safer place, everything is possible. As Abe Lincoln said, "Let us have faith that right makes might, and . . . let us, to the end, dare to do our duty as we understand it." And, that duty can be done every day by making easy, green choices that add up to eminent, great change.

# 25 Ways to Go Green

Here are 25 simple ways to be greener. Start small. Start anywhere. It feels good because it's the right thing to do—and that's contagious.

## A Greener Home

**1. Clean kindly.**

- Use plant-based, biodegradable soaps and detergents.
- Use all-purpose and surface cleaners that contain plant-based solvents, and use ammonia-free glass cleaners.
- Lose cleaners that contain chlorine.
- If the ingredients are not fully disclosed on a product label (or you can't pronounce them), choose a product you can trust!

**2. Be wise with laundry.**

- Wash full loads to get the most out of water and energy use.
- Rinse laundry with cold water. Eighty-five to 90 percent of the energy used to wash clothes goes to heat the water.[1]
- Use plant-based, biodegradable detergents that don't have chemical fragrances or dyes.
- Opt out of using chlorine bleach. Choose oxygen bleach instead—it's color safe, fabric friendly, and eco-brilliant.

- Line dry what you can. It saves energy and money and extends the life of your clothes.

*Next Green Step:* When you're looking for a new washer or dryer, look for high-efficiency models to save a bundle of energy, water, and money in the long run. (See Chapter 6 for details, tips, and products.)

**3. Choose natural personal care products and cosmetics.**

Choose pure products made with pronounceable, plant-based ingredients. Opt for natural beauty and grooming products that don't have petroleum-based chemicals and synthetic ingredients—especially paraben preservatives (such as methylparaben, propylparaben, sodium lauryl sulfate, and sodium laureth sulfate), and synthetic or vaguely identified fragrances or colorants. It will do your body and the planet a gorgeous world of good.

- Choose soaps and body washes that are plant based and free of synthetic fragrances and colors. They are naturally biodegradable, which is better for you and the planet.
- Use face and body moisturizers made with pure, plant-based, and botanical ingredients to keep your skin hydrated and healthy without chemicals and synthetic preservatives.

- For lustrous locks, choose natural hair care products that are sans petrochemical foaming agents and paraben preservatives.
- Go for naturally effective deodorants and duck away from those that contain aluminum and other chemicals.
- Attention, ladies! Choose organic, nonchlorine-bleached feminine products. It's a wise, health-savvy, eco-smart move for your precious body and the planet. (See Chapter 5 for the in-depth scoop on personal care products.)

**4. Go for recycled, naturally bleached toilet paper, paper towels, and tissues.**

Majestic trees are too precious to put in the toilet. (See number 11, on page 6, for more on trees.) Buy postconsumer recycled paper goods. I am not suggesting that you use sandpaper-grade toilet paper on your hindquarters; there are fluffy recycled papers that are made snowy white with safe oxygen bleach instead of dastardly chlorine (see "Dioxins," on page 42, and "Green Solution: Oxygen Bleach," on page 244, for more on bleach). Ditto for paper towels and tissues. (See "Green Thumb Guide: Toilet Paper and Facial Tissues" on page 165 for a guide to products.)

**5. Use unbleached coffee filters for a dioxin-free cup o' joe.**

Some great things come in small packages. Choosing unbleached coffee filters is a grand act that requires little effort. Bleaching paper with chlorine—coffee filters included—is a notorious source of truly malevolent dioxins, which are some of the most toxic substances on the planet.

And dioxins migrate! Studies clearly show that brewing coffee with chlorine-bleached filters leaches detectable amounts of dioxins into the coffee—up to 24 percent of the dioxins migrate into your cup of java.[2] This means that if you drink coffee brewed with conventionally bleached filters, you will definitely ingest dioxins.[3] According to the Environmental Protection Agency (EPA), the use of chlorine-bleached coffee filters gives you enough dioxins to exceed a lifetime of "acceptable levels."

*Next Green Step:* Procure a reusable coffee filter or French press to opt out of using disposable filters.

*Note:* Buy "fair trade" coffee to stay on socially and environmentally sound ground. Fair-trade products ensure fair terms for farmers, adhering to internationally agreed-upon standards for wages, labor rights, and conditions and minimum prices to protect farmers and promote sustainable production methods. It's feel-good java for drinkers and farmers alike.

**6. Install a water filter.**

Clean, safe water without all the waste: Brilliant. You'll use fewer plastic water bottles, which means using less energy and fewer resources to make the bottles and less fuel to ship them around for delivery, and creating less waste. Fresh, clean water is a necessity, not a luxury.

More than half of Americans drink bottled water, and more than a third of us do it on a regular basis[4][5]—that adds up to billions of gallons of bottled water and more than $15 billion in sales annually. A majority of bottled-water drinkers do so out of concern about the healthfulness and safety of tap water,[6] and for good reason—more than 60 percent of municipal facilities across the country violate their Clean Water Act permits,[7] meaning that the water supplied by these facilities may contain contaminants and chemicals. In fact, the EPA estimates that more than 2,100 known contaminants and toxic chemicals are in our drinking water, several of which are known poisons and carcinogens.[8]

Bottled water might be cleaner, but boy, does it produce a mountain of waste, and golly, is it expensive. Though the demand for recycling is pretty high, the actual rate of recycling water bottles is dismally low (about 12 percent in 2003).[9] The result is that 40 million bottles *every day* are thrown in with the rubbish. That's a lot of plastic. Installing a water filter simply makes a lot of sense.

**7.** **Get a low-flow toilet, or make your existing toilet low flow.**

Old-school toilets guzzle water like it's going out of style. About a third of the water used at home is flushed down the toilet.[10]

Older standard toilets swallow 3.5 to 7 gallons per flush. New, low-flow toilets send away as little as 1.6 gallons per flush, for a savings of 54 to 77 percent of water used for the john (which can mean a savings of 16 to 23 percent of total water use at home).

You can easily retrofit any toilet for lower-flow efficiency without compromising performance by displacing water in the toilet's reservoir. Install a toilet dam (a water displacement device), or simply submerge a full plastic water bottle or two in the tank. Save water and the planet one flush at a time. See "Low-Flow Toilets: Save Water, Save Money!" on page 162 for details.

**8.** **Don't be a drip—fix leaky faucets and toilets.**

A leaky faucet or shower that loses water at the rate of one drip per second can waste 3,000 gallons of water a year.[11] Don't be a drip; save money and water resources by fixing it!

A leaky toilet can waste 200 gallons of water a day.[12] Talk about flushing away money and resources! The traditional test to find out if a toilet is leaking is to add food dye to the tank (I've used unsweetened cranberry juice to avoid using chemicals). If the toilet is leaking, color will appear in the bowl within 15 minutes. Most replacement parts are cheap, readily available, and easily installed. *Note:* Flush as soon as the test is done to avoid staining the tank and bowl.

## 9. Kick off your shoes.

Removing your shoes at the door is not just a pleasant custom, it also prevents you from tracking a host of unwanted things like pesticides and herbicides into your home. Other shoe hitchhikers include synthetic lawn fertilizers, lead, toxic cleaners used on outdoor surfaces like decks and patios, and wood preservatives. Yikes!

It's just common sense, like washing your hands before eating or covering your mouth when sneezing. Taking off your shoes is an especially good idea if your floors are clad in carpeting, which can rub all that nasty stuff off your soles and accumulate it.

Scientists suspect that exposure to dangerous pesticides from the "tracked in" route might trump the most well known source—conventionally grown fruits, vegetables, and animal products.[13] That's pretty serious, especially for families with young kids, where everything on the floor eventually ends up in the little 'uns mouths.

Get a welcome mat. A doormat outside and an entryway rug inside also help to collect toxins that are tracked in and prevent these substances from migrating throughout the house. Doormats are simple and smart, and they look nice, too.

## 10. Bring in houseplants!

Houseplants literally grow fresh air by producing clean, fresh oxygen and absorbing carbon dioxide and chemicals such as formaldehyde and benzene.

The EPA estimates that indoor air is 2 to 10 times more polluted than outdoor air.[14] The culprits? Synthetic materials found in furniture, carpeting, plywood, adhesives, mattresses, and shower curtains; chemical cleaning products; plastics; and chlorinated water are just a few.

Two small plants or one medium-size plant per 100 square feet will provide fresh air and healthy, mold-free humidity in any room so everyone can breathe deeply with ease. See page 71 for more on the benefits of houseplants.

## 11. Plant a tree every year.

Trees are the lungs of the planet. They heroically remove carbon dioxide from the atmosphere, storing it as cellulose in their woody parts, and generously release oxygen in its place. That is a sophisticated service that makes our very lives possible and has the potential to offset and reverse the currently rising levels of greenhouse gases. About half of the greenhouse gases that are causing global warming are carbon dioxide emissions.

## 12. Opt out of getting junk mail.

Do you know anyone who likes junk mail? Me neither. More than 62 billion pieces of junk mail are delivered to American mailboxes every year[15]—that's about 41 pounds a person.[16] About 100 million trees and 28 billion gallons of water[17] are used annually to produce the 5.8 million tons of catalogs and unsolicited wads of preap-

# How Trees Help to Keep Our Air Clean

- A single mature tree can absorb almost 50 pounds of carbon dioxide a year and produce enough oxygen to sustain two adults.[18]
- If every American family planted just one tree a year, it would remove more than a billion pounds of carbon dioxide from the atmosphere annually—which in 1992 was about 5 percent of the worldwide output.[19]
- Trees absorb all kinds of pollutants, such as gaseous pollutants like sulfur dioxide from coal-burning power plants, nitrous oxides from vehicle exhaust, and particulate pollutants from burning fuel, especially diesel fuel. A mature tree can absorb 120 to 240 pounds per year.[20]
- Urban areas that are well planted with trees have up to 60 percent less street-level particulate pollution.[21]
- Trees are natural air conditioners that keep cities cooler. Just one large, healthy tree has a cooling effect that is equivalent to 10 room-size air conditioners running for 20 hours a day.[22]
- Tree cover can reduce asphalt temperature by as much as 36°F and the interior temperature of parked cars by more than 47°F.[23]
- Trees reduce noise pollution by absorbing sound.
- Trees reduce storm water runoff and erosion by up to 7 percent. In urban areas, this can save some of the tax dollars spent every year on installation, materials, cleanup, and maintenance of water drainage systems.[24] Rainwater runoff collects pollutants as it flows, and much of it eventually ends up in streams and other freshwater bodies, which are common sources of drinking water, so managing and reducing runoff are important. Just 100 mature trees can catch about 100,000 gallons of rainfall per year, reducing runoff to keep surface water cleaner.[25]
- Trees increase property values. Studies show that homes that are well landscaped, especially with trees, have a value that's 5 to 9 percent higher than that of equivalent homes that don't have good landscaping.[26,27]
- Commercial real estate in wooded areas is more valuable.
- Apartments and offices surrounded by trees have higher occupancy rates.[28,29]

proved credit card offers and other junk[30] that arrive at our homes—44 percent of which are thrown away unopened.[31] But there are ways to reduce the onslaught, and therefore the wasting of the trees and the energy that is needed to truck around these mountains of mail.

- Stop credit card offers. Go to www. optoutprescreen.com, where the consumer credit report industry lets you opt out of receiving preapproved and prescreened credit card offers. You can also phone your request to 888-567-8688.

- To get off mailing and telemarketing lists, contact the Direct Marketing Association. Register online at www.dmaconsumers.org/consumerassistance.html. Another way to get off telemarketing lists is to sign up for the government's National Do Not Call Registry, which registers your phone number for free. The ban stays in effect for 5 years, after which you will need to reregister. Register online at www.donotcall.gov.

- Stop your name from being sold. When you order something online or over the phone, you can specifically request that your name not be lent, sold, or traded. Create a form letter asking that your name be removed from mailing lists when you're renewing subscriptions and don't fill out warranty cards, which are commonly used to gather names for mailing lists—most products are covered by the manufacturer's warranty even if you don't fill out the warranty card. When you make purchases online, note in the comment box that you don't want your name shared for any purpose without your authorization. A little persistent effort pays off, and the forests and ice caps will thank you.

- Green Dimes will do it for you. This nonprofit organization will reduce the amount of marketing materials delivered to your home, help maintain your privacy, and plant trees on your behalf. For less than a dime a day

($36 a year), it will stop what you want it to stop—meaning that you can still get the catalogs you like—and contact the Direct Marketing Association to nip the output of national and direct marketers in the bud. It will plant five trees for you when you sign up, and also plant a tree for each of the first five catalogs you stop. Its representatives are on call seven days a week to answer your questions and provide help. Go to www.greendimes.com for details.

**13.** **Go veggie 1 day a week**
Beyond being a solid source of a full spectrum of good stuff—vitamins, nutrients, minerals, antioxidants, and phytonutrients—a plant-based diet requires a lot less energy and water to produce than a meat-based diet. Meat is the least-energy-efficient food on the planet, requires a serious amount of water, and is a major polluter. Beef requires 35 calories of energy for every 1 calorie it provides.[32] That doesn't sound like a very good investment—imagine someone asking you to invest $35 for a $1 return. Cows are thirsty: producing just 1 pound of beef requires 2,500 gallons of water—that's 40 times more water than it takes to produce a pound of potatoes.[33]

Get this: Eating just 2 to 4 pounds less meat a year will save as much water as not showering every day for a year. *Note:* These figures are based on these two calculations:

- A 5-minute shower with a water-conserving showerhead (2.5 gallons per minute) × 365 days = 4,562.5 gallons per year (2 pounds of meat = 5,000 gallons water)
- A 5-minute shower with an ordinary showerhead (5 gallons per minute) × 365 days = 9,125 gallons per year (4 pounds meat = 10,000 gallons water)

Plus, livestock produce a massive amount of waste—130 times the waste generated by humans![34] Eleven billion pounds of manure, sludge, and slurry waste are produced by livestock every year.[35] All that waste in turn emits VOCs (volatile organic compounds),[36] hydrogen sulfide,[37] ammonia,[38] and endotoxins.[39] One VOC is methane (the number-two greenhouse gas causing global warming, with 20 times the heat-trapping ability of carbon dioxide[40]). The livestock industry alone is responsible for almost 20 percent of the methane in the atmosphere.[41] Adopting a more-plant-based diet, or even going veggie just 1 day a week, is a powerfully green choice. Your body, the freshwater supplies, and ice caps everywhere will rejoice.

## Greener Energy

**14.** **Energy-efficient lightbulbs save energy, money, and emissions.**
Lighting sucks up about 20 percent of the energy used at home, which adds up on utility bills and causes literally tons of carbon dioxide to be spewed into the air by our overburdened power plants. Standard incandescent bulbs waste 90 percent of the energy they draw in creating heat, not light.

Energy-efficient lightbulbs like compact fluorescent lightbulbs and light-emitting diodes have come a long way, baby! Producing just as much light as incandescent bulbs but using a fraction of the energy, there are a bevy of bulbs available in all shapes, sizes, brightnesses, and light qualities to fit every socket and then some. That's something to get lit up about! (See Chapter 8 for details on lightbulbs.)

**15.** **Turn the thermostat down 2°F.**
During the cold months, set the thermostat at 68°F (20°C) during the day and 60°F (15°C) at night.
- Turning the thermostat down 5°F to 10°F at night will save you 5 to 10 percent on your heating bill. It is also helpful to all of the houseplants that are busy cleaning and filtering your indoor air—most of them like this kind of temperature drop at night! When you're going to be away for a full day or weekend, turn the thermostat down to 55°F (13°C); you will save money and energy, and don't worry, your pipes will not be at risk for freezing.

During the warm months, set the air conditioning at 78°F (25°C).

*Next Green Step:* Install an automated setback thermostat. Available for most gas- and oil-fueled central heating systems, setback thermostats automatically turn down the heat at night and turn it back up before you wake up. Some even allow you to set two schedules, which can be timed to turn down the heat when you leave for work or school and back up before you get home!

**16.** **Set your water heater at 120°F (49°C).**

You'll find that 120°F (49°C) is piping hot! Most water heaters are set at 140°F (60°C), which is simply a waste—it's really too hot for household needs. Turning the temperature down just 10°F will prevent each and every household from producing about 600 pounds of carbon dioxide a year for an electric water heater or 440 pounds for a gas water heater.[42]

## GREEN TIP

If every American household turned the water heater down by just 10°F, it would prevent 45 million *tons* of carbon dioxide from entering the environment each year. That equals the entire amount of carbon dioxide emitted by Kuwait or Libya.[43]

*Next Green Step:* Insulate your water heater. Insulating your water heater will reduce the heat lost by 25 to 45 percent, saving you 4 to 9 percent of the cost for the energy to heat your water. Precut insulating jackets for water heaters run only about $10 to $20.

*Next Green Upgrade:* On-demand water heaters more efficiently save both money and energy.

**17.** **Smarten your fridge and freezer. Turn their thermostats up and make sure the seals are snug.**
Set the fridge at 37°F (3°C).
Set the freezer at 3°F (−16°C).

## GREEN TIPS for Maintaining Your Fridge and Freezer

- Maintain a tight seal on the doors of your fridge and freezer. Here's a quick way to test your seals: a dollar bill should be held snugly when the door is shut.

- Vacuum the fridge and freezer coils regularly. Every 4 to 6 months, depending on how dusty they get, simply vacuum the coils at the back of your fridge and freezer for optimal performance and to extend the life of the appliance.

- If you don't have a self-defrosting or no-frost freezer, defrost your freezer regularly. An iced-up freezer doesn't work well and requires a lot more energy to keep it cold. Most newer refrigerators have self-defrosting or no-frost freezers with a built-in mechanism that prevents ice from building up. However, if you have an older model or a non-self-defrosting freezer, defrost it by turning the thermostat to the warmest setting (take everything out first!). Depending on how quickly ice builds up, defrost it every other month.

**18.** **Use power strips and unplug appliances.**

Power strips are our friends. Save energy and money by plugging your electronics into power strips that can be turned off when the components are not in use. TVs, stereos, game consoles, computers, and accessories all have a hefty "phantom" draw of energy (called *idle current*) even when they're turned off—about the same amount of energy as a 60-watt lightbulb burning continuously.[44] That really adds up on individual electric bills and, collectively, on power plant output.

*Green Bonus Step:* Look for "smart" power strips, which have advanced circuitry that senses the flow of electricity and automatically shuts off components that are consuming idle current (find them at www.smarthomeusa.com and www.amazon.com).

**19.** **Choose green residential energy service options.**

Utility companies across the country offer renewable energy options that generate electricity with wind, solar, biomass, and geothermal sources. Choosing clean energy is cheap and easy; for a small premium, based on how much energy your home draws, you can opt for green energy and feel like an eco-hero.

If we want it, they will make it. In the United States about 97 percent of electricity is generated from nonrenewable resources, including petroleum (40 percent), coal (23 percent), natural gas (22 percent), and nuclear energy (8

percent).[45] These sources pollute our air, spoil our water, and devastate the atmosphere. Coal mining involves open-pit or strip mining or in-situ leach mining, and nuclear energy produces radioactive effluent that will stick around for at least 10,000 years. Renewable energy provides only about 7 percent of our needs, from sources such as biomass (3 percent), hydroelectric (3 percent), and geothermal, solar, and wind (1 percent),[46] but every household that pays an electric bill can change that. Just think of what would happen if just 10 or 20 percent of us put a few bucks in the pot for this future. We could change the world.

For information on green power options available in your state through your utility provider, visit www.epa.gov/greenpower/locator/index.htm.

## Green on the Go

**20.** **Buy local.**

Buying locally grown food means fewer fossil fuels are used to truck it to you. That's a good thing, because these days food isn't just shipped around the country, it's shipped all over the world! The average morsel of food travels about 1,300 to 1,500 miles from farm to plate in the United States.[47] [48] That's some well-traveled food! Some experts estimate that it takes almost as much energy to ship food as it does to grow it.[49] [50] That's a lot of energy. In addition, the jury is out on the exact figure, but it's said to take more energy (in calories) to produce and ship food today than we actually get from eating it.[51] [52] [53] Buying locally grown food is a simple way to change that equation for the better and get the most for your money. The bottom line is that local food is fresher, tastes better, and saves energy. Everybody wins.

**21. Go organic!**

Buying and eating organically grown food is one of the single most powerful green choices, period.

**22. Take a cloth bag or basket to the store.**

In New York City, just *one less* grocery bag per person would prevent *5 million pounds* of waste and save $250,000 in disposal costs.[54]

If every American used just *one less* grocery bag, it would prevent *187.5 million pounds* of waste and save millions of dollars in disposal costs.

**23. Inflate your car's tires to their proper pressure to save gas and money.**

Properly inflated car tires can improve gas mileage by more than 3 percent[55] and extend the life of the tires. Underinflated tires experience more rolling resistance, which directly affects fuel economy and can cut the tread life in half![56] If every American simply kept his or her car's tires properly inflated, it would save 2.8 billion gallons of gas a year, saving billions of dollars and helping to curb global warming.[57]

Tires lose pressure naturally over time, like a balloon, so check their pressure regularly.

- The proper pressure varies from car to car. Check the owner's manual to find out where to find the recommended tire pressure—it is often printed on the pillar of the driver's door, in the glove compartment, or on the fuel door.
- Check the pressure when the tires are cool and have not been driven for more than a few miles.

## More Auto Tips

- **Lighten up on the pedals.** Avoid flooring the gas pedal and mashing the brake pedal for massive fuel economy gains. The standard advice is to drive like there's an egg under the gas pedal. Moderating your driving techniques can save gas and improve mileage by as much as a whopping 37 percent![58]
- **Clean the air filter.** Replacing a car's air filter regularly can boost your gas mileage by 10 percent.[59]
- **Get tuned up.** Regular tune-ups can hike your miles per gallon by an impressive 4 to 40 percent, depending on the type of car and how badly it needed to be tuned up.[60]
- **Recycle motor oil.** Motor oil can be recycled, rerefined, and used again. If you change your own oil, many service stations are used motor oil collection centers, as are local and county recycling centers. If you have someone else change it, ask around and take your car to a service center that recycles its used oil.

**24.** **Get a travel mug!**

In 2005, we Americans used and disposed of 14.4 billion paper coffee cups.[61] Yes, that's enough to circle the Earth 55 times if placed end to end. Most paper coffee cups are not only bleached with devastating chlorine, they are also lined with a thin film of plastic to prevent leakage. That has a significant impact on the waste stream and uses enough petroleum to heat 8,300 homes.[62]

**25.** **Recycle your cell phone.**

According to the *Washington Post*, the 128 million Americans who have cell phones upgrade to a new one an average of every 18 months. Many recycling programs will take your old cell phones.

What happens to phones that are recycled?

- If they work, the devices are simply given a second life by worthy charities. If they need work, they are refurbished and returned to service.

- If the phone can't be reused or refurbished, some of its components, like plastics and precious metals, are still valuable and can be recovered and recycled into new products ranging from kitchen counters and cabinets to circuitry boards. Cell phones and other electronics also contain toxic heavy metals that should not be sent to landfills, which is another good reason to recycle them.

Before recycling your phone:

- Terminate your service.

- Clear the phone's memory of its contacts, address book, and other stored information.

- Remove the SIM card, if it has one. If you don't know how to remove it, contact your service provider.

- Choose a domestic recycling program. There are growing concerns about old American electronics being sent to countries where standards may not protect workers from being exposed to all kinds of toxic stuff.

Organizations that recycle cell phones:

- CTIA—The Wireless Association, www.recyclewirelessphones.com. This nationwide, voluntary program implemented by the wireless industry facilitates environmentally sound production and recycling of wireless devices. The central Web site links to all participating CTIA members' recycling information.

- Eco-Cell, www.eco-cell.org. This company purchases cell phones from fund-raisers, paying up to $15 per phone for refurbishing or recycling.

- GRC Wireless Recycling, www.grcrecycling.com, offers socially responsible cell phone recycling opportunities that benefit charities.

- Recycle for Breast Cancer Program, www.recycleforbreastcancer.org. This program's goal is to keep toxic electronic wastes out of the environment to reduce the incidence of breast cancers caused by environmental pollution.

# 7 Green Office Moves

Green living is not just relegated to the home. Making a few basic green office moves collectively adds up to great change. Here are seven simple ways to be greener in your workplace and feel like an eco-hero.

I. **Print on recycled paper.**
The higher the percentage of postconsumer content, the better. Using recycled paper is so smart. Paper made from recycled fibers instead of virgin fibers conserves loads of trees, energy, and water, and it prevents air pollution because it requires less energy to produce.

Try looking at it this way: According to Environmental Defense and Conservatree, it takes about 24 trees to make a ton (2,000 pounds) of standard (20-pound) virgin printer/copy paper,[63] which is 40 cartons of paper. One carton weighs 50 pounds. That means that 1 tree yields 83 pounds, and that each tree produces only 1⅔ cartons of paper!

According to the EPA's municipal solid waste figures for 2005, Americans use 14 million tons of printer/copy paper a year (that's 28 billion pounds).[64] That breaks down to about 93 pounds for every person in the United States. That's a lot of paper. Some offices use more paper and others, less. For instance, according to the American Bar Association, a large law firm might go through two cartons of paper per lawyer per year,[65] which is more than a whole tree per person every year. How much paper does your office go through?

## COMPARISON OF RESOURCES USED AND POLLUTANTS GENERATED IN PRODUCING 1 TON OF PAPER

| | VIRGIN PAPER | 30% POSTCONSUMER RECYCLED PAPER | 100% POSTCONSUMER RECYCLED PAPER |
|---|---|---|---|
| Trees used* | 3 tons (24 trees) | 2 tons (saves 7 trees) | 0 tons (saves 24 trees) |
| Total energy used | 38 million BTUs | 33 million BTUs (13% less) | 22 million BTUs (42% less) |
| Wastewater produced | 19,075 gallons | 16,450 gallons (14% less) | 10,325 gallons (46% less) |
| Solid waste produced | 2,278 pounds | 1,941 pounds (15% less) | 1,115 pounds (51% less) |
| Greenhouse gases produced | 5,690 pounds | 5,058 pounds (11% less) | 3,582 pounds (37% less) |
| Particulate pollution produced | 12 pounds | 11 pounds (8% less) | 7 pounds (42% less) |
| Volatile organic compounds produced | 6 pounds | 4 pounds (33% less) | 2 pounds (67% less) |

\* The figure for trees per ton of paper assumes a mix of hardwoods and softwoods 6 to 8 feet in diameter and 40 feet tall[66]

*Source:* Based on calculations from Environmental Defense. "Paper Calculator." http://www.environmentaldefense.org/papercalculator/incompat.cfm.

The first step to being green with printer/copy paper at your office is to choose the recycled paper that has the highest postconsumer content available. The next step is to reduce how much you use (see number 2, below), and to recycle as much of the used paper as possible. The good news is that 62.6 percent of printer/copy paper gets recycled (8.24 billion pounds in 2005)![67] Go, team. Keep it up!

Look at the table on the opposite page to see what can be saved by using 1 ton of recycled paper instead of 1 ton of virgin paper, and the difference between 30 percent and 100 percent postconsumer recycled content.[68] It's major.

**2.  Print on both sides of the paper.**

Many computer printers allow double-sided printing. If yours doesn't, but your software allows you to print alternating pages, figure out how your printer pulls pages from the paper tray. Then, print the odd-numbered pages of your document first, properly reorient the printed pages and replace them in the paper tray, and print the even-numbered pages on the back. Done!

A lot of photocopiers also have a double-sided option—use it.

**3.  Recycle ink and toner cartridges.**

Most office supply stores will happily take empty ink and toner cartridges off your hands, and some offer free paper or discounts on future purchases in exchange. But used cartridges are valu-

able enough that companies and recycling organizations will buy them back. *Ch-ching!* Or, to practice socially responsible recycling, donate empty cartridges to support a good cause—there are many out there that need help.

Here are a few organizations to contact.

- eCycle Group, www.ecyclegroup. com. This recycling company will pay you for your used printer and fax cartridges and cell phones.
- FreeRecycling, www.freerecycling. com. This recycler also pays for ink cartridges and cell phones. A new program offers a route for recycling CDs and DVDs, too.
- Recycle for Breast Cancer Program, www.recycleforbreastcancer.org. This program accepts a variety of electronic items as well as printer cartridges nationwide. It'll even take large things like computers and television sets at its San Ramon, California, recycling center.

**4.  Use your computer's power-saving or energy-saving mode by setting it to "sleep" when it will not be used for a short period of time.**

According to the US Department of Energy, turning off a typical computer when it's not in use can save $186 a year in electricity and prevent 1½ *tons* of carbon dioxide emissions. *Note:* Screen savers are not energy savers—a screen saver uses more energy than the sleep mode does.[69]

## COMPARISON OF ANNUAL ENERGY USE
## FOR DESKTOP AND LAPTOP COMPUTERS

| | POWER ON, ACTIVE MODE | POWER ON, SLEEP MODE | POWER OFF |
|---|---|---|---|
| Desktop computer | 126 watts (320% more than a laptop) | 11.2 watts (60% more than a laptop) | 2.9 watts (21% more than a laptop) |
| Laptop computer | 30 watts (76% less than a desktop) | 7 watts (37% less than a desktop) | 2.4 watts (17% less than a desktop) |

*Source:* US Environmental Protection Agency and US Department of Energy. "Summary of Assumptions for EPA Energy Star Savings Estimates: Energy Star Preliminary Draft Computer Specification (Version 4.0)." 2005. http://www.energystar.gov/ia/partners/prod_development/revisions/downloads/computer/Assumptions_Prelim_Draft_Comp_Spec.pdf.

### 5. Use a laptop computer.

A laptop computer uses about one-quarter of the energy that a desktop does.[70] Check it out in the table above.

### 6. Rely on Smart Strip power strips.

Computers and their peripherals—like printers and scanners—eat up energy even when they are turned off. It is called *idle current*, and it can draw up to 40 percent of full power. The US Department of Energy estimates that nationwide, the idle current of electronics adds up to the output of 17 power plants annually.[71] Smart Strip power strips save time, money, and energy by preventing this drawing of idle current.

Smart Strip power strips have advanced circuitry that can "sense" the flow of the electrical current to any device, like a computer, that is plugged into it. A Smart Strip can tell when you turn off your computer and will automatically shut off the peripherals that are also plugged into it, damming the flow of "idle current" electricity. Smart Strip power strips also offer excellent power surge protection and line noise filtering, and they're excellent for TVs and entertainment equipment, too. The manufacturer, BITS, says a Smart Strip will pay for itself in electricity savings in as little as 6 weeks. Now that's smart!

Find more information at www.bitsltd.net/ConsumerProducts/index.htm. Buy Smart Strips at www.smarthomeusa.com or www.amazon.com.

### 7. Go for recycled and eco-friendly office supplies.

Look for pens made with recycled plastics or bioplastics, pencils made with Forest Stewardship Council–certified wood from sustainably managed forests, paper clips and mouse pads made with recycled content, and scissors with recycled plastic handles. You can find these items and more at www.thegreenoffice.com.

# 10 Green Home Maintenance Measures

There are many green measures to maximize the efficacy of maintaining a home. Here are some smart green ideas that will save energy and money and improve the value of your home.

### 1. Weather-strip it.

Save energy on heating and cooling by weather-stripping around windows and doors. Weather-stripping will save you a bundle—when done right, it can save 10 percent of home energy costs.[72] Other places to weather-strip and seal are around plumbing and electrical lines and ducts (sealing and insulating them can improve efficiency by as much as 20 percent);[73] the attic door; and air conditioners. It's easy to do yourself. However, sealing your home for energy efficiency is a good reason to choose safe, green interior paints and home furnishings like carpets, couches, mattresses, and shower curtains over synthetic materials that may emit VOCs (volatile organic compounds; see Chapter 9 for information). Houseplants will also help keep the indoor air clean by producing fresh oxygen and filtering out chemicals emitted by synthetic materials. Lastly, consider replacing screens with storm windows for winter months.

### 2. Shade your air-conditioning unit and clean the filters regularly.

- An air-conditioning unit in the shade uses up to 10 percent less energy than one in the sun.[74] Planting bushes or trees on the south side of the unit will do the trick. Just be sure they don't block airflow.
- Clean the filters regularly. Check them once a month, especially during heavy-use months in the height of summer. At a minimum, change the filters every 3 months for maximal performance. Dirty filters slow down airflow, making units work harder and waste energy. A clean air-conditioning filter can cut the unit's energy use by 5 to 15 percent[75] and prevent dust buildup, which will also save cash on maintenance and premature system failure in the long-term.

### 3. Use green paints.

Once upon a time—not that long ago—many house paints contained lead, which is highly toxic, especially to young children, who find a way to put everything in their mouths, including paint flakes. Today's house paints don't contain lead, but they do contain a lot of other nasty stuff. Most paint is made with a slew of petrochemicals that emit toxic fumes. On the manufacturing side, paint can create up to 10 times its weight in toxic waste.[76] On the wall, it releases noxious VOCs, like formaldehyde, that are no good to breathe. VOCs are solvents that allow the paint to dry, and some evaporate quickly, with acutely toxic fumes, while others degrade more slowly, with long-term, low-level toxic emissions. VOCs also cause chemical reactions in the atmosphere that produce ground-level pollution and smog that can cause breathing problems and nervous system and kidney damage.[77] [78] Who wants that at home or on the planet? Fortunately, there are other alternatives.

Green paint to the rescue! Natural paints, zero-VOC paints, and low-VOC paints—finishes too!—are the smart green options. Thanks to consumer demand and environmental regulations, most paint manufacturers now offer one or more types of low-VOC or zero-VOC paint. Made with plant oils and resins instead of petroleum, they're durable, cost-effective, and less harmful to humans and the planet. (See Chapter 9 for details, products, and tips.)

### 4. Install rheostatic light dimmers to create ambience and save energy and money.

Dimmers save energy on lighting by allowing you to control the brightness of lightbulbs with a dial or slide. They're inexpensive and easy to install. Create ambience with a soft glow or radiant brightness with eco-savvy style, saving energy and money at the same time.

### 5. Install reflective window films and tints.

South-facing windows can turn living spaces into veritable saunas in the summer months, fading furniture, rugs, and artwork. Protective window film can cut cooling costs and improve the general quality of life. Tinted film was once the only option for controlling the amount of sun shining through windows, but the new generation of reflective films are much more effective and hardly influence the color of the light passing through the panes. Reflective film can reduce 50 percent of the total solar heat for cooler indoor temperatures and lower cooling costs and cut out 98 percent of the UV light that fades home interiors.[79] Most are scratch resistant and have a lifespan of 20 years. It's recommended that you have reflective film installed by a professional who can gauge your needs and give you optimally smooth results.

*Next Green Step:* Install double-pane windows.

### 6. Go for a natural gas on-demand water heater for tankless water heating.

Heating water on demand with natural gas is one of the most efficient means around. These systems use loads less energy, offering instantly hot water at a fraction of the cost of water heaters that store hot water in a tank. Consider that the water heater is one of the biggest energy hogs at home. While hot water storage tanks fueled by natural gas are

## COMPARISON OF WATER HEATERS

| WATER HEATER TYPE | ENERGY SAVINGS ON MINIMUM FEDERAL STANDARDS | EXPECTED LIFETIME | ENERGY COST SAVINGS OVER EQUIPMENT LIFETIME | ADVANTAGES |
|---|---|---|---|---|
| High-Efficiency Storage Tank | 10–20% | 8–10 years | Up to $500 | Lower initial cost |
| On-Demand (Tankless) | 45–60% | 20 years | Up to $1,800 | Unlimited supply of hot water |
| Solar (with electric backup)* | 70–90% | 20 years | Up to $2,000 | Huge savings |

\* Solar water heaters are a good choice in warm to hot regions only.

*Source:* US Environmental Protection Agency. "High Efficiency Water Heaters: Provide Hot Water for Less." http://www.energystar.gov/ia/new_homes/features/WaterHtrs_062906.pdf.

much more efficient and much less polluting than electric water-storing heaters, on-demand water heating trumps storage heating by 30 percent.[80] You can save a bundle, and because it's available on demand, your tank of hot water will never run out because there isn't one![81] Some on-demand water heaters cost more initially than conventional storage models, but their lower operating costs can more than offset the higher purchase price.

To sum it up, go for a high-efficiency water heater: on-demand is better than storage, and solar is the best of all if you live in an area where operating one is feasible.

*Next Green Step* (in very hot regions): Consider a solar water heater. Some states and utilities even offer rebates on installation.

### 7. Insulate your roof with reflective insulation.

Insulating the inside surface of a home's roof is a simple, effective way to keep a home cooler in the summer and warmer in the winter.

Reflective insulation, or a radiant barrier, is a new, eco-smart way to reduce cooling costs during the summer by up to 10 percent[82] and heat loss in the winter. It literally shields energy, keeping hot air out or warm air in depending on the season. Usually made of a sheet of thin metal or foil applied to one or both sides of a substrate material, a radiant barrier is designed to block heat transfer across open spaces, like attics. It can be installed directly on rafter framing or simply over insulation. During construction of a roof, it can also be laid over the tops of the rafters before the roof deck is put on.

*Next Green Step:* Consider reflective paint and roofing materials. Reflective paint and roofing will keep the house cool and comfy in hot months, reducing cooling demands by 10 to 15 percent.[83] Visit www.energystar.gov for more information.

### 8. Choose sustainable materials.

If and when the time comes for home renovation, go for eco-friendly materials for beautiful sustainable flooring, counters, tiles, carpets, insulation, wallpaper, and more. Choose from green-savvy materials like bamboo, cork, reclaimed wood, and recycled glass tiles for *Architectural Digest*—worthy digs with planet-friendly endorsement. See Chapter 9 for more.

**9. Plant shade trees.**

Big, beautiful trees not only improve property value by 5 to 9 percent,[84] [85] they also offer energy savings on heating and cooling costs year-round. According to the US Forest Service, houses with trees use 20 to 25 percent less energy than houses in wide-open areas.[86] As few as three wisely positioned trees can save the average home owner between $100 and $250 every year in heating and cooling costs.[87] Plant summer shade trees (two on the west side of a house and one on the east side) to save up to 30 percent of your home's air-conditioning costs.[88] For winter protection, plant trees on the north side of the house (or on whatever side the prevailing winds come from in the winter) to save up to 25 percent on winter heating costs.[89] For a winter windbreak, put a row of trees between your house and the prevailing winds; a windbreak slows the force of wind behind it for a distance of 10 times its height, and two to three times its height in front of it.

**10. Purchase energy-efficient appliances.**

A substantial chunk of monthly utility bills goes to feeding the major appliances in your home—fridge, washing machine, dryer, dishwasher. Older models are energy hogs; refrigerators and washing machines more than 12 years old can use twice the operating energy of today's energy-efficient models. Over the years, federal energy-efficiency standards have been tightened to ensure better performance while using less energy, so today's appliances are better for your pocketbook and better for the planet.

When the time comes to replace appliances, look for the most efficient models to save energy and money. Here are some guidelines for getting the most bang for your buck.

- Energy Star—rated models are the most energy efficient in any category—they exceed federal energy-efficiency minimums. In some regions, utilities and state governments up the ante by offering rebates on Energy Star models. Visit www.energystar.gov for more information.

- Look at ENERGYguide labels. New appliances must have an ENERGYguide label, either on the appliance itself or on the packaging. This yellow and black label will allow you to compare the skinny on operating costs and annual energy consumption. It will let you judge how much energy can be saved by choosing the most efficient models.

- Choose the right-size model for your needs—oversize fridges, air conditioners, washing machines, and water heaters not only waste energy and money, in many cases they don't perform as well as smaller models.

- Some of the most energy-efficient appliances cost more up front, but will save you a bundle in energy costs in the long run. Considering that most major appliances will last for 10 to 20 years, a very energy-efficient model will pay for itself quickly by lowering monthly utility bills and more than offset a higher price tag.

# What Labels Really Mean

Reading labels is a simple, effective way to find out what's in a product, whether it's food, a household cleaning product, paper, a home appliance, or office equipment. Learning what's behind the label is a key piece in making an informed decision about how green a product really is. Some labels carry more clout than others and are backed up by defined standards that are regulated and enforced by trustworthy organizations. For instance, food labeled *Certified Organic* must be grown in accordance with USDA standards, which prohibit the use of chemical pesticides, synthetic fertilizers, hormones, genetically modified organisms, added sulfites, and artificial colors and flavors. Though there is concern among consumers and producers that these standards are being eroded as organic foods become big business, in general, the certified-organic label can be trusted to mean that the product is congruent with these standards. On the other hand, labeling food *Natural* has little to no meaning. Though the US Food and Drug Administration (FDA) does not allow artificial colors or flavors to be included in foods that are labeled *Natural*, highly refined ingredients like high fructose corn syrup can be considered natural. Hmm.

When it comes to paper products, understanding labels is a fundamental tool for choosing the greenest product, whether it's printer paper, toilet paper, tissues, or coffee filters. Learning to differentiate *recycled* content paper (which may be virgin content that was recovered from disposal) from *postconsumer recycled* content paper (which was recovered after use and repulped into new paper), as well as how it is bleached (*processed chlorine-free*, which means that no chlorine was used in processing, versus *elemental chlorine-free*, which may be processed with chlorine derivatives), is essential for making the greenest consumer choice when browsing store shelves.

For household cleaning products, learning to look on labels for important words such as *biodegradable*, *phosphate free*, and *VOC free*, and learning what those words mean, will help you choose the most eco-friendly and human-safe products on the market.

With the help of this section, you will be on your way to making smart green choices. Information is powerful and liberating, and becoming informed about what labels really mean makes it easier than ever to go green!

## Produce and Packaged Products

**The label says:** CERTIFIED ORGANIC

**It means:** As clean and good as it gets

**Standards:** Certified by the USDA to be grown or raised without chemical pesticides, synthetic fertilizers, hormones, or genetically modified organisms. The product may not contain added sulfites or artificial colors or flavors. Some added enzymes, acids, and waxes are permitted. Packaged food labeled *Certified Organic* must contain at least 95 percent organic ingredients, not including water and salt, but may contain up to 5 percent nonorganic agricultural ingredients that are "not commercially available in organic form."

**Who certifies it:** USDA certifying agents (paid outside auditors)

**Be aware of:** Food products that are labeled *Made with Organic Ingredients*, which is not the same as *Certified Organic*. Look for the USDA organic seal.

**The label says:** MADE WITH ORGANIC INGREDIENTS

**It means:** Made with *mostly* organic ingredients

**Standards:** These products must contain at least 70 percent organic ingredi-

ents, not including water and salt. They must not contain added sulfites, although wine is an exception.

**Who certifies it:** USDA certifying agents (paid outside auditors)

**Be aware of:** Look out for nonorganic ingredients, such as corn and soy, which are likely to be genetically modified.

**The label says:** NATURAL

**It means:** Not too much

**Standards:** No legal standards. The FDA allows products that don't contain artificial flavors or colors to be labeled *Natural*. Products that include highly refined and adulterated ingredients, including high fructose corn syrup, can qualify as natural.

**Who certifies it:** No one. But there are federal penalties for companies that make false claims on their labels.

**Be aware of:** Vaguely identified *natural flavor* among the ingredients. All sorts of weird stuff, including chemically treated substances, passes under this name.

**The label says:** DEMETER CERTIFIED BIODYNAMIC

**It means:** Beyond organic. The Demeter biodynamic agricultural method is one of the oldest and most ecologically self-sustainable methods of farming, founded on a holistic approach to nature and the seasons. Crops are planted in cycles set by the sun and moon, and the soil is fortified and replenished organically.

**Standards**: Strict and detailed standards began to be established in 1924 by Rudolf Steiner and an agricultural research group. To apply for Demeter biodynamic certification, farmers must submit a 10- to 20-year history of the land and then keep adequate records that are reviewed annually. No synthetic fertilizers, pesticides, herbicides, fungicides, growth regulators, or genetically engineered substances may be used, ever. Serious soil fertility management is also required, and farms must establish a detailed baseline soil analysis. No chlorinated or fluoridated water can be used for irrigation. Produce must be guarded from contact with conventional or other produce during shipping.

**Who certifies it**: Third-party evaluation and enforcement by the Demeter Association; farmers must also submit annual reports

**Be aware of**: The *Demeter Certified Biodynamic* standard is applied to all kinds of foods—fruits, veggies, dairy products, eggs, meats, and wines. Once you taste the difference and read the standards, you will want to eat nothing else.

🍂

**The label says**: TRANSITIONAL or CERTIFIED TRANSITIONAL

**It means**: The produce is from growers who are transitioning their crops from conventional to organic methods. There may or may not be chemical residues in the food, depending on how far along in the process the farm is.

**Standards**: This label is granted to growers after at least 1 full year of production while meeting certified-organic standards. The full transition from conventional to organic takes 3 years (prior to the USDA organic standards taking effect, it was a 7-year transition).

**Who certifies it**: USDA certifying agents

**Be aware of**: Transitional food is not certified organic, though it is safer and cleaner than conventionally grown good. The "transitional" standard creates an incentive for growers to convert to organic farming.

🍂

**The label says**: GMO (Genetically Modified Organism) FREE or GE (Genetic Engineering) FREE

**It means**: The product has not been *knowingly* genetically manipulated or engineered by producers and manufacturers.

**Standards**: GMO-free and GE-free labels are voluntary, and there are no federal regulations or enforcement of claims. These labels imply that manufactured products do not knowingly contain GMOs, though there are no guarantees because of widespread genetic engineering of crops like corn and soy and the fact that pollen from a GMO plant can be carried to a non-GMO field nearby to cross-pollinate and contaminate those plants.

**Who certifies it**: No one

**Be aware of:** Corn and soy products and ingredients that are not certified organic; otherwise, they are highly likely to be GMO.

✦

**The label says:** FAIR TRADE

**It means:** The product was produced and traded in a socially responsible way. Suppliers of fair-trade food and products must meet internationally agreed-upon standards.

**Standards:** Fair-trade standards for social responsibility are set by Fairtrade Labelling Organizations International. The group sets clear minimum and developmental criteria and objectives for social, economic, and environmental sustainability, including wages, working conditions, and the rights of workers. The standards stipulate that buyers must pay a minimum price to producers, as well as a Fair Trade Premium that producers must then invest in projects that enhance local social, economic, and environmental development.

**Who certifies it:** TransFair USA, a private, nonprofit organization

**Be aware of:** Look for the insignia— the International Fair Trade Certification Mark—and be mindful of big manufacturers that adopt the label to "greenwash" their not-so-fair acts in the past.

## Animal Products

A number of labels are used for animal products, such as eggs, dairy products,

poultry, and meat, to indicate the manner and conditions in which the animals are raised, including whether they have access to the outdoors, what they're fed, and if antibiotics or hormones are administered. Ultimately, these conditions influence not only the animal's quality of life, but also the quality of the food they provide. Fish are sort of in their own category, with labels that nod at more sustainable fishing practices. Some labels for animal foods have more credence, authority, and enforcement backing them up than others. Here's a look at some of the labels to look for and what they actually mean.

### Dairy and Eggs

**The label says:** CAGE FREE (eggs)

**It means:** The chickens that produced the eggs were not restrained in battery cages.

**Standards:** Egg-laying hens cannot be caged, though that doesn't ensure treatment that meets any other humane standards or access to the outdoors. Hens may still be crowded inside a structure their whole lives, with their wings, feet, and beaks clipped to prevent them from causing a ruckus. *Certified Humane Raised and Handled* eggs are subject to higher standards (see the opposite page).

**Who certifies it:** No one, really

**Be aware of:** This is a pretty misleading label. Instead, look for eggs produced to other standards, such as *Certified Humane Raised and Handled* and *Certified Organic*.

✦

**The label says:** CERTIFIED HUMANE RAISED AND HANDLED (eggs, poultry, beef, pork, lamb)

**It means:** The animals were treated humanely in a safe, healthy living environment.

**Standards:** *Certified Humane Raised and Handled* follows strict standards set by Humane Farm Animal Care, a nonprofit organization. They include a nutritious diet free of antibiotics and hormones and sufficient shelter and space to engage in natural behaviors from birth through slaughter.

**Who certifies it:** Verified and enforced by third-party inspectors who have expertise in animal care, with voluntary audits to confirm compliance with the International Organization for Standardization

**Be aware of:** Check that all five words are on the label. Products that simply say *Humane* may not comply with these standards.

**The label says:** HORMONE FREE, rBGH FREE, or rBST FREE (dairy)

**It means:** The dairy products came from cows who were not pumped full of hormones.

**Standards:** Dairy products from cows who have not been injected with synthetic recombinant bovine growth hormone (known as rBGH, rBST, and Prosilac) to stimulate excessive milk production can be labeled *Hormone Free*. Though the FDA approved the hormone in 1993, alleging it was safe, much evidence has challenged its safety since then. rBGH has been banned by many governments, including the European Union, Japan, Canada, Australia, and New Zealand, but it is widely used in the United States.

**Who certifies it:** USDA enforces that certified organic dairy products come from animals that are not given growth hormones

**Be aware of:** Milk by nature contains some hormones. But dairy products are among the foods it is most important to choose in organically produced form to ensure that you're not getting recombinant hormones, period.

**The label says:** ANTIBIOTIC FREE (ABF) PROCESS VERIFIED (dairy, eggs, pork, poultry, beef)

**It means:** The animals were not given antibiotics as a preventive measure, only for real illnesses.

**Standards:** Antibiotics are not given in "subtherapeutic" amounts to prevent illness.

**Who certifies it:** The USDA, through annual on-site inspection and evaluation

**Be aware of:** Look for the USDA Process Verified seal or the ABF stamp; it's the only USDA-verified program for antibiotic-free production.

## Fish and Seafood

**The label says:** DOLPHIN SAFE (tuna)

**It means:** No drift gill nets were used and no intentional chasing or netting of dolphins occurred during fishing for the tuna.

**Standards:** International agreements require five standards to be met to label tuna *Dolphin Safe*, including no intentional or accidental killing of or serious injury caused to dolphins in any nets set; no drift gill nets allowed; and no dolphin-safe tuna may be mixed in the same boat well with tuna caught by other methods. Independent observers may be required to be on board to attest to compliance. Thanks to dolphin-safe standards, dolphin mortality has dropped by more than 97 percent in the past 10 years, and more than 90 percent of the world's tuna canners now meet dolphin-safe standards.

**Who certifies it:** The Earth Island Institute; visit www.earthisland.org for more information about this great organization

**Be aware of:** Look for the Dolphin Safe logo on the tuna you purchase.

**The label says:** MARINE STEWARDSHIP COUNCIL CERTIFIED

**It means:** The fishery that produced the food follows environmentally managed, socially beneficial, and economically viable fishing practices worldwide.

**Standards:** These are an internationally recognized set of environmental principles for assessing well-managed, sustainable fisheries based on the Marine Stewardship Council's standards that ensure there are enough fish to sustain the fishery; examine the effects of the fishing on the immediate environment and on nontargeted fish, marine mammals, and seabirds; and evaluate the company's rules and procedures to ensure that the fishery remains sustainable and that its impact on the marine environment is minimal.

**Who certifies it:** Independent certifiers from the Marine Stewardship Council, an independent, nonprofit organization

**Be aware of:** Don't take a product's word for it—look for the Marine Stewardship Council logo. Visit www.msc.org for more information on what types of fish are certified sustainable and where to buy them (you might be surprised by how many places there are).

## Poultry and Meat

**The label says:** FREE RANGE (poultry)

**It means:** The bird had outdoor access at least once a day, though the producer may be an industrialized farm, not a mom-and-pop operation.

**Standards:** The *Free Range* label is regulated by the USDA for use on poultry only (not eggs). The bird must have had access to the outdoors, but for "an undetermined period each day"—5 minutes of open-air access is enough to get the label. However, it doesn't guarantee that the animal got to go outside; if she didn't see that the door was open during that time or chose not to go out, she can still be considered free range.

**Who certifies it:** The USDA; not independently verified

**Be aware of:** Poultry is the only animal product that can be labeled *Free Range*; this label has no meaning on eggs or meat.

**The label says:** FREE RANGE, FREE ROAMING, or PASTURE RAISED (beef, lamb, and pork)

**It means:** Not much. It's a nice idea, but there is no regulation; until pending USDA standards are approved, it's up to producers to support their claims.

**Standards:** There are no federal criteria for nonpoultry products, which means there are no requirements for the size or quality of the "range" or how much space each animal is given. The USDA has proposed standards that include breeding, antibiotic, and grain-fed claims and define the standard as "livestock that have had continuous and unconfined access to pasture throughout their life cycle" (pigs will be okayed for 80 percent of the production cycle). Current proof of "free range" relies "upon producer testimonials to support the accuracy of these claims."[90]

**Who certifies it:** No one; USDA-proposed standards are pending as of this writing.

**Be aware of:** The only way to know the truth is to ask the producer. There are trustworthy producers out there, so go for it! It's worth caring about.

❦

**The label says:** GRASS-FED BEEF

**It means:** Pending standards will ensure that 99 percent of a ruminant animal's food source for the creature's entire life is forage from pasture grass or harvested grass.

**Standards:** Currently there are no standards, though the USDA has proposed minimum requirements to certify grass-fed beef. As it stands, the proposed standard looks like it will read "a grass or forage-based diet that is 99 percent or higher . . . for the lifetime of the ruminant specie, with the exception of milk consumed prior to weaning."[91] Vitamin and mineral supplementation are permitted.

**Who certifies it:** Will be verified by independent auditors

**Be aware of:** It's not yet law, so the only way to know is to look into producers' practices. Smaller and local producers are generally easier to approach.

❦

**The label says:** NO HORMONES ADMINISTERED (beef)

**It means:** It may be accurate, it may be a marketing ploy—no organization checks to make sure the claims are true.

**Standards:** There are currently no standards for this claim. According to the USDA, the term *No Hormones Administered* may be used for beef products if the producer can provide sufficient documentation that no hormones were used in raising the cow from birth to harvest.[92]

**Who certifies it:** The USDA is supposed to.

**Be aware of:** Big companies touting this claim may be as porous as the standard. Look into smaller or local producers who can be trusted.

## Household Products, Cleaners, and Solvents

**The label says:** BIODEGRADABLE (cleaning products and personal care products)

**It means:** The product breaks down into elements found in nature within a reasonable amount of time.

**Standards:** There must be competent and reliable scientific evidence to prove a substance will decompose in a reasonably short period of time after customary disposal,[93] though that period of time is not defined. It is illegal to misrepresent a product or packaging as being biodegradable, though it remains unregulated.

**Who certifies it:** No one, really. The Federal Trade Commission can slap a company with a lawsuit if it chooses to look into a producer's claims and finds them deceptive.

**Be aware of:** Products marked *Degradable* or *Biodegradable* without any other information or qualification to back it up. Look for products that explain the testing they have done and disclose their ingredients on their labels.

---

**The label says:** NONTOXIC (cleaning products, personal care products and cosmetics, paints, finishes, and arts and crafts supplies)

**It means:** Supposedly, this stuff won't kill you right off or cause long-term adverse effects on humans or the ecosystem.

**Standards:** There are no federal standards. *Toxic* means harmful or deadly when exposure exceeds a certain limit (depending on the chemical). Anything that doesn't meet the Federal Hazardous Substances Act's or the Consumer Product Safety Commission's definition of toxic can technically be labeled *Nontoxic*.

**Who certifies it:** No one

**Be aware of:** Products that are not plant-based and make this claim. Be very wary if this claim is made with no supporting information.

---

**The label says:** PHOSPHATE FREE (detergents and soaps)

**It means:** The product contains no phosphates per se. Plant-based alternatives are ideal, but synthetic phosphates may be used, which may be just as harmful in the environment in different ways. (See "What's the Deal with Phosphates?" on page 240 for details.)

**Standards:** Some states have banned phosphates and manufacturers are complying, but there is no federal regulation for enforcement.

**Who certifies it:** It's a little vague; because no official standards exist for this term, it's unclear who's responsible for verifying it.

**Be aware of:** Products that are labeled *Phosphate Free* but contain synthetic phosphates. To be sure of their safety, look for products made with fully disclosed, plant-based ingredients by companies you trust.

**The label says:** Not Tested on Animals (personal care products, cosmetics, household products, cleaning products)

**It means:** The company that made the product does not conduct any animal testing, though products and ingredients that have been tested on animals in the past may be used in their manufacture.

**Standards:** Rigorous standards were developed by an international organization of nongovernmental agencies in cooperation with industry. In order to use the leaping bunny seal, companies must submit a written commitment to stop animal testing in perpetuity.

**Who certifies it:** An international coalition that includes the Humane Society, along with independent private auditing every 3 years

**Be aware of:** Products that don't have the leaping bunny symbol; claims of *Cruelty Free* and *Not Tested on Animals* may not have been verified for products that don't have it

**The label says:** No VOCs or Low VOCs (paints, paint strippers, solvents, cleaning products, personal care products, arts and crafts supplies, building materials, carpeting)

**It means:** The product contains concentrations of volatile organic compounds (VOCs) that are below the legal limit or tests negative for VOCs

**Standards:** VOCs are smog- and cancer-causing chemicals.[94] There is no federal definition for *No VOCs* or *Low VOCs*,

but the EPA governs the use of these labels. They are based on outdoor environmental standards, not indoor health standards. Also see "Volatile Organic Compounds" on page 46 for more on VOCs.

**Who certifies it:** The EPA

**Be aware of:** Products with vaguely identified ingredients. For paint, choose latex over oil-based products. For other products, choose water-based over solvent-based materials.

**The label says:** PVC Free (plastic goods, such as food containers and packaging, office and arts and crafts supplies, building materials, toys, sports shoes, and clothing accessories)

**It means:** The product does not contain polyvinyl chloride (PVC) or vinyl. For information on the bad effects of PVCs, see page 120.

**Standards:** PVCs have received so much negative attention that the federal government has issued regulations and warnings, and companies are responding to the public outcry. PVC-free goods cannot contain polyvinyl chloride or vinyl, period. However, the packages these products come in are not subject to this regulation and the products may pick up phthalate residues from the packaging.

**Who certifies it:** Governed by federal regulation by the EPA. NASA even banned PVCs from use in space vehicles because the plasticizers they emit coat optical equipment.

**Be aware of:** Avoid plastic whenever possible, especially in food containers, shower curtains, building supplies, and children's toys. For a great list of safe goods, check out www.pvcfree.org.

🍃

**The label says:** GREEN SEAL (cleansers, paints and stains, papers, newsprint, windows, and doors)

**It means:** The product is eco-friendly throughout its life cycle.

**Standards:** Products are evaluated thoroughly for their environmental impact throughout their life cycle, including raw material extraction, manufacturing, use, and disposal. Manufacturing facilities are subject to annual monitoring for quality control.

**Who certifies it:** Green Seal is an independent, nonprofit science-based organization; its primary research partner is the University of Tennessee's Center for Clean Products and Clean Technologies. See "4 Green Standards to Look for in Sustainable Products and Services" on page 312 or visit www.greenseal.org for more information.

**Be aware of:** Make sure the product has the symbol and the words *Green Seal*.

🍃

**The label says:** OZONE SAFE or OZONE FRIENDLY (anything in an aerosol can, such as cleaning products, air fresheners, personal care products; air conditioning units of all types; refrigeration units)

**It means:** The product contains no chemicals that deplete atmospheric ozone or cause ozone pollution at ground level.

**Standards:** Clear standards set by the EPA's Stratospheric Protection Division and published in the *Code of Federal Regulations*[95]

**Who certifies it:** The EPA

**Be aware of:** Aerosols in general; avoid them altogether to be safe. Use pump sprays instead.

🍃

**The label says:** CO-OP AMERICA APPROVED FOR PEOPLE AND PLANET (a wide variety of goods and services, such as baby products, building materials, clothing, papers, pet products, wood, toys, and more)

**It means:** The businesses and products with this seal have demonstrated a firm commitment to social and environmental responsibility.

**Standards:** Businesses are carefully screened by Co-op America and must demonstrate[96] social and environmental responsibility in sourcing, manufacture, and marketing; use of the business as a tool for positive social change; and commitment to helping workers, communities, customers, and the environment.

**Who certifies it:** Co-op America. For more, check out www.coopamerica.org and the organization's *National Green Pages*, which can be found on the site.

**Be aware of:** How cool this certification is!

## Paper Products

**The label says:** RECYCLED (printer/copy papers, tissues, toilet papers, paper towels, stationery)

**It means:** The paper is made from recovered fibers (which can mean they have preconsumer or postconsumer content). *Recycled paper* may be scraps leftover from producing new paper. *PCW* (postconsumer waste) is paper that has been used and is repulped to use again.

**Standards:** There is no regulation on minimum content or sourcing. There is no federal definition of recycled paper. The EPA does mandate that all federal and state government agencies and many companies receiving federal funding use paper that is 50 percent postconsumer recycled content.

**Who certifies it:** The Federal Trade Commission guides responsible marketing with its "Guides for the Use of Environmental Marketing Claims,"[97] though it's vague about who enforces anything. Products that make false claims may incur liability.

**Be aware of:** Recycled products with no PCW content—it's better than virgin paper, but PCW is the greenest. Look for recycled paper that has been processed without chlorine.

**The label says:** PCW CONTENT (printer/copy papers, tissues, toilet papers, paper towels, stationery)

**It means:** PCW recycled paper is truly recycled, having been made from paper that was used in a finished product, separated from the waste stream for recovery, and repulped into new paper. This means that if you recycle your printer paper through a municipal program, it may come back as new PCW recycled paper.

**Standards:** PCW recycled paper must be made from finished paper products and cannot include scrap materials or overruns from new paper processing or over-issue publications.

**Who certifies it:** The EPA defines *postconsumer materials* and the Federal Trade Commission enforces accurate marketing.

**Be aware of:** Look for recycled paper products with the highest percentage of PCW available; it ranges from 10 to 100 percent. Look for paper that has been processed chlorine free.

**The label says:** TREE FREE (printer/copy papers, tissues, toilet papers, paper towels, stationery)

**It means:** Tree-free paper is exactly what it says it is—paper made from nonwood plants like cotton, kenaf, hemp, and bamboo.

**Standards:** Standards for tree-free paper are up to the manufacturer. There are no specifications regarding the minimum tree-free content for the paper to be marketed as such—products range from 10 to 100 percent alternative fibers—or for the source of the fibers. There is no standard on using recycled content in tree-free products, though many companies producing tree-free papers use recycled content.

**Who certifies it:** There are no federal regulations, though tree-free paper manufacturers are typically forthcoming about the products' content, sources, and processing.

**Be aware of:** Check the content of the paper—look for blends that contain PCW recycled content if they aren't 100 percent tree free. Look for tree-free paper that has been processed chlorine free.

## Chlorine-Free Paper

**The label says:** PROCESSED CHLORINE FREE

**It means:** The paper was processed without chlorine *and* it contains PCW recycled content!

**Standards:** No chlorine or chlorine compounds can be used in processing; instead, the paper is bleached with oxygen, ozone, or hydrogen peroxide. The paper must contain a minimum of 30 percent PCW recycled content. The paper mill must use sources of PCW content that meet EPA guidelines. Virgin fiber content must come from certifiable sustainably managed forests—no old-growth timber can be used for virgin pulp. The mill cannot have any current or pending federal environmental permit violations.

**Who certifies it:** The Chlorine Free Products Association (CFPA)

**Be aware of:** There's a difference between *Recycled* and *PCW* content—the latter is much better. However, processed chlorine-free paper may have content that was bleached with chlorine in its original incarnation. This is the best of what's around.

**The label says:** TOTALLY CHLORINE FREE

**It means:** The paper is totally chlorine free, but made with virgin paper.

**Standards:** No chlorine or derivatives are used in manufacture, and bleaching is done with oxygen, ozone, or hydrogen peroxide. Virgin paper is used; if the product contains recycled paper, it will be called *Processed Chlorine Free*. The virgin fiber must come from certifiable sustainably managed forests—no old-growth timber can be used for virgin pulp. The mill cannot have any current or pending federal environmental violations.

**Who certifies it:** The CFPA

**Be aware of:** Nonchlorine bleaching is a great thing. The virgin content is not ideal; recycled is the way to go!

**The label says:** ELEMENTAL CHLORINE FREE (ECF)

**It means:** The paper was supposedly not bleached with elemental chlorine, but chlorine derivatives may have been used. Since elemental chlorine gas is required to make some chlorine derivatives, this may not be true.

**Standards:** Although no elemental chlorine (chlorine gas) is supposed to be used, chlorine derivatives, such as chlorine dioxide (which releases toxic elemental chlorine as a by-product), may be used. The result may be the release of more chlorine than in papers processed with conventional (elemental) chlorine bleaching. The paper is made with virgin content, so it contains no recycled materials. EFC papers are not necessarily less toxic than papers processed with elemental chlorine There is no guarantee that ECF papers generate less dioxins as by-products.

**Who certifies it**: No one.

**Beware of**: This is a pretty misleading label. ECF processing is becoming the industry standard and a way for some mills to avoid making the full step to chlorine-free processing. It may be a smidgen better than conventional chlorine bleaching, but there are no standards to guarantee that EFC papers have a lower environmental impact.

## Appliances and Products

**The label says**: ENERGY STAR RATED (household appliances, office machines, commercial appliances, electronics, building materials)

**It means**: The product meets strict federal energy-efficiency guidelines.

**Standards**: Products are evaluated for how efficiently they consume energy or whether they reduce energy use (such as windows and insulation). Products that get the Energy Star meet minimum energy-efficiency standards. On average, Energy Star products use about one-third less energy[98] than nonrated models.

**Who certifies it**: The EPA and the Department of Energy

**Be aware of**: Look for the Energy Star symbol and the ENERGYguide sticker that lists the product's energy use—don't settle for less.

**The label says**: GREEN-E (green energy products offered by utilities, greenhouse gas offset certificates, and a wide variety of consumer products)

**It means**: A company that is certified by Green-e gets a minimum of 2 to 10 percent of its energy from renewable sources.

**Standards**: Green-e is a nationally recognized symbol applied to products and companies that use certified renewable energy. Eligible renewable energy sources include wind, solar, and biogas. Visit www.green-e.org for more information.

**Who certifies it**: The nonprofit Center for Resource Solutions

**Be aware of**: Products that claim to be manufactured with renewable energy but don't have the Green-e logo attached.

**The label says**: EPA GREEN POWER PARTNERSHIP (companies, products, municipal governments, and schools)

**It means**: A certified group has opted to use renewable energy from sources such as solar, wind, geothermal, biogas, and biomass for some percentage of its energy needs.

**Standards**: This voluntary program has no standards for minimum use.

However, the eligible green energy sources must produce electricity with zero emissions and have a superior environmental profile compared to conventional power generation. An impressive number of companies (including Fortune 500 companies), colleges and universities, and municipal and state governments have joined; you can see the full list at www.epa.gov/grnpower/partners/index.htm. Visit www.epa.gov/grnpower for more information.

**Who certifies it:** The EPA

**Be aware of:** "Greenwashing" companies that use the mark, but use a very low percentage of renewable energy. It's a start, but it can be misleading.

❧

**The label says:** RECLAIMED, RECOVERED, or SALVAGED (wood products, such as furniture, furnishings, building materials, and flooring)

**It means:** The wood was previously used or reclaimed from various sources.

**Standards:** Reclaimed wood can be from various sources,[99] including demolition projects; dead, fallen, or nuisance trees; orchards where unproductive trees are cut for replacement; trees recovered from rivers and lakes; and wood reclaimed from landfill or as a by-product. Most reclaimed wood is high grade.

**Who certifies it:** Third-party certification is done by the Rainforest Alliance (www.ra-smartwood.org); there is no federal certification.

**Be aware of:** The definition is broad and a little vague. There is no regulation, so ask the manufacturer or supplier for full details.

❧

**The label says:** SUSTAINABLE FORESTRY CERTIFIED (wood products, including furniture, furnishings, building materials, and flooring; and paper products such as printer/copy papers, toilet papers, tissues, and paper towels)

**It means:** The product was made with virgin wood harvested from sustainably managed stands run by foresters that have responsible long-term forest and soil productivity management and protect special sites and biological diversity.

**Standards:** Standards are based on 13 objectives developed by professional foresters, conservationists, and scientists that involve sustainable forest management, the productivity and procurement of wood and fiber, public reporting, continuous improvement, and mitigation of illegal logging. The program is a partnership among landowners, wood and pulp producers, contractors, and purchasers.

**Who certifies it:** The Forest Stewardship Council (www.fscus.org) provides independent auditing and enforcement.

**Be aware of:** Products without the seal of approval. *Note:* 100 percent recycled products don't need the seal because they are not made with virgin trees.

# Reduce, Reuse, Extend, Recycle

We Americans love our stuff. That's not inherently bad, but lots of stuff sure does produce *a lot* of rubbish. Mountains of it. It's called municipal solid waste (MSW)—otherwise known as garbage or trash.

Altogether, we produce a little more than half a billion pounds of MSW a year.[100] That means that each of us throws out more than 4½ pounds of garbage a day—a 50 percent increase from 20 years ago.[101] In other words, we each generate our own body weight in trash in about a month.[102] Have mercy!

The big questions are: Where is it all coming from? Where is it going? What can we do about it?

## Municipal Solid Waste: What Is It?

Taking a look at what kinds of materials make up the waste we create can help us figure out how to first reduce its volume and then how to reuse or recycle it. The biggest contributor to the solid waste stream is paper products; it accounts for 33.9 percent of municipal solid waste.[103] Therefore, recycling paper products whenever possible will reduce the waste stream by diverting the paper to be used again. Yard waste makes up the next largest segment at 12.9 percent[104] and food scraps are after that at 12.4 percent,[105] both of which can be composted into valuable materials to fortify soil. Take a look at the table to see what else goes into our waste stream and in what proportions.[106]

## Where's It Going?

Fortunately, more and more waste is being recovered for recycling! Almost one-third of the materials destined for landfills are now recycled through curbside programs, drop-off centers, buy-back programs, and deposit systems.[107] According to the EPA, in 2006 almost 164 billion pounds[108] of stuff (including composting) were diverted from landfills.[109] That's 4.8 million pounds more than the year before,[110] and about double the amount from 10 years ago. By recycling that 164 billion pounds of waste, we conserved the equivalent of 10

### MUNICIPAL SOLID WASTE— WHERE IS IT COMING FROM?

502.6 billion pounds generated annually*
4.6 pounds per person/day

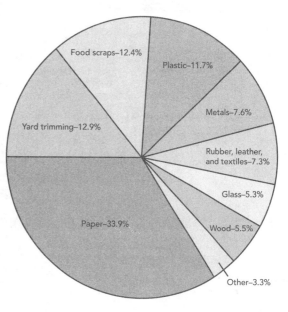

Food scraps–12.4%
Plastic–11.7%
Metals–7.6%
Yard trimming–12.9%
Rubber, leather, and textiles–7.3%
Glass–5.3%
Paper–33.9%
Wood–5.5%
Other–3.3%

*Total weight of waste generated before recovery for recycling

billion gallons of gasoline,[111] which correlates to removing almost 40 million cars from the road every year.[112] Go, team!

## 4.6 Pounds per Person per Day

On average, each of us produces about 4.6 pounds of garbage every single day. That's almost 150 pounds of rubbish for each of us in one month's time. Yowser!

Where's it all going, you may ask. About one-third of garbage is recycled (1.5 pounds per person per day) and a smidgen of it is composted, while the rest ends up in a landfill (2.5 pounds per person per day) or is incinerated (0.6 pounds per person per day).

### RECYCLED AND RECOVERED GOODS

To check out how to improve our noble efforts, let's take a look at what we're recycling versus what ends up in a landfill.

Total Recovery of Goods = 163.3 billion pounds per year (32.5% of total garbage produced)

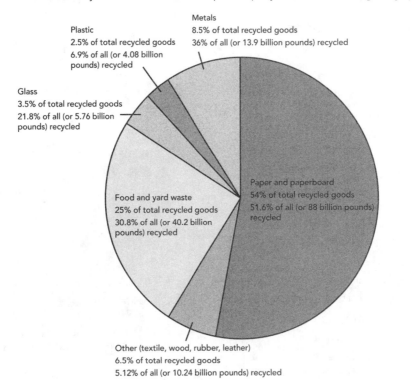

Plastic
2.5% of total recycled goods
6.9% of all (or 4.08 billion pounds) recycled

Metals
8.5% of total recycled goods
36% of all (or 13.9 billion pounds) recycled

Glass
3.5% of total recycled goods
21.8% of all (or 5.76 billion pounds) recycled

Food and yard waste
25% of total recycled goods
30.8% of all (or 40.2 billion pounds) recycled

Paper and paperboard
54% of total recycled goods
51.6% of all (or 88 billion pounds) recycled

Other (textile, wood, rubber, leather)
6.5% of total recycled goods
5.12% of all (or 10.24 billion pounds) recycled

# Recycling Rates

In 2006, US citizens recycled: 99 percent of auto batteries; 62 percent of yard trimmings; 51.6 percent of all paper and paperboard; 88 percent of newspapers; 72 percent of corrugated cardboard; 66 percent of office paper; 40 percent of magazines; 36.3 percent of metals; 62.9 percent of steel cans; 45.1 percent of aluminum beverage cans; 34.9 percent of tires; 25.3 percent of glass containers; 10 percent of all plastics; 31 percent of plastic milk and water bottles; and 30.9 percent of plastic beverage bottles.[113]

The overall trends are improving every year. We are generating less waste and recycling more of it. Good job, team. But we can do even better!

## How Much Gets Recycled?

Americans recycle about a third (32.5 percent) of our waste,[114] which is more than ever—almost 1½ pounds per person per day, including materials recovered for composting.[115] Still, about 55 percent of our waste stream ends up in landfills,[116] and 12.5 percent is incinerated with energy recovery.[117] Of the 502 billion pounds of waste,[118] 164 billion pounds are recycled,[119] while about 338 billion pounds end up in landfills or incinerators.[120]

Thanks to the 8,660 curbside recycling programs,[121] 48 percent of Americans recycle from home,[122] and more of us have access to the almost 13,000 drop-off centers and 3,470 community composting programs[123] in the United States.[124]

## Containers and Packaging: Paper and Plastic

The products we buy come in containers and packages. A lot of them. Containers and packaging make up 31.7 percent of the waste generated in the United States,[125] to the tune of 159.2 billion pounds a year.[126] The good news is that almost 40 percent of it is being recovered for recycling,[127] and the numbers are growing (it was only 26 percent in 1990).[128]

Paper and plastic are the two most popular materials used for containers and packaging. Using less packaging overall is the greener choice to make. Look for products that are not shrink-wrapped and do not have layers of packaging, such as trays inside a box. We can't avoid packaging entirely, so choosing wisely is a smart green step.

When wrestling with whether paper or plastic is better, consider a few things. Waste is measured by weight, not volume. Paper is heavier by weight than plastic. Although by weight we use a lot more paper than plastic, by volume we use a lot of darn plastic.

- Paper is made from a renewable resource, trees. Plastic is made from a nonrenewable resource, petroleum.

- Paper is biodegradable; plastic is not.
- Though we use more paper than plastic, we recycle a lot more paper—51.6 percent of all paper and paperboard, as opposed to 10 percent of plastic.[129]

So, reducing the use of packaging is the best green move, and choosing paper packaging over plastic is another green step.

## Recycling More Paper

Paper can be a greener material when it's chosen and used wisely—it's versatile, renewable, biodegradable, and easy to recycle. However, we Americans use an excessive amount of it—almost 570 pounds of paper per person per year.[130] That's a touch more than $1\frac{1}{2}$ pounds each and every day! It can take a serious toll on the environment. But because so many Americans have access to recycling programs, 51.6 percent of all the paper we use is recovered for recycling[131]—three-quarters more than in 1990![132]

Recycling more paper is a heroically green trend because virgin paper is seriously hostile to the environment. The virgin paper industry is one of the most eco-destructive industries, logging timber from pristine, ecologically rich habitats and polluting waterways like there's no tomorrow. The virgin paper industry is the third largest industrial emitter of global warming pollution. The recycled paper industry, on the other hand, is much more sustainable. Manufacturing paper from recycled pulp uses 64 percent

### AMOUNT OF PAPER PRODUCTS RECOVERED FOR RECYCLING IN THE UNITED STATES IN 2006

| PAPER PRODUCT | % OF ALL PAPER SENT FOR DISPOSAL | % OF DISPOSED PAPER THAT'S RECYCLED | PAPER PRODUCT | % OF ALL PAPER SENT FOR DISPOSAL | % OF DISPOSED PAPER THAT'S RECYCLED |
|---|---|---|---|---|---|
| Corrugated Boxes | 39% (62 billion pounds) | 72% (44.6 billion pounds) | Tissue Products | 4.4% (6.9 billion pounds) | less than 0.05% |
| Newsprint | 15.7% (24.7 billion pounds) | 88.1% (21.8 billion pounds) | Magazines | 3.2% (5.1 billion pounds) | 40.5% (2 billion pounds) |
| Commercial Printing | 8.4% (13.3 billion pounds) | 21.1% (2.8 billion pounds) | Bags and Sacks | 1.7% (2.7 billion pounds) | 25.4% (686 million pounds) |
| Printer and Copy Paper | 8% (12.6 billion pounds) | 65.7% (8.2 billion pounds) | Paper Plates and Cups | 1.5% (2.4 billion pounds) | less than 0.05% |
| Paperboard Cartons | 8% (12.5 billion pounds) | 16% (2 billion pounds) | Books | 1.4% (2.2 billion pounds) | 25.7% (565 million pounds) |
| Mail | 7.5% (11.8 billion pounds) | 38.7% (4.6 billion pounds) | Phone Books | 1% (1.4 billion pounds) | 19.1% (260 million pounds) |

Individual figures may not add up to the total due to rounding.

Source: US Environmental Protection Agency. "Municipal Solid Waste in the United States: 2006 MSW Characterization Data Tables: Table 4: Paper and Paperboard Products in MSW, 2006." http://www.epa.gov/epaoswer/non-hw/muncpl/pubs/06data.pdf.

# 4 Golden Rules for Curbing Waste

Producing rubbish is part of life. But, there are ways to reduce the heap.

It adds up: Choosing well-made products that use high-quality materials and have less packaging and taking care of our stuff so it lasts longer are small efforts that can have significant effects over time if we all get on board. There are four golden rules for reducing how much waste we generate: reduce, reuse, extend, and recycle.

## 1. REDUCE: CHOOSE PRODUCTS WISELY

- Less packaging = less waste
- Choose high-quality products with fewer packaging materials:

    Made with *recycled materials*

    Made with *less toxic materials*

    Made with *reclaimed materials*

    Made with *biodegradable materials*

## 2. REUSE: CHOOSE REUSABLE GOODS

- Favor cloth over paper
- BYOB—bring your own bag
- BYOC—bring your own cup
- Use refillable water bottles
- Use reusable coffee filters
- Use refillable pens and pencils
- Use cloth shower curtains instead of plastic

## 3. EXTEND: TAKE CARE OF PRODUCTS TO MAXIMIZE THEIR LIFE SPAN

- Maintain products—care for clothing and cars kindly
- Maintain household appliances, such as washers, dryers, fridges, freezers, and air-conditioning units

## 4. RECYCLE AND COMPOST: JUST DO IT!

- Recycle containers and packaging
- Compost everything you can
- Recycle or donate electronics for reuse, repair, and repurposing
- Recycle or donate appliances

# AMOUNT OF PLASTIC PRODUCTS RECYCLED
## AND DISPOSED OF IN THE UNITED STATES, 2006

| PLASTICS | TOTAL GENERATED: 58 BILLION POUNDS A YEAR<br>RECYCLED: 5.7% (3.3 BILLION POUNDS)<br>DISPOSED OF: 54.7 BILLION POUNDS* |
|---|---|
| **Containers and Packaging**<br><br>Generated: 47% (of total plastics generated) (24.7 billion pounds)<br><br>Recycled: 9.4% (of total plastic containers and packaging generated) (2.6 billion pounds)<br><br>Disposed of: 22.1 billion pounds | **Plastic Bottles (water, soft drinks, milk)**<br><br>6% of plastic generated = 3.4 billion pounds<br><br>Recycled: 31.5% (1.1 billion pounds)<br><br>Disposed of: 2.2 billion pounds<br><br>**Bags, Sacks, and Plastic Wrap**<br><br>16% of plastic generated = 9 billion pounds<br><br>Recycled: 5.2% (5 million pounds)<br><br>Disposed of: 8.5 billion pounds<br><br>**Other (packaging, caps and lids, closures, trays, shapers, etc.)**<br><br>15% of plastic generated = 8.8 billion pounds<br><br>Recycled: 2% (180 million pounds)<br><br>Disposed of: 8.6 billion pounds |
| **Disposable Goods**<br><br>Generated: 23% (13.2 billion pounds)<br><br>Recycled: less than 0.05%<br><br>Disposed of: 13.2 billion pounds | **Trash Bags**<br><br>4% of plastic generated = 2.2 billion pounds<br><br>Recycled: 0%<br><br>Disposed of: 2.2 billion pounds<br><br>**Plastic Plates and Cups**<br><br>3.5% of plastic generated = 1.9 billion pounds<br><br>Recycled: 0%<br><br>Disposed of: 1.9 billion pounds<br><br>**Other (utensils, diapers, shower curtains, etc.)**<br><br>15.5% of plastic generated = 8.8 billion pounds<br><br>Recycled: 0%<br><br>Disposed of: 8.8 billion pounds |
| **Durable Goods**<br><br>Generated: 30% (19.5 billion pounds)<br><br>Recycled: 4.2% (800 million pounds)<br><br>Disposed of: 18.7 billion pounds | Durable goods last 3 or more years (appliances, carpeting, electronics casing and other, furniture, etc.) |

Individual figures may not add up to the total due to rounding.

* Most plastic is disposed of in landfills; some is incinerated.

*Source:* US Environmental Protection Agency. "Municipal Solid Waste in the United States: 2006 MSW Characterization Data Tables: Table 7: Plastics in Products in MSW, 2006." http://www.epa.gov/epaoswer/non-hw/muncpl/pubs/06data.pdf.

less energy[133] and creates 35 percent less water pollution[134] and 74 percent less air pollution.[135] Even the government is getting on board—the EPA has mandated that all federal and state government agencies and many companies that receive federal funding must use paper with a minimum of 50 percent postconsumer recycled content.[136] But paper is not without its costs to the environment. To be green, choose and use paper wisely. Here's how:

- Limit your use of disposable paper products like paper napkins, paper towels, paper plates, and paper cups. Use cloth and reusable plates and cups instead.
- Limit magazine subscriptions (you can now read many magazines online) or share subscriptions with a friend (have some delivered to you, others to him or her, and trade after a week or two).
- Use nonrecyclable paper (like slick paper inserts and glossy paper) as packing material.
- Look for items with packaging made with recycled materials. (See "25 Ways to Go Green" on page 3 and "7 Green Office Moves" on page 14 for more ways to be green with paper.)
- And *recycle* every shred possible![137]

## Persistent Plastics

Plastics have fast become a persistent material in our lives. They're ubiquitous and tough to ditch. Americans toss *59 billion pounds* of plastic disposables, containers, packaging materials, and durable goods every year[138]—that's a little more than 197 pounds per person per year[139]—and only 10 percent of it is recycled.[140] Part of the problem is that only a few kinds of plastic are widely accepted for recycling—like water and soda pop bottles and, in some places, plastic bags.[141] The rest of it ends up in the landfill and isn't going anywhere anytime soon. What can we do about it? A lot. Check out Chapter 3 for information on how to scale down, dodge the most dangerous plastics, and choose safer bioplastics, and Chapter 4 for details about opting for cloth shower curtains.

# Widespread Hazardous Materials to Avoid

Among the hazardous materials to watch out for are a few outstanding offenders—dioxins, persistent organic pollutants, and volatile organic compounds. They are widespread worldwide and show up in lots of household items, from chlorine-bleached paper products to cleaners to nonstick pans to plastic packaging to foods. Forewarned is forearmed, so familiarize yourself with this stuff and take precautions to reduce your exposure to them and to help lessen their impact on the planet.

# Dioxins

Dioxins are a by-product of industrial processing (such as making chlorine bleach, bleaching paper with chlorine, and manufacturing pesticides) and waste incineration (generated by burning plastics, wood treated with pentachlorophenols, and bleached paper).

Dioxins have a nasty proclivity to accumulate in the fatty tissues of humans and animals—a process called *bioaccumulation*[142]—and also to *biomagnify*, meaning that they travel up the food chain.[143] Once in the body, they stay there—our bodies have a hard time getting rid of them. And because they stay in our bodies, exposure to even small amounts is dangerous because they add up over a lifetime. There is no safe level of dioxins.[144] According to the EPA, the use of bleached coffee filters alone is enough to exceed a lifetime of "acceptable levels" of dioxins.

## What Dioxins Do

Dioxins affect us in three ways. They are known teratogens,[145] [146] which cause malformations in fetal development; they are mutagens,[147] which cause genetic mutations, some of which cause cancer; and they are suspected of being human carcinogens,[148] meaning that they may cause cancer. Dioxins mess with the growth regulation of our cells—inducing or blocking cell death—and may cause tissue underdevelopment, overgrowth, or tumors.[149]

Dioxins have been proven to cause cancer in animals; the effect appears to occur in humans, too, with dioxins acting as complete carcinogens that don't require another chemical to have the effect.[150] Dioxins appear to cause tumors[151] and increase the risk for all cancers, according to the World Health Organization and the National Institute for Occupational Safety and Health.

In addition, dioxins mess with estrogen receptors,[152] may be toxic to growth and development,[153] and cause liver damage,[154] nerve damage,[155] and glandular changes.[156] In addition, dioxins are suspected of causing respiratory tract and prostate cancers[157] and type 2 diabetes.[158]

## How We Are Exposed

According to the Agency for Toxic Substances and Disease Registry, dioxins have been found in virtually *all* samples of tissues and blood from people with no known direct exposure.[159]

More than 90 percent of our intake of dioxins is from food because they bioaccumulate in fatty tissues and travel up the food chain.[160] Diet accounts for 96 percent of our total dioxin exposure,[161] and it comes from these sources:

- Animal fats in meat
- Full-fat dairy products
- Fatty fishes like herring, mackerel, salmon, sardines, trout, and tuna
- Produce laden with pesticides

We are also exposed by food that is contaminated when it comes in contact with containers that have dioxins, such as bleached paper products like paper plates, food containers, and milk cartons. We can also absorb dioxins from products like bleached feminine products that are in intimate contact with our bodies (tampons, for instance).

Dioxins can enter our bodies from the air when we breathe in gases, vapors, and emissions from municipal, medical, and hazardous waste incinerators, or from industrial plants like paper mills, cement plants, and metal smelting plants.

Finally, dioxins can also come from exposure to waste sites. Chronic low-level exposure can occur from living or working near hazardous waste sites, and there are currently 126 Superfund sites in the United States that contain dioxins.[162]

### How to Avoid Exposure

Although dioxins have permeated the far reaches of the globe and the near corners of our bodies, there are ways to reduce our own exposure and nip planetary contamination in the bud. Here are some things we can all do.

- Choose paper products wisely. Opt for unbleached or naturally bleached (oxygen-bleached) products, especially for products that come in contact with food and our intimate body tissues—coffee filters, paper towels and napkins, facial tissues and toilet paper, and feminine products (tampons and sanitary pads).
- Choose organic, low-fat, sustainably raised animal products, including low-fat or nonfat dairy products and lean,

grass-fed meats (more than 90 percent of dioxin exposure is from food, particularly fatty foods higher on the food chain like meat,[163] and studies show that vegetarian mothers have fewer dioxins in their breast milk than mothers who eat a diet rich in meat).[164] Better yet, lean toward a plant-based diet, like choosing olive oil over butter.

## Persistent Organic Pollutants

Yes, you might call your dad POP affectionately, but other POPs that aren't quite as nifty are a brand-new category of pollutants, *persistent organic pollutants*. They are a particularly nasty bunch—they are highly toxic, persist in the environment, and bioaccumulate up the food chain. POPs are linked to seriously adverse effects on humans and the environment. They have a nasty proclivity to migrate and travel far from their source of origin. The United Nations Environmental Programme officially adopted the name POPs, and the EPA finds it fitting, too. The EPA also descriptively calls them PBTs, which stands for *persistent, bioaccumulative, and toxic.*

POPs are revolutionary because they are the first group of compounds to be categorized together based on their behavioral similarities. All other materials under the sun are classified according to what they're made of—their molecular similarities. Because of their unique ability to spread and persist in the environment, POPs get their own club. They are

## Mad as a Hatter

The phrase *mad as a hatter* came about because of bioaccumulation. The traditional processing method for stiffening the felt used to make dapper and debonair hats used mercury. Now, mercury is a fat-loving compound that bioaccumulates in the body and brain. The hatters who worked with the stuff went mad as a result of mercury poisoning.

showing up ubiquitously in breast milk and marine life, even at the poles.

They are everywhere and they are not going away.

POPs include a horde of household and industrial chemicals, including pesticides, and by-products of manufacturing and waste incineration.

To officially achieve the status of a POP, a chemical must:

- Persist stubbornly in the environment (have a long environmental half-life)[165]
- Accumulate in body fat (*bioaccumulate*) at greater concentrations as it travels up the food chain, a process called *bioconcentration* or *biomagnification*[166]
- Travel quickly and easily into water systems and/or the atmosphere[167]
- Be acutely toxic in its own right,[168] without the interaction of any other chemicals
- Be associated and linked with acute hormonal, immunological, neurological, and/or reproductive disorders

POPs both bioaccumulate and biomagnify. Let's take mercury as an example (in honor of the hatters; see "Mad as a Hatter," above) because many folks are worried about eating it in fish. Mercury is pervasive at low levels in the ocean. There, algae absorb it rather innocently but quite efficiently. Some hungry plankton snack on the algae for lunch and then a small fish eats the plankton for dinner. Since mercury accumulates in tissues with ease but is slow to be eliminated, it starts to add up. Anything that comes along to feast on the small fish will be eating all the mercury the algae, plankton, and small fish have accumulated. Therefore, when a larger predatory fish like a swordfish or tuna comes along for a banquet meal, it gets a hefty accumulation of mercury. Animals raised for meat, milk, and eggs on land don't go fishing themselves, but ground-up fish in their feed is standard. Guess who's at the top of the food chain, getting the brunt of the bioaccumulative burden? The humans who eat those (or the products of those) critters that eat mercury.

## POPs Worldwide

POPs are a very big deal worldwide because they know no boundaries. One of the properties of persistent pollutants is their ability to travel far from their source of origin—typically from temperate regions toward the equator and the poles, ending up in far-flung places where they have never been used. Because of this trait, the effort to eliminate POPs must be global.

After all, once POPs are manufactured, it is impossible to keep them from escaping and causing irreparable harm. They just don't go away, and even minute amounts of them can be extremely harmful,[169] causing cancer,[170] developmental and reproductive disorders,[171] and damage to the nervous and immune systems.[172] Not nice. But international cooperation is leading a charge to reduce and eliminate POP-releasing activity globally.

## COMMON POPS AND POP-LIKE CHEMICALS

| POP OR CHEMICAL WITH POP-LIKE BEHAVIOR | USED FOR | FOUND IN | HEALTH AND ENVIRONMENTAL EFFECTS |
|---|---|---|---|
| Polybrominated diphenyl ethers | Fire and flame retardants | Carpeting, furnishings, polyurethane foam in furniture and mattresses, car interiors, plastics for TVs and computers | Persistent and mobile in the environment, they are found in Arctic animals[173] and in human breast milk[174][175] and tissue.[176][177] They bioaccumulate.[178] They are endocrine disrupters,[179] and are linked to cancer[180] and reproductive damage.[181] Children at much more at risk than adults.[182] |
| Perfluorooctane sulfonate and perfluorooctanoic acid | Nonstick coatings and stain-resistance coatings | Nonstick cookware, soil- and stain-resistant fabrics, cosmetics, electronics, firefighting foams | They are very persistent and mobile and they bioaccumulate.[183] They are linked to cancer, liver damage, and developmental and reproductive effects.[184] They are found in virtually all humans tested.[185] |
| Polychlorinated naphthalenes | Plasticizer, insulation, heat transfer, preservative | Cable insulation, wood preservatives, engine oil additives, hair dye intermediates, flame retardants, capacitor fluids | Much like dioxins, they are persistent, migrate, and bioaccumulate.[186] They are linked with cancer,[187] endocrine disruption,[188] and reproductive and developmental effects.[189] They are highly toxic to fish and mammals.[190][191] |
| Polybrominated dioxins and bromo-chloro dioxins | By-products generated by the combustion of brominated products (fire retardants) | By-products | They are persistent[192] and bioaccumulative.[193] They are suspected carcinogens[194] and endocrine disrupters.[195] |

Besides mercury, POPs include the pesticides aldrin, chlordane, DDT, dieldrin, endrin, heptachlor, hexachlorobenzene, mirex (also used as a fire retardant), and toxaphene; industrial by-products such as dioxins and furans; and various other chemicals, including polychlorinated biphenyls, polybrominated diphenyl ethers (PBDEs), perfluorooctane sulfonate, perfluorooctanoic acid, and polychlorinated naphthalenes. These chemicals are found in all sorts of household products, from plastic goods to paints, weatherproofing, carpeting, upholstered furniture, cookware, electronics, and cosmetics. More details appear throughout this book.

## Some POPs to Beware Of

There are lots of POPs being produced, both purposefully and as accidental by-products. They're lurking in oodles of consumer products, posing as fire retardants and nonstick coatings. They are also being produced en mass as unwanted, yet pervasive industrial by-products, like dioxins produced by bleaching paper with chlorine or burning plastics.

The table on page 45 lists a few common POPs, or chemicals with POP-like behavior, that are generated by everyday items. Use your consumer dollars, choices, pressure, and support to help stop the generation of these persistent nightmares. Seek out products that don't contain these chemicals—you'll find plenty of recommendations in the rest of this book.

## Consumer Power: How to Avoid POPs

When it comes to issues as big as POPs, it's easy to feel small. Given that you and I are not personally creating them, as consumers we can only avoid buying products that produce POPs. Supply follows demand.

### Here's what you can do

- **Buy organic produce.** While the worst POP pesticide offenders have been banned, there are still plenty of others roaming around conventional fields.
- **Buy organic cotton.** Conventional cotton is one of the most pesticide-intensive crops, and those that are used include POP and POP-like chemicals.
- **Buy an organic or natural mattress not treated with fire-retardant PBDEs.**
- **Avoid nonstick pots and pans.**
- **Eat lower on the food chain.** Because POPs bioaccumulate and biomagnify, animal products have higher concentrations of POPs that are passed on to you.
- **Avoid stain-resistant clothing.**
- **Recycle computers and TVs.** They contain brominated fire retardants that, if incinerated, can form highly brominated dioxins, polybrominated dioxins, and furans.[196]

## Volatile Organic Compounds

Volatile organic compounds (VOCs) are a pesky bunch of gases emitted by a variety of synthetic chemical liquids and solids.

They just won't stay put. Put them in a liquid or solid and they evaporate like our tax dollars at work. A huge number of chemicals are VOCs, and they have differing degrees of short- and long-term adverse effects on humans and the planet.

They're especially destructive to the lungs and the atmosphere. Indoors, the concentration of many VOCs is consistently higher (up to 10 times higher) than outdoors.[197]

Outdoors, VOCs are a menace, too—part of what defines a VOC is that it can evaporate right into the atmosphere, which isn't any good at all. They also react to sunlight and chemicals in the atmosphere and cause ground-level smog, big time.

## Effects on Humans and the Environment

VOCs cause adverse acute and chronic effects on humans and the environment. VOCs are wickedly dangerous and damaging to breathe. They are severely irritating to the eyes, lungs, and delicate tissues in the nose and throat; and can damage the liver, kidneys, and central nervous system with repeated exposure.[198] Some VOCs are known to cause cancer in humans[199] and others are suspected to because they have been shown to cause cancer in animals.[200] Many are suspected reproductive and developmental toxicants.[201]

Classic symptoms from exposure to VOCs include headache; allergic skin reaction; eye, nose, and throat irritation;

shortness of breath; fatigue; dizziness; and memory impairment.[202]

Environmentally, VOCs are a major contributor to air pollution and a key component in smog. VOCs can also have serious effects on wildlife and plants, and pollute the water and soil.

## Where VOCs Come From

VOCs are born from thousands of products. When you hear the term *off-gassing*, that's VOCs at work.

VOCs are emitted by a wide array of products, including solvent-based materials and plastics. A huge proportion of household, building, and office products and materials are classic, common culprits. Solvent-based household commodities that give off VOCs include cleaning products and cosmetics, aerosol sprays and air fresheners, conventionally dry-cleaned clothing, moth repellents, and lawn and garden pesticides. VOCs also come from building and furnishing materials like paints and lacquers, paint strippers, treated wood and particleboard, furnishings, upholstery, and carpet backing. Office equipment such as copiers and printers, correction fluids, and carbonless copy paper; hobby and arts and crafts supplies; glues and adhesives; and permanent markers are other sources of VOCs.

## How to Avoid Them

There are no standards for controlling the use of VOCs outside of industrial settings. Yikes! While the Occupational

Safety and Health Administration regulates one VOC, formaldehyde, as a carcinogen,[203] it's up to savvy consumers to make choices that will reduce and eliminate their VOC exposure. Here are some things you can do.

- **Source control.** Get rid of products that have high levels of VOCs and purchase new products that have low or zero VOCs.
- **Ventilate.** If and when using products with high VOCs, keep air circulating by opening doors and windows or running a fan.
- **Filter air.** In offices, VOCs emitted by printers and photocopiers can be removed by a charcoal-filter air purifier.
- **Plants, plants, plants.** Plants have the ability to absorb VOCs, namely formaldehyde and benzene. Ahhh.
- **Choose eco- and lung-friendly plant-based products,** especially all-purpose cleaners, stain removers, floor cleaners, air fresheners, and heavy-duty cleaners. See Chapters 3 and 4 for recommendations.
- **Avoid aerosol products,** across the board, period.
- **Choose natural cosmetics and personal care products** that don't contain formaldehyde-releasing preservatives. See page 173 for the scoop.

- **Choose low-VOC or zero-VOC paints, finishes, and stains** as well as nontoxic paint strippers. See page 316 for green products.
- **Opt out of using particleboard and pressed wood.** Choose natural, untreated materials for shelving, cabinets, desks, and other furniture. Particleboard contains formaldehyde, a known carcinogenic VOC.[204]
- **Choose cloth or PVC-free plastic shower curtains.** See page 155 for details.
- **Use less plastic all around.** Plastics emit VOCs. The less of it there is around, the better it is all around.
- **Go for a natural or organic mattress.** Opt out of getting a synthetic chemical foam mattress, which can emit VOCs throughout its lifetime. See page 277 for better choices.
- **Choose natural and organic sheets.** Most conventional bedsheets are treated with a formaldehyde finish for wrinkle-free "easy care." See page 271 for the skinny.
- **Ditch synthetic carpeting.** Synthetic carpeting, backing, and adhesives are notorious sources of VOC emissions. Natural fiber carpets or sustainably harvested bamboo, hardwood, or cork; tile; and stone floorings are natural, emission-free options for a house and world of good. See page 325 for some ideas.

CHAPTER 2

# Green Cleaning Basics

**Clean** *adjective*

**1.** free from dirt, pollutants,
or harmful substances (*Oxford English Dictionary*)

The definition of "clean" is very straightforward. Ironically, however, the vast majority of cleaning products do, in fact, pollute both our homes and the environment and are laden with harmful substances. What's the deal, and when did *that* happen?

Up until 60 years ago, all households used a handful of simple, basic materials to keep everything spic-and-span. Stuff like soap, baking soda, salt, vinegar, washing soda, alcohol, and cornstarch were used to lift stains, scour surfaces, polish wood, repel pests, and deodorize and disinfect every surface, nook, and cranny.

The dawn of the chemical age followed quickly on the heels of World War II, instigated by war-related research and a host of "new and improved" products like chemical cleaners, plastics, and disposable goods that quickly became symbols of American prosperity and modern luxury, along with advertising slogans like "better living through chemistry." Vinegar and soap were out, chlorine and synthetic, petroleum-based detergents were in. The modern marvel of petrochemical wonders made domestic chores a breeze. Who needs elbow grease when chemicals will do the work for you? As America's economy bloomed, so did the dizzying array of cleaning products on supermarket shelves, backed by big business's muscle and marketing genius, and tried-and-true methods were subjugated to the products of a chemical revolution. Synthetic products came of age in a time well before the words *ecology* and *environment* were in the common vernacular. But today, these words are part of a growing standard of eco-friendly products and practices that is fueling a new kind of revolution for better living.

In physics, Newton's third law of motion states, "For every action, there is an equal and opposite reaction." Synthetic and chemical cleaning products provide action. The reaction to them arrives in human and ecological terms in acute and chronic effects that compromise the most precious things we have, things like health, clean air, and fresh water. Immediate and long-term human and environmental danger, damage, and contamination are big prices to pay when other cleaning products that would preserve our own health and well-being, as well as those of our children and the planet, could be used instead. Choosing to use effective cleaning products that interact more kindly with the soft tissues of humans and with the environment is the right thing to do. It's not just about saving the fish and the birds and the bees, it's about enjoying a quality of life and health that are worth passing on to succeeding generations. May our demands and practices as consumers rise to the challenge and be the change that is so deeply needed on the planet. If cleanliness is next to godliness, then the devil is in the details and we've got work to do!

## Green Thumb Guidelines

The "Green Thumb Guides" in this chapter will help you choose nontoxic cleaning products that are eco-smart and human-friendly for every corner, nook, and cranny at home.

Here are some guidelines for choosing effective, eco-friendly household products every time. Look for these words and details on product labels.

- Full disclosure of ingredients. Products that do not have a comprehensive list of ingredients are always suspect for harboring nasty chemicals that are no

# 10 Basics of Green Cleaning

There are 10 basic products that will cover cleaning just about everything at home. Choosing green products is a cinch when you know what to look for. Look for these words on product labels for help with choosing wisely and being green.

- Plant based
- Biodegradable
- Chlorine free
- Ammonia free

- Solvent free
- Phosphate free
- No synthetic fragrances or dyes

Here's what to look for in the 10 basic products. In this chapter and later ones, you'll find specific recommendations for these and other green products.

*All-purpose surface spray:* chlorine free, ammonia free, solvent free

*Window and mirror spray:* ammonia free, no synthetic fragrances or dyes

*Liquid dish soap:* plant based, biodegradable, no synthetic fragrances or dyes

*Dishwashing detergent:* plant based, biodegradable, phosphate free, chlorine free, no synthetic fragrances or dyes

*Laundry detergent:* plant based, biodegradable, phosphate free, chlorine free, no synthetic fragrances or dyes

*Oxygen bleach:* chlorine free

*Stain remover:* plant based, biodegradable, chlorine free, solvent free

*Toilet bowl cleaner:* plant based, biodegradable, chlorine free, ammonia free

*Surface scrub:* plant based, biodegradable, chlorine free, no synthetic fragrances or dyes

*Concentrated citrus cleaner:* plant based, biodegradable, no synthetic fragrances or dyes

good for humans and the environment. If a product does not have an ingredient list, look for one that does so you'll know what you are getting. Look for products with labels that explain ingredients such as "plant-based" surfactants or "natural" fragrances. The more description there is, the better. Non-toxic, eco-friendly products will boast about their attributes on their labels.

- Plant and mineral based
- Biodegradable
- No synthetic fragrances or colors
- Chemical free; use products that include no solvents, chlorine, ammonia, or phosphates

# COMMON INGREDIENT HAZARDS:
## ALL-PURPOSE CLEANERS AND GLASS CLEANERS

*All-purpose cleaners are broadly useful, but conventional products are laden with toxic chemicals that you may not be aware of. Here are some examples.*

**Alkyl dimethylbenzyl ammonium chloride, aka quaternary ammonium compound.** This compound has acute and chronic hazards and is an irritant of the eyes, skin, and lungs. Prolonged inhalation may cause loss of motor skills and disorientation.[1]

**Ammonia.** Ammonia is toxic. It's a severely corrosive alkaline that is extremely dangerous to the eyes. It may cause permanent damage,[2] can burn the skin,[3] and is very harmful to inhale.[4]

**Butyl cellusolve, aka 2-butoxyethanol.** It's an irritant of the eyes, skin, and lungs, and can be absorbed through the skin.[5] Prolonged or chronic exposure can damage the liver, kidneys, lymphatic system, blood, and blood-forming organs.[6]

**Chlorine.** This toxic substance is a severe irritant of the eyes, skin, and lungs,[7] as well as a severe corrosive of those same organs.[8] It's very harmful to inhale it,[9] and it may cause permanent lung damage or chemical-induced asthma.[10] It can convert into hypochlorous acid, which can penetrate cells and react with cytoplasmic proteins to destroy cell structure.[11] Children are at greater risk for sustaining injury than are adults.[12] It is also acutely toxic to aquatic life.[13]

**Diethanolamine.** This severe irritant of the eyes, skin, and lungs is harmful if absorbed through the skin.[14] Chronic exposure may affect the blood.[15] Prolonged or repeated exposure may cause liver or kidney damage.[16]

**Dipropylene glycol monobutyl ether.** This compound is an irritant of the eyes, skin, and lungs.[17] Chronic exposure may cause nausea, dizziness, and headache.[18]

**Ethylene glycol.** This highly toxic substance is an irritant of the skin and lungs[19] and a severe irritant of the eyes.[20] It is very harmful to inhale[21] and it is a reproductive hazard.[22] It's also hazardous in the environment.[23]

**Glycol ether.** Chronic exposure to this irritant of the eyes and skin may cause liver and kidney lesions and damage.[24]

**Hydroxyacetic acid,** aka glycolic acid. This acid is extremely corrosive—it will burn the skin.[25] It's also a severe irritant that will burn every area of skin contact.[26] Inhaling it can burn the lungs,[27] and even its vapors can burn the lungs.[28]

**Naphtha.** This substance is toxic. It's an irritant of the eyes, skin, and lungs[29] that is very harmful to inhale.[30] Chronic exposure may cause skin damage, including defatting and dermatitis.[31] A possible carcinogen, it may contain benzene, which is a known carcinogen.[32] Naphtha is found in all-purpose glass and surface cleaners.

**Petroleum distillates.** These toxic substances are irritants of the eyes, skin, and lungs.[33] They may damage the central and peripheral nervous systems and the respiratory system.[34] Very harmful to inhale, petroleum distillates may cause dizziness and loss of coordination and act like a narcotic.[35] Repeated skin contact may cause defatting.[36]

**Phenols.** These compounds are toxic. They're severe irritants of the eyes, skin, and lungs[37] and severe corrosives of the eyes and skin.[38] They may cause an allergic skin reaction.[39] Acutely toxic in the environment, especially to aquatic organisms,[40] phenols also cause long-term harm to the environment.[41]

**Sodium hydroxide.** This severe irritant of the eyes, skin, and lungs[42] may cause a skin rash.[43] It is severely corrosive, causing skin burns. Topical contact with sodium hydroxide may have a delayed effect,[44] and may result in permanent eye damage.[45] Inhaling it causes severe irritation of the respiratory tract, burns, and, possibly, coma.[46]

**Sodium hypochlorite (chlorine bleach).** Chlorine bleach is a severe irritant of the eyes, skin, and lungs. A corrosive, it may cause burning of the skin and irreversible eye injury.[47] Inhalation may cause severe lung damage.[48] If mixed with ammonia, it will create deadly fumes!

**Triethanolamine (TEA).** This compound is a severe irritant of the eyes, skin, and lungs. It may cause an allergic skin reaction.[49] Inhalation of TEA mist may cause respiratory tract irritation.[50] Chronic exposure may cause liver and kidney damage.[51] Prolonged or repeated contact may cause skin necrosis or ulceration.[52]

# The Dirt on Cleaning Products

Cleaning house should be an honest chore, not one that is riddled with unpronounceable chemicals that can literally make your head spin, undermine your central nervous system, and contaminate the ecosystem. The solution to these problems is simple: go for a green all-purpose cleaner to tackle tons of household tasks.

The trouble is that it's terribly tough to find out what's really in a lot of regular all-purpose cleaners. Manufacturers simply aren't required to list ingredients on household cleaning products, and those that do often cloak chemical ingredients in vague terms like *fragrances* and *color* or in unrecognizable names and don't warn users about their possible ill effects. Cleaning has become a dirty business. It's true that miraculous modern cleaning products leave sparkle and shine, and assault you with their "clean" smell. But they can leave behind quite a bit of other stuff that is much less desirable. Check out a few of the many ingredients that may be hazardous and harmful to humans and the planet and are lurking undisclosed on labels. The jury is out on how much exposure for how long is necessary for damage to be done to people and the environment, but even small amounts of dangerous materials can add up to trouble over a lifetime. Less is better and none is the best.

# Green All-Purpose Surface and Glass Cleaners to the Rescue!

All-purpose surface and glass cleaners are the two products used in every room at home. Many conventional all-purpose products contain one or more of a trio of chemicals—most commonly ammonia, bleach, and toxic solvents. None of them are good to be in close quarters or direct contact with, and all are linked with a sliding scale of serious health and environmental effects. Therefore, going green by choosing an all-purpose cleaner and a glass cleaner with nontoxic ingredients is essential for a healthy home. Cleaning and chronic health effects do not go hand in hand in this book, nor does sparkling, spanking clean involve noxious fumes or chemical residues. There are nontoxic options that produce all-purpose cleaning action and sparkling mirrors to boot. Eco-friendly products to the rescue!

An all-purpose surface spray that is sans chemical effluvium is the cornerstone of green cleaning and a multitasking champion. It's the one-stop shop for a wide spectrum of surfaces, from counters and cabinets to stovetops and sinks, and even for soap dishes coated with stubborn soap scum. A naturally effective all-purpose spray will fulfill its promises with a lot of punch and is a formula no household can clean without.

Glass cleaners are another essential for a smudge-free house. Green glass cleaners make mirrors, windows, glass tabletops, and shower doors sparkle, delivering flatteringly reflective and crystal clear results without noxious fumes.

## Scouring Scrubs and Powdered Surface Scrubs

Every now and again, a thorough scouring is called for. Surfaces like sinks, basins, tubs, tile, and others subject to built-up gunk benefit from the use of an old-school remedy: scouring powder.

Conventional multipurpose scouring scrubs are packed with chemicals that are

## SAVING THE PLANET ONE SPRAY AT A TIME

According to the Seventh Generation company, if every household in the United States replaced just one 32-ounce bottle of petroleum-based all-purpose cleaner with a plant-based, biodegradable product, it would save 6,800 barrels of oil—enough to power hundreds of homes for a year.[53]

# 6 Basics For Homemade Cleaning Formulas

Homemade cleaning formulas are cheap, easy, and green to a T. To whip up a medley of your own green cleaners, you will need a handful of easy-to-find ingredients.

1. White distilled vinegar
2. Baking soda
3. Castile soap or another eco-friendly liquid soap
4. Oxygen bleach powder and/or hydrogen peroxide
5. Antiseptic essential oils: cinnamon, clove, lavender, lemon, lemongrass, lime, oregano, rosemary, tea tree, and thyme (see page 64 for information on these)
6. Grapefruit seed extract (available at most natural markets and online)

tough on not only grime, but also on human skin and lungs and the ecosystem later on. They commonly include toxic surfactants that allow oil and water to mix, such as sodium dodecylbenzene sulfonate, which is a severe irritant[54] and extremely corrosive.[55] It can burn skin that comes in contact with it and burn the lungs when its fine dust is inhaled. It's also noted for having long-term adverse effects in the ecosystem,[56] which obviously is no good at all. Chlorine bleach is often thrown into surface scrub powders for good measure. Chlorine is hazardous to breathe[57] or touch[58]—it can actually penetrate skin and damage cells[59]—and it is broadly hazardous in the environment,[60] throwing water ecosystems out of whack and poisoning wildlife and soil. All of that makes reaching for nontoxic, natural scouring scrubs a choice green pick for your paws, your lungs, and the planet.

Natural scouring scrubs use the power of plants, minerals, and oxygen bleach to scour and slough off dirt and stains. Check out the "Green Thumb Guide" on page 58 for clean, green surface scrub options. For more information, and some nifty homemade soft scrub and frosting scrub formulas, see Chapter 4.

*When you are in the market for effective, green all-purpose and glass cleaners and powdered surface scrubs, look for these products for safe, eco-friendly cleaning action.*

# ALL-PURPOSE AND GLASS CLEANERS

## BIOKLEEN

### All Purpose Spray
32-ounce trigger spray bottle

*Ingredients:* All ingredients are disclosed. The spray is plant based, nontoxic, chemical free, and biodegradable. Its fragrance is derived from citrus. It is not tested on animals.

*Uses:* Use to clean all washable surfaces and fabrics, appliances, mirrors, walls, vinyl, stainless steel, porcelain, painted surfaces, and more.

### Glass Cleaner
32-ounce trigger spray bottle

*Ingredients:* All ingredients are disclosed. The cleaner is plant based, nontoxic, chemical free, ammonia free, and biodegradable. It has no fragrances or dyes, and no fumes. It is not tested on animals.

*Uses:* It cleans glass, mirrors, chrome, and hard, shiny surfaces.

*Available:* at natural markets and select supermarkets and online

www.biokleenhome.com

## CALDREA

### Countertop Cleanser
16-ounce trigger spray bottle

*Ingredients:* This nontoxic, plant-based, chlorine- and solvent-free biodegradable spray includes naturally antiseptic Birch Bark Extract and Vegetable Protein Extract for added cleaning potency. It's available in five lovely fragrances such as Italian Cypress Pear and Citrus Mint Ylang Ylang from naturally derived sources and some well-researched, biodegradable, human-safe synthetic sources.

*Uses:* Safe for nonporous surfaces such as finished wooden and tile floors, countertops, walls, porcelain, bathroom fixtures, sealed granite, stainless steel, and more

### All-Purpose Cleanser
32-ounce screw-top bottle

*Ingredients:* This highly concentrated cleaner uses plant-based surfactants and naturally antiseptic Birch Bark Extract. No chemical solvents, chlorine or artificial colorants. Available in five fantastic scents such as Ginger Pomelo and Lavender Pine derived from natural fragrances including essential oils and some well-researched, biodegradable, human-safe synthetic sources.

*Uses:* For cleaning nonporous surfaces including sealed wooden floors, cupboards, tile, sealed granite and marble countertops, and stainless steel

### Window Spray
16-ounce trigger spray bottle

*Ingredients:* This spray is biodegradable and contains no harsh ammonia or synthetic ingredients. It's available in 4 enticing fragrances such as Green Tea Patchouli and Basil Blue Sage from natural and well-researched, biodegradable, human-safe synthetic sources.

*Uses:* It works wonders on all glass, mirrors, and hard shiny surfaces.

*Available:* in select home stores such Sur la Table, Smith & Hawkin, and online

www.caldrea.com

## CITRA-SOLV

### Natural Cleaner and Degreaser
22-ounce trigger spray bottle

*Ingredients:* All ingredients are disclosed. The spray is plant based, nontoxic, ammonia free, solvent free, and 100 percent biodegradable. It has citrus peel strength.

*Uses:* Use on countertops, stoves, floors, walls, upholstery, carpets, bathroom surfaces, showers, stainless steel, wood, and porcelain.

*Available:* at natural markets and select supermarkets and online

www.citra-solv.com

## EARTH FRIENDLY PRODUCTS

### Parsley Plus All-Surface Cleaner
22-ounce trigger spray bottle

*Ingredients:* All ingredients are disclosed. This spray is plant based, nontoxic, chlorine free, solvent free, ammonia free, glycol free, and biodegradable with a fresh parsley scent.

*Uses:* It's great for all washable hard surfaces, including countertops, ovens, appliances, sinks, walls, floors, ceramic tile, clothing, painted surfaces, vinyl, linoleum, metal, porcelain, and wood.

*Available:* at natural markets and select supermarkets and online

www.ecos.com

## ECOVER

### All-Purpose Cleaner
32-ounce screw-top bottle

*Ingredients:* All ingredients are disclosed. This cleaner is plant based, nontoxic, chlorine free, free of synthetic fragrances and dyes, and biodegradable. It has a natural lemon fragrance and is not tested on animals.

*Uses:* For all washable surfaces, including counters, cabinets, floors, tile, and wood.

### Glass and Surface Cleaner
16-ounce trigger spray bottle

*Ingredients:* All ingredients are disclosed. This cleaner is plant based, nontoxic, chlorine free, free of synthetic fragrances and dyes, and biodegradable. It has a plant-based fragrance.

*Uses:* It's good for all washable surfaces, including counters, cabinets, floors, tile, and wood.

*Available:* at natural markets and select supermarkets and online. To find a store near you, call 800-449-4925.

www.ecover.com

## METHOD

### All Purpose Surface Cleaner
28-ounce trigger spray bottle

*Ingredients:* This cleaner is nontoxic and contains naturally derived surfactants. It is biodegradable. It uses nontoxic, natural fragrances (not all are plant based), but the Go Naked variety has no dyes or perfumes.

*Uses:* It's safe for virtually any surface in the home.

*Available:* at grocery stores and retail chains and online

www.methodhome.com

## MRS. MEYER'S CLEAN DAY

### All Purpose Cleaner
32-ounce screw-top bottle

*Ingredients:* All ingredients are disclosed. The cleaner is plant based, nontoxic, chlorine free, and biodegradable. Its natural fragrances are derived from essential oils. The formula is concentrated and should be diluted for use.

*Uses:* Great for all nonporous surfaces, such as finished wood, tile, countertops, walls, porcelain, bathroom fixtures, and sealed natural and synthetic stone.

### Countertop Spray
16-ounce trigger spray bottle

*Ingredients:* All ingredients are disclosed. The spray is plant based, nontoxic, chlorine free, and biodegradable. It has a special vegetable protein to combat odors, and its natural fragrances are derived from essential oils.

*Uses:* It's great for all nonporous surfaces, such as finished wood and tile floors, countertops, walls, vinyl, concrete, porcelain, bathroom fixtures, sealed natural and synthetic stone, and more.

### Window Spray
20-ounce pump spray bottle

*Ingredients:* All ingredients are disclosed. This window cleaner is plant based, nontoxic, ammonia free, solvent free, and biodegradable. Its natural fragrances are derived from essential oils. It's not tested on animals.

*Uses:* Use it for cleaning mirrors, glass, and windows.

*Available:* at natural markets, select supermarkets, and grocery stores and online

www.mrsmeyers.com

*(continued)*

## PLANET

### All Purpose Spray Cleaner
22-ounce trigger spray bottle

*Ingredients:* This product is nontoxic, phosphate free, free of fragrances and dyes, and biodegradable. It is not tested on animals and comes in bottles made with recycled content.

*Uses:* It cleans most surfaces, including countertops, painted wood and metal, plastic, carpets, vinyl floors, ceramic tiles, porcelain, sinks, tubs, and fiberglass.

*Available:* at grocery stores and retail chains and online

www.planetinc.com

## SEVENTH GENERATION

### Free and Clear All Purpose Cleaner
32-ounce trigger spray bottle

*Ingredients:* All ingredients are disclosed. This cleaner is plant based, nontoxic, chlorine free, free of fragrances and dyes, and biodegradable. It leaves no residue on cleaned surfaces and generates no fumes. It's not tested on animals.

*Uses:* This product cleans most hard surfaces inside and outside the home. It can be used for wet mopping, but it's not recommended for wood floors. It is suitable for heavy-duty use.

### Glass and Surface Cleaner
16-ounce trigger spray bottle

*Ingredients:* All ingredients are disclosed. This cleaner is plant based, nontoxic, and biodegradable. It contains no fragrances, dyes, volatile organic compounds (VOCs), alcohols, ammonia, or solvents and will produce no fumes. It is not tested on animals.

*Uses:* Use it for cleaning glass, mirrors, chrome, and hard surfaces around the house.

*Available:* at natural markets and select supermarkets and online

www.seventhgeneration.com

## POWDERED SURFACE SCRUBS

## BON AMI

### Polishing Cleanser
14-ounce shake canister

*Ingredients:* All ingredients are disclosed. Bon Ami is nontoxic, plant and mineral based, and 100 percent biodegradable. It contains no chlorine, perfumes, dyes, or harsh abrasives, so it won't scratch surfaces.

*Uses:* Cleans appliances, sinks, bathtubs, pots and pans, tile, china, grout, grills, and more.

*Available:* at grocery stores and natural markets and online

www.bonami.com

## CALDREA

### Powdered Scrub
11-ounce shake canister

*Ingredients:* This scrub is plant and mineral based and contains no chlorine, phosphates, dyes, or harsh abrasives. It's available in five inviting scents such as Ginger Pomelo and Citrus Mint Ylang Ylang, from naturally derived and some well-researched, biodegradable, human-safe synthetic sources.

*Uses:* On virtually any surface in your bathroom or kitchen

*Available:* in select home stores such Sur la Table, Smith & Hawkin, and online

www.caldrea.com

## MRS. MEYER'S CLEAN DAY

### Surface Scrub
11-ounce shake canister

*Ingredients:* All ingredients are disclosed. It's nontoxic, mineral and plant based, and 100 percent biodegradable. It contains oxygen bleach and fragrances from essential oils.

*Uses:* On countertops, stoves, floors, walls, upholstery, carpets, bathroom surfaces, showers, stainless steel, wood, porcelain

*Available:* at natural markets and select supermarkets and online

www.mrsmeyers.com

## Homemade Master Formulas

Homemade cleaning formulas are cheap, effective, and a breeze to whip up using basic ingredients found in the pantry. These homemade formulas offer primo punch for everyday cleaning.

*Note:* Some very effective homemade formulas for heavy-duty jobs call for heavy-duty ingredients like borax and washing soda. Both are very alkaline substances that caustically cut grease and grime with a vengeance, but are a little stronger than I generally like to use. I am a loyal enthusiast of do-it-yourself domesticity, but some stuff I am happy to leave to the pros—such as making nontoxic products formulated for all-purpose heavy-duty cleaning. If you are a dedicated homemade maven and want to make your own heavy-duty cleaners, I recommend checking out *Better Basics for the Home*, by Annie Berthold-Bond, for detailed formulations that will combat just about every household cleaning task.

# Lavender–Lemon Disinfecting Spirits Spray

*This spray is a disinfecting dream sans chlorine and solvents. Hydrogen peroxide and vodka both deliver strong antiseptic disinfection without noxious fumes or toxic residue. The spray works superbly for giving surfaces a quick once-over after deep or light cleaning, and it's commendable for cleaning cutting boards. It's for general use, but may not destroy all bacteria from raw meat and poultry. The scent of alcohol will quickly dissipate, leaving sanitary conditions in its wake. Adding essential oils provides extra disinfecting power as well as a lovely smell. Salute!*

**YIELD: ABOUT 1 PINT**

¼ cup vodka (not the Belvedere, darling, a cheaper one will do)

½ cup 3 percent hydrogen peroxide (yup, the stuff from the drugstore)

1 cup water

5 drops grapefruit seed extract (optional)

10 drops essential oil of lavender (optional)

5 drops essential oil of lemon (optional)

In a spray bottle, combine all the ingredients and swirl to mix them. Do not shake the bottle vigorously or the active oxygen in the hydrogen peroxide will go flat and lose its action.

Spray the surface and wipe it, or spray it and let it dry.

It will keep indefinitely.

# All-Purpose Citrus Spray

*This spray is a grand all-purpose formula that will beat all kinds of grime, and it's cheap as beans! Tried-and-true vinegar has been used for generations to naturally deodorize and disinfect. It has a pretty strong smell, but it dissipates quickly, neutralizing odors in the process and leaving a fresh, clean scent in its wake. A wee bit of concentrated citrus cleaner can go the extra mile to cut grime and lift stains. Essential oils boost the antiseptic action, and their pleasant scent will linger after the vinegar evaporates. Yum.*

*Use this spray on all washable surfaces in the kitchen and bathroom (especially sinks, countertops, tubs, and tiled areas). It's highly effective against mineral stains, hard-water deposits, and soap scum.*

**YIELD: 1 PINT**

½ cup white distilled vinegar
1 tablespoon Citra-Solv Cleaner and Degreaser concentrate (see page 56)
½ teaspoon liquid dish soap or castile soap
1½ cups warm water
½ teaspoon total antiseptic essential oils (see note at right)

In a spray bottle, combine all the ingredients and shake well to mix.

Spray and wipe as you go.

The solution will keep indefinitely.

*Note:* Customize your formula with the essential oils of your choice. A number of essential oils will naturally boost the antiseptic abilities of a homemade cleaning formula. Keep your cleaning fresh and exciting by mixing and matching the essential oils of cinnamon, clove, lavender, lemon, lemongrass, lime, oregano, rosemary, sweet orange, tea tree, and thyme. I recommend starting with one or two essential oils and going from there, because too many competing scents can be just too much, plus essential oils are concentrated and very strong, so a little goes a long way. Follow your sense—your nose knows!

# All-Purpose Deodorizing Basic Soda Spray

*This alkaline formula is tough on dirt and stains. Baking soda and club soda are chock full of alkaline minerals, which cut grime, lift soil, and naturally deodorize. Baking soda is a little abrasive, but it won't scratch surfaces. Castile soap is one of the oldest and most effective cleansers around. Together, they make a safe substitute for solvent-based cleaners. The essential oils both disinfect and refresh with their alluring aromas. Life is too short not to smell good.*

*Use this spray on all washable surfaces in the kitchen and bathroom. It's especially good for lifting stains, dissolving grease, and neutralizing odors. This spray is best for areas in the kitchen and bathroom that can be wiped off after applying it, because the baking soda can leave a wee bit of residue.*

**YIELD: 1 PINT**

½ teaspoon baking soda

½ teaspoon castile soap (scented or unscented)

½ teaspoon total rosemary and sweet orange essential oils (or other antiseptic essential oils of your choice)

1 cup very warm water

1 cup club soda

In a clean spray bottle, combine the baking soda, soap, essential oils, and water. Screw on the top and shake the bottle well to dissolve the ingredients. Add the club soda and swirl the bottle gently to mix it in. If pressure builds up from the carbonated club soda, unscrew the bottle's top to release the gas.

Spray the cleaner on the surface and rub it with a sponge or rag. Wipe it off and admire the view.

For tough spots, spray it on and let it stand for a few minutes before scrubbing and wiping.

If the baking soda settles, shake the bottle before each use and release any remaining gas from the club soda.

# All-Purpose Oxygen Bleach Spray

*Oxygen bleach is a powerhouse cleanser. Commonly used in laundry detergents to boost the detergents' action and effectively lift stains (and it's not just for white fabrics, it's safe for colored garments too!), oxygen bleach powder can be mixed with water to make a fabulous all-purpose spray for cleaning all kinds of surfaces in the kitchen and bathroom, as well as applying to laundry stains. Like chlorine bleach, it disinfects. Unlike chlorine bleach, it is nontoxic and safe for the environment and humans. Essential oils add a nice scent for surface cleaning, but don't use a solution that includes them on laundry stains.*

*It's best to make a small batch of this spray because the active oxygen will dissipate in a day or two. Cut the recipe in half if you don't plan to use it all at once.*

**YIELD: ABOUT 1 PINT**

2 tablespoons oxygen bleach powder

2 cups warm water

¼ teaspoon antiseptic essential oils of your choice (optional; see page 64)

Place the oxygen bleach powder and warm water in a spray bottle. Gently swirl to mix and dissolve the oxygen bleach powder. Add the essential oils and swirl again. Don't shake this mixture vigorously or the active oxygen will dissipate. For general cleaning, spray the cleaner on the surface and let it stand for 1 to 2 minutes, then wipe with a sponge or rag for the most effective action. For laundry stains, spray it directly on the stain until it is thoroughly damp. Let it stand for 10 to 15 minutes before washing.

# Clear and Clean Glass Spray

*Vinegar is the protagonist in this recipe for squeaky-clean glass and mirrors. It's a fine alternative to the offensive fumes from the ammonia and toxic solvents found in commercial cleaners, and it's a thrifty deal to mix up, too. Adding a wee bit of liquid soap will help it cut though grimy film for sparkly, streak-free results. This is one of the simplest formulas to whip up to save money and avoid chemicals.*

**YIELD: 1 QUART**

¼ cup distilled white vinegar

½ teaspoon liquid soap (dish soap or castile soap)

1¾ cups water

8 drops essential oils of your choice (optional; see "Essential-Oil Aroma Combos" on page 64 for ideas)

In a spray bottle, mix together all of the ingredients.

Spray the cleaner on glass, windows, and mirrors and wipe until clear and dry. (Newspaper is the cat's meow for wiping glass; see below.)

## GREEN TIPS for Streak-Free Glass and Mirrors

When switching from ammonia-based products, you might see streaks after the first application of an ammonia-free product. These streaks are residue from the previously used products.

To get rid of the streaks, clean the glass or mirror two or three times with the ammonia-free product to remove the buildup. I know, it's a little extra effort, but you will have to do it just this once. It's worth it!

Newspaper is absolutely the best for cleaning windows, glass, and mirrors. It works brilliantly because, unlike cloths or rags, it simply has no lint to leave behind to besmirch the clarity. And it's a fine way to use fewer paper towels (saving money, trees, and pollution). Dandy.

When the task is complete, you can still recycle the newspaper. Now that's news that's fit to print.

# Essential Oils for Cleaning

For eons, essential oils derived from plants have been valued for their medicinal and therapeutic properties. Modern science has verified the value of many traditional oils, especially their antiseptic, antibacterial, antimicrobial, and antiviral qualities. The most notable essential oils in this regard are cinnamon,[61] clove,[62] [63] lavender,[64] lemon,[65] lemongrass,[66] orange,[67] oregano,[68][69][70] rosemary,[71] thyme,[72][73][74] and tea tree.[75]

Pure essential oils are available at most natural markets and from online sources. They aren't cheap, but one bottle can easily last a year.

Here's a guide to some essential oils that are effective cleaners. They work as well as they smell, which is wonderfully.

**Cinnamon** (*Cinnamomum verum*)
*Properties:* antiseptic; said to stimulate the body and mind
*Aroma:* warm, sweet, invigorating, fresh, spicy wood

**Clove** (*Syzygium aromaticum*)
*Properties:* antiseptic; repels ants
*Aroma:* warm, spicy–fruity, penetratingly sweet, woody; very strong scent, use moderately

**Lavender** (*Lavandula augustifolia*)
*Properties:* antiseptic, antifungal; traditionally used to heal skin and clean cuts
*Aroma:* floral, herbal, sweet

**Lemon** (*Citrus limon*)
*Properties:* antibacterial, antiseptic, deodorizing
*Aroma:* fresh, bright, citrusy, refreshing

**Lemongrass** (*Cymbopogon citratus*)
*Properties:* antiseptic; repels insects
*Aroma:* fresh, sweet, lemony, grassy, floral

**Lime** (*Citrus aurantiifolia*)
*Properties:* antibacterial, antifungal, antiseptic
*Aroma:* fresh, sweetly citrusy

**Oregano** (*Origanum* species)
*Properties:* antibacterial, antiviral
*Aroma:* spicy, woody, sweet, savory

**Rosemary** (*Rosmarinus officialis*)
*Properties:* antiseptic
*Aroma:* clean, herbal, balsamic, woody, minty

**Sweet Orange** (*Citrus sinensis*)
*Properties:* disinfectant
*Aroma:* fresh, juicy, sweetly citrusy

**Tea Tree** (*Melaleuca alternifolia*)
*Properties:* antiseptic, disinfectant, antifungal
*Aroma:* strong, camphorlike

**Thyme** (*Thymus vulgaris*)
*Properties:* antiseptic, disinfectant, antibacterial, antimicrobial
*Aroma:* spicy, woody, sweet, sharp

## ESSENTIAL-OIL AROMA COMBOS

Try making your own fragrance combinations. Here are a few scent combinations you can find in commercial blends.

*Citrus Blend:* lemon, sweet orange, and lime
*Lavender and Lemongrass*
*Clean Spice:* thyme, oregano, and rosemary
*Winter Spice:* cinnamon, clove, and sweet orange
*Sweet Woods:* thyme, rosemary, and cinnamon
*Sweet Citrus Fields:* lavender, lemon, lemongrass, and sweet orange

# Floor Cleaners

Wood, tile, linoleum, vinyl, stone, bamboo, carpet: Floors serve our every step. Whether you opt to clean your floors with a mop, a sponge on a stick, or a sponge wielded while on your hands and knees, keeping floors clean with green, nontoxic products is a wise, winning move.

There are two types of floor cleaners: solvent based and water based. Most conventional floor cleaners are the solvent-based variety. They effectively cut grimy dirt, but because they are also harmful to delicate lung tissue and skin, they're really dangerous to touch or breathe.[76] [77] [78] [79] Petrochemical solvents aren't biodegradable, period. Nonbiodegradable products like floor cleaners don't contaminate just some far-flung river over yonder, they also build up and contaminate our homes. We're talking about really nasty chemicals that accumulate in our kitchens, bathrooms, and intimate spaces. Unless you are sealed in a spacesuit, it's inevitable that you will breathe and touch the stuff when you're cleaning floors. That's a big deal, especially if you look at what some of the chemicals can do.

Using my cunning investigative skills,

I looked at what was lurking behind the labels of about a dozen conventional name-brand floor cleaners. I tell you, this was no simple task. The labels of household products don't have to include an ingredient list, which is astounding considering the possible health effects associated with them. As I had expected, I found that solvents are widely used, but I was shocked by which chemical solvents are being used so casually.

The most common solvents I found in floor cleaners were dipropylene glycol methyl ether, 2-butoxyethanol, monoethanolamine, and ammonium hydroxide. In addition, I found heavy-duty surfactant detergents such as nonylphenol polyethoxylate. All of those are extremely nasty and toxic; these substances are harmful to inhale and to touch, and they may damage organs. Now, think about applying that to your floor, walking around on it, then getting into bed—not a cuddly thought. Think about the kids playing on the floor and putting everything that's been on the floor in their mouths. That's *really* not a cuddly thought.

## Green Floor Cleaning

Keeping floors spic-and-span with non-toxic products keeps everything green inside and out. Green floor cleaners pack the power of plant-based surfactants for spiffy floors made of any material. Water-based products are a safe alternative to chemical-solvent cleaners, and for heavy-duty jobs, citrus-based solvents wield grime-busting muscle.

High-traffic carpeted areas that become dull, dirty, or stained can be cleaned with nontoxic green solutions without leaving the harmful residues that accompany conventional products. Having carpets professionally steam cleaned from time to time is the most effective deep-cleaning method, but for do-it-yourself cleaning and taking care of spots and stains, these products will keep carpet and rug fibers at their best so you can breathe easier.

## COMMON INGREDIENT HAZARDS: FLOOR CLEANERS

*Here are just a few of the nasty ingredients commonly found in conventional floor cleaners and their possible ill effects. With this in mind, choosing nontoxic products for cleaning every floor makes a world of sense.*

**Dipropylene glycol methyl ether.** This highly toxic compound is a severe irritant of the eyes, nose, and throat,[81] and neurotoxic.[82] It may have reproductive and developmental effects,[83] as well as possibly damaging the central nervous system.[84] It's also hazardous in the environment.[85]

**2-Butoxyethanol.** A highly toxic substance, it's also an irritant that may cause respiratory problems and/or damage the lungs.[86] It also may damage red blood cells[87] and the liver,[88] and it may cause reproductive disorders and birth defects.[89]

**Monoethanolamine.** This is an irritant of the eyes, skin, and lungs,[90] and it's harmful to inhale.[91] Corrosive to the eyes, skin, and lungs,[92] it may cause dermatitis.[93] Repeated exposure may affect the liver or kidneys.[94] It's also toxic to fish.[95]

**Ammonium hydroxide.** An irritant of the eyes, nose, throat, skin, and lungs,[96] this substance causes irreparable damage to the respiratory tract.[97] It may cross the placental barrier in pregnant sheep[98] and is hazardous to aquatic ecosystems.[99]

**Nonylphenol polyethoxylate.** This irritant of the eyes, skin, and lungs[100] is a skin sensitizer and may cause allergies and dematitis.[101] [102] It also disrupts the endocrine system,[103] and may affect the kidneys and liver.[104] It's acutely toxic to aquatic life.[105]

*For green, nontoxic, spic-and-span floor cleaning, check out these eco-friendly products.*

# FLOOR CLEANERS

## BONA

### Swedish Formula Hardwood Floor Cleaner
32-ounce trigger spray bottle, 1-gallon screw-top bottle

*Ingredients:* This cleaner is nontoxic, biodegradable, and solvent free.

*Uses:* It's good for all finished wood floors.

*Available:* at hardware stores and online

www.bonakemi.com

## CITRA-SOLV

### Natural Cleaner and Degreaser
8-, 16-, and 32-ounce screw-top bottles

*Ingredients:* Citra-Solv is a nontoxic, natural citrus solvent.

*Uses:* Diluted, it will clean most floors.

*Available:* at natural markets, grocery stores, and hardware stores and online

www.citra-solv.com

## EARTH FRIENDLY PRODUCTS

### Floor Kleener
22-ounce trigger spray bottle

*Ingredients:* This nontoxic cleaner has naturally derived surfactants and is biodegradable and solvent free.

*Uses:* It's good for all floors, including wood and wood laminates.

*Available:* at natural markets and online

www.ecos.com

## ECOVER

### Floor Soap
32-ounce screw-top bottle

*Ingredients:* A nontoxic, plant-based, biodegradable soap, it is also solvent free. Its natural fragrances come from plants, and its saponified oils will fill the pores of the floor.

*Uses:* Use it on all untreated floors, such as tile, marble, concrete, and linoleum, but not on sealed wood floors.

*Available:* at natural markets and online

www.ecover.com

## METHOD

### Omop Floor Cleaner
25-ounce squeeze-top bottle

*Ingredients:* Omop is nontoxic, plant based, biodegradable, and solvent-free. It gets its natural fragrances from plants.

*Uses:* All-Floor Lemon Ginger is for all floor types except wood. "Wood for Good" Almond is for wood floors.

*Available:* at grocery stores and retail chains and online

www.methodhome.com

## OLD TYME 1881

### Super Pine Cleaner
16-ounce screw-top bottle

*Ingredients:* This highly concentrated nontoxic cleaner has pine-oil surfactants and is biodegradable and solvent free. The pine oil is tapped from pine trees like maple syrup is from maple trees, so it's a renewable resource.

*Uses:* It deodorizes and sanitizes all floors, including wood. It can also be used as an all-purpose cleaner for all hard surfaces, even garbage cans.

*Available:* at natural markets and online

www.gaiam.com

*(continued)*

## PRO SHOT

**Industrial Re-Newing Floor Restorer and Finish**
32-ounce screw-top bottle

*Ingredients:* This product is nontoxic and petrochemical free.

*Uses:* The industrial-strength formula fills in scratches and goes on like wax to rejuvenate and protect sealed wood, vinyl, linoleum, terrazzo, concrete, marble, and slate floors.

*Available:* at select hardware stores and online

www.proshotcorp.com

# CARPET CLEANERS

## BEGLEY'S BEST

**Household Cleaner and Carpet Spot Remover**
24-ounce trigger spray bottle, 1-gallon screw-top bottle (concentrate)

*Ingredients:* It's plant based, nontoxic, biodegradable, and contains no harsh chemicals, chlorine, solvents, or phosphates. I have used this on really dingy car floor mats and they came out looking brand-new.

*Uses:* This is one of the ultimate all-purpose stain removers for laundry, carpets, and upholstery, and it's from actor Ed Begley Jr.'s company; thank you, Ed!

*Available:* at some natural markets and online

www.begleysbest.com

## CITRA-SOLV

**Citra-Spot**
22-ounce trigger spray bottle

*Ingredients:* This plant-based, nontoxic, biodegradable spot remover has natural enzymes and bacterial cultures.

*Uses:* It's good for removing organic stains (blood, pet stains, grass stains, and more) and odors.

*Available:* at natural markets and online

www.citra-solv.com

## EARTH FRIENDLY PRODUCTS

**Carpet Shampoo**
40-ounce screw-top bottle

*Ingredients:* This product is nontoxic, biodegradable, all natural, and free of harsh chemicals, chlorine, solvents, and phosphates. The concentrated formula includes extracts of bergamot and sage.

*Uses:* Use it with hot- or cold-water extraction machines.

**Everyday Stain and Odor Remover**
22-ounce trigger spray bottle

*Ingredients:* This product is nontoxic, biodegradable, all natural, and free of harsh chemicals, chlorine, solvents, and phosphates. The formula contains enzymes and natural lemon oil, and it is safe on colors.

*Uses:* Use it with hot- or cold-water extraction machines.

*Available:* at natural markets and online

www.ecos.com

## ECOVER

**Stain Remover**
6.8-ounce bottle with built-in brush

*Ingredients:* It's plant based, nontoxic, and biodegradable.

*Uses:* Designed for treating laundry stains, it also removes all kinds of stains (grass, blood, mud, oil, and food) from carpets and upholstery.

*Available:* at natural markets and online. For a list of stores in your area, call 800-449-4925.

www.ecover.com

## MRS. MEYER'S CLEAN DAY

**Odor Removing Carpet Cleaner**
22-ounce trigger spray bottle

*Ingredients:* Nontoxic, plant and mineral based, and biodegradable, this cleaner gets its natural fragrances from plants and essential oils.

*Uses:* It's excellent for removing spots and stains.

*Available:* at natural markets and online

www.mrsmeyers.com

## SEVENTH GENERATION

**Natural Citrus Carpet Cleaner**
32-ounce trigger spray bottle

*Ingredients:* This carpet cleaner is nontoxic, has all natural ingredients, and is biodegradable. It contains no harsh chemicals, chlorine, solvents, or phosphates.

*Uses:* Use its hydrogen peroxide and citrus stain-removing power for removing grease and oil.

*Available:* at natural markets and some grocery stores and online

www.seventhgeneration.com

# Heavy-Duty Formula for Floors

*This floor formula is quick to mix up and less expensive than store-bought products. Citra-Solv is a concentrated citrus solvent that can cut through the toughest dirt, grease, and grime. Vinegar disinfects and deodorizes, and the naturally derived surfactants in liquid dish soap round out the formula to lift dirt with ease. The essential oil of lavender is optional, but it's an antiseptic and leaves a lovely smell after the vinegar has dissipated. For heavy-duty action on nonwood floors, wet the floor with this formula and let it stand for 10 to 15 minutes before mopping. Don't let it sit on wood floors, however.*

2 gallons warm water

½ cup white vinegar

¼ cup Citra-Solv Natural Cleaner and Degreaser (undiluted)

2 tablespoons biodegradable liquid dish soap

½ teaspoon essential oil of lavender (optional)

Mix all of the ingredients in a bucket. Mop to your heart's content.

# Air Fresheners

Who doesn't love a fresh-smelling room? The difference between a fresh smell and a toxic chemical mist is a very blurry line in the conventional air-freshening-product world. Most air fresheners are laced with artificial perfumes—unfriendly chemicals that actually pollute the air. That doesn't make very much sense. Chemical fragrances and perfumes in air-freshening products can be pretty hazardous, causing sensitization,[106] allergies,[107] respiratory problems,[108] and cellular damage.[109] The trouble is that on a product label, *fragrance* can mean just about anything, because a fragrance can contain as few as 10 chemicals or as many as hundreds. Ninety-five percent of chemicals used in fragrances are synthetic petrochemicals.[110] They include benzene derivatives, aldehydes, and other well-known toxins and sensitizers that have been linked to cancer, central nervous system damage, birth defects, and allergic reactions.[111] Phthalate compounds are among the favored chemicals for fragrances because of their ability to make a smell stick around. They stick around, all right. Phthalates are neurotoxins[112] that accumulate in the tissues of humans and wildlife[113] and are linked to endocrine disruption,[114] [115] developmental and reproductive disorders,[116] [117] and cancer.[118] [119] They're also wickedly toxic in the environment.[120] Yikes! All in the name of fresh air?

Chemicals like these are anything but fresh.

## The Deal with Aerosols

Aerosol sprays are possibly the most chemically insulting air fresheners. While ozone-devouring chlorofluorocarbons have been banned in aerosols for a long time, commonly used hydrofluorocarbon propellants like propane, butane, and isobutane are pretty dodgy on their own, let alone when used to mist a fine vapor of chemicals throughout a room. I looked at publicly registered Material Safety Data Sheets for a passel of aerosol room sprays that contain mist propellants and consistently came across warnings about an "aspiration hazard"—meaning that they're dangerous to breathe. That doesn't sound very compatible with fresh air.

Nonaerosol pump sprays are a healthy, green option for room freshening. Pure products with plant-based fragrances and essential oils are an eco-friendly, human-safe way to freshen rooms naturally so everyone can breathe easier.

## Naturally Fresh

Natural air-freshening products tap into the purifying power of plants and essential oils to resuscitate stale air in a nontoxic way.

# Air-Purifying Plants!

Plants are perhaps the most sophisticated air-purification systems around. Plants are not simply aesthetically agreeable companions flush with ambience, they are also cosmopolitan air filters that wick away indoor air pollutants and produce fresh, clean oxygen. It's a pretty good deal. A constant, silent battle goes on in homes and offices everywhere, with oxygen duking it out in a fight for space with the volatile chemicals emitted by synthetic materials.

The US Environmental Protection Agency currently ranks indoor air pollution near the top of a handful of constant threats to human health.[121] Indoor air is commonly two to five times more polluted than outside air,[122] even in urban areas, and the volume of volatile organic compounds (VOCs) is consistently 10 times higher indoors than outdoors,[123] and sometimes even 100 times higher.[124] Oh my. While removing and reducing the use of the causes of indoor air pollution—chemical cleaners, synthetic carpets, plastic shower curtains, and the like—are fine, wise moves, populating the inside scene with plants is a brilliant, green way to improve the atmosphere.

The most effective plants for purifying indoor air include bamboo palm, Chinese evergreen, corn plant (*Dracaena massangeana*, not edible corn), dragon tree, chrysanthemum, English ivy, peace lily, pothos, philodendron, and snake plant.

Here are a few prodigious benefits all plants provide.

- They manufacture fresh oxygen and remove carbon dioxide.
- They reduce airborne chemicals and VOCs[125] emitted by formaldehyde, benzene, and ammonia.[126]
- They cultivate healthy levels of humidity.[127]
- They enhance the indoor environment, perceptibly reducing stress[128][129] and increasing productivity.[130][131]

For the full scoop on and a great guide to more than two dozen superhero houseplants, including a 1-to-10 ranking of how effectively they clean the air and information on how to care for them, and how hard it is to kill them with neglect, check my last book, *The Balanced Plate* (Rodale, 2006).

You can choose from a bouquet of naturally revitalizing, eco-friendly air fresheners delivered via nonaerosol sprays, vaporizing diffusers, reed stick diffusers, and candle lamps. Pick your potion, not your poison.

## Room Diffusers

Room diffusers are a lovely way to infuse enticing natural aromas from essential oils into a stuffy, stale room. There are a few basic types of room diffusers. Check them often to make sure they don't go dry—they can be a fire hazard when they're plugged in but empty.

- **Electric vaporizer or diffuser.** This is a small unit that stands alone or plugs directly into an electrical outlet to diffuse essential oils by using a wee bit of heat to keep the aroma going.

- **Candle lamp.** This is a stone or pottery dish holding essential oils that is set over a small tealight candle to warm and diffuse the oils, filling the room with naturally good smells. Just be sure not to leave lit candles unattended.
- **Car diffuser.** This small unit plugs into a car's cigarette lighter and diffuses essential oils for good smells on the go.
- **Reed sticks.** Long, thin reed sticks are placed in a glass jar or vase that is filled with natural plant and essential oils, generating a gentle, natural fragrance. *Note:* Be sure to choose products that have oils derived from plant sources; many contain artificial fragrances and perfumes.
- **Lamp ring.** This is a simple metal ring that is set atop the lightbulb in any lamp to diffuse essential oils via the heat of the bulb.

# Home Spray:
# Grapefruit Lavender or Vanilla Orange

*This simple spray will freshen stale rooms in a jiffy. The alcohol preserves the spray for a longer shelf life and deodorizes the air, leaving a light, lingering fragrance.*

**YIELD: 1 CUP**

½ cup filtered or distilled water
½ cup vodka
10 drops essential oil of lavender and 8 drops essential oil of grapefruit
  *or*
1 teaspoon pure vanilla extract and 4 drops essential oil of sweet orange

Mix the ingredients in a spray bottle. Shake well before using. Spray several times in rooms that need freshening.

*When you're in the market for a natural air freshener or room diffuser, look for these products with safe, clean ingredients.*

# AIR FRESHENERS

## CITRA-SOLV

**Air Scense**
7-ounce nonaerosol pump spray bottle

*Varieties:* Orange, Lime, Vanilla, Lavender

*Ingredients:* These fresheners are nontoxic and made with all-natural, plant-based ingredients. Orange and Lime use a citrus peel base carrier, whereas Vanilla and Lavender use a solution of grain alcohol and water. All get their fragrances from plant oils.

*Available:* at most natural markets and online

www.citra-solv.com

## EARTH FRIENDLY PRODUCTS

**Eco Breeze Fabric Refresher**
22-ounce trigger spray bottle

*Varieties:* Lavender Mint, Lemongrass, Citrus

*Ingredients:* These nontoxic fresheners are made with all-natural, plant-based ingredients.

**Uni-Fresh Air Freshener**
4.4-ounce nonaerosol pump spray bottle

*Varieties:* Cinnamon, Citrus, Lavender, Vanilla, Parsley

*Ingredients:* These fresheners are nontoxic and made with all-natural, plant-based ingredients.

*Available:* at most natural markets and online

www.ecos.com

## ECCO BELLA

**Ecco Mist**
8-ounce nonaerosol pump spray bottle

*Varieties:* Citrus, Lavender, Summer Fruit

*Ingredients:* Ecco Mists are nontoxic and made with all-natural, plant-based ingredients—pure essential oils, emulsifier, and water.

*Available:* at most natural markets and online

www.eccobella.com

## MIA ROSE

**Air Therapy**
2.2- and 4.6-ounce nonaerosol pump spray bottles

*Varieties:* Original Orange, Key Lime, Silver Spruce, Spearmint, Vibrant Vanilla

*Ingredients:* Nontoxic and 100 percent natural, this product is made from the purest essential oils and nothing else.

*Available:* at most natural markets and online

www.miarose.com

## MRS. MEYER'S CLEAN DAY

**Room Freshener**
8-ounce nonaerosol pump spray bottle

*Varieties:* Lavender, Lemon Verbena, Geranium

*Ingredients:* These fresheners are nontoxic and made with all-natural, plant-based ingredients, including fragrances from essential oils.

*Available:* at most natural markets and online

www.mrsmeyers.com

*(continued)*

## ORANGE MATE

### Mate Mist

3.5- and 7-ounce nonaerosol pump spray bottles

*Varieties:* Grapefruit, Lemon, Lime, Orange

*Ingredients:* They're nontoxic and made with all-natural, plant-based ingredients.

*Available:* at most natural markets and online

www.orangemate.com

## PUNATI

### Smells Begone

12-ounce nonaerosol pump spray bottle

*Varieties:* Calming Rain, Energizing Citrus, Fragrance Free, Soothing Breeze

*Ingredients:* These fresheners are nontoxic, nonstaining, safe for fabrics and pets, and made with a proprietary blend of natural ingredients and plant-based fragrances.

*Available:* at select natural markets and online

www.punati.com

# ROOM DIFFUSERS

*Most large natural markets (like Whole Foods) stock air-freshening accoutrements in the vitamin and beauty aisles. A bouquet of options are also available online from places like www.amazon.com or any of the companies listed below.*

## AURA CACIA

Aura Cacia is among the best and most widely available sources of pure essential oils and aromatherapy products. Committed to using organic ingredients and sourcing them carefully, Aura Cacia offers a wide selection of high-quality essential oils and ready-to-use aromatherapy products.

Products include an aromatherapy vaporizer, a diffuser that plugs into a wall outlet, a car diffuser, candle lamps, and lamp rings.

*Available:* at natural markets and online

www.auracacia.com

## NATURA ESSENTIALS

Natura Essentials carries a wide selection of pure essential oils and aromatherapy products sourced from around the world. The company's products include a portable battery-operated diffuser and an assortment of architectural candle diffusers—simple or ornate metal diffusers with a copper well that holds the essential oils and is warmed by a tealight candle.

*Available:* at select stores and online

www.naturaessentials.com

## RED FLOWER

### Organic Room Diffusers

Red Flower's four organic room diffusers contain Demeter-certified biodynamic blends of plant and essential oils that are diffused through reed sticks. The scents on offer are Cardamom Amber Resin, Cherry Blossom, Jasmine Grandiflorum, and Orange Blossom. Long wood palm stems that poke from the recycled Spanish glass vase will diffuse the aroma for months. Absolutely divine.

*Available:* at select stores and spas and online

www.redflower.com

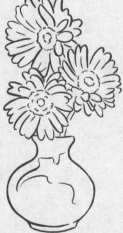

CHAPTER 3

# 5 Steps to a Green Kitchen

**Essential** *adjective*

**1**: fundamental; central **2**: absolutely necessary (*Oxford English Dictionary*)

**Environment** *noun*

**2**: The natural world, especially as affected by human activity (*Oxford English Dictionary*)

**1**: The circumstances, object, or conditions by which one is surrounded **2.** The complex of physical, chemical, and biotic factors (as climate, soil, and living things) that act upon an organism or ecological community and ultimately determine its form and survival (*Merriam-Webster's Collegiate Dictionary*)

In many ways, the kitchen is the heart of the home. It's a place to congregate, cook, and create, and certainly one room of the house that requires upkeep. Greening your kitchen is an essential part of a healthy, happy home, and these five steps will help you on your way: first, opt for nontoxic, biodegradable dishwashing products; second, tackle nontoxic cleaning for ovens and appliances; third, choose green, safe cookware; next, take inventory of safer plastics; and last, use recycled paper towels and napkins when you need them.

# step 1 Nontoxic, Biodegradable Dishwashing 1-2-3

There are two main types of dish cleansers: soap and detergent. Among those, there are synthetic (petroleum based) or natural (plant based) dishwashing products. In this section, we'll take a good look at both kinds of dish cleaners and at why choosing green products is the way to go.

## The Surfactant Conundrum

Let's face it, soap is at odds with itself. Part of what makes up soap is water loving (*hydrophilic*, meaning that it amorphously bonds with water), whereas the other part is repulsed by it (*hydrophobic*, literally meaning water fearing). Together these properties make soap a *surfactant*, a wetting agent that lessens the surface tension of water so it can spread out and get underneath grime to clean it away.

Surfactants in soaps and detergents are great. They clean stuff. For the sake of keeping the planet clean, it's essential that the surfactants biodegrade when they've done their job in the sink. Once upon a time, all soaps were biodegradable because they were rendered from plant or animal oils. Scarcity of these oils during and after World War II drove chemists to figure out how to make soaps and detergents, along with a legion of other products like plastic, from petroleum derivatives. Because of the surging interest in petroleum's

many possibilities, tried-and-true natural soap was steadily abandoned for cheap, synthetic products. The results swept the nation with reckless abandon and dominate the market to this day. That's beginning to change as we wake up to the effects of synthetic products and, consequently, great green products become more widely available. Synthetic soaps and detergents work well for cleaning dishes, clothes, and skin, but they are very harsh to the skin and their ecological side effects are not so great.

## Synthetic Soap and Detergent

It seems odd that we use the same stuff that fuels cars and makes plastics for washing dishes, but that's the case with conventional soap and detergent. Petroleum is an ubiquitous and versatile material that can be made into an effective surfactant for sudsy cleaning action. It's cheap, but also very persistent in the environment and slow to break down, even in a liquid form like dish soap. Petroleum products have an enormous ecological impact, beginning with extracting the petroleum from the ground, continuing through processing and using the products made with it, and ending with the way we dispose of the waste and end products. None of it is very friendly for humans, either.

# Dish Soap Epiphany

Liquid dish soap has been a major catalyst in my life. In one moment, it put everything in perspective for me. In a friend's kitchen years ago after a lovely dinner, as the good guest I seek to be, I approached the sink to wash some dishes. A bottle of unnaturally bright liquid dish soap stood at the ready. Squeezing out a potently perfumed dab, I sudsed up my plate dutifully, then felt the dawning of a major epiphany. In that moment, as I looked at the bottle of soap, I realized that this one act of dishwashing with petrochemical soap was undoing so many of the eco-smart, health-promoting efforts I genuinely embrace—like eating organic food; using recycled printer and copy paper, toilet paper, and tissues; and little things like using a cloth bag to tote things from the grocery store. As the suds disappeared down the drain, it dawned on me that it wasn't disappearing at all, really. Made with petroleum and chemicals that lent it its bright color and artificial fragrance, that soap will take a long time to biodegrade and it will be years before it completely goes away.

Ultimately, this soap would contaminate the very water I was washing with. The same water I shower in, wash food with, water the plants with, and filter to drink. The same water used to grow the very food I had just eaten. It was major. The simple act of washing a dish kicked wind into my sails and planted the seeds that ultimately led to my writing this book. Dishwashing is a universal domestic activity, one that can be clean, green, and eco-heroic. The next time I was invited for dinner, I brought my hosts a basket of eco-friendly cleaning products, including liquid dish soap scented with lavender, which is now their house standard. Being green is contagious, and it starts with just one act.

Synthetic automatic dish detergents also generally include a mishmash of chlorine bleaches for sterilization. They do the trick all right, though the fumes that powdered chlorine gives off when hot water hits it are pretty poisonous, not to mention the residue that's left behind on dishes and the contamination of the ecosystem from dishwasher wastewater.

## Natural Soap and Detergent

The difference between natural and synthetic soap is kind of like the difference between cotton and nylon. Natural soap and cotton are produced from plants, a renewable resource, with relatively little modification. Synthetic soap and nylon, on the other hand, both require major chemical production processes. Natural soap is made with plant oil mixed with a water-soluble alkali salt to *saponify* it—that is, to make it into soap. Simple. It's made pretty much the same way today as it was ages ago. Synthetic soap, on the other hand, is a modern marvel made in a chemical factory. One way to make synthetic soap from petroleum is to take a bunch of propylene, a petrochemical waste product that used to be burned off as a

# Green Rule of Thumb: Product Labels

Reading ingredient lists is the single most effective way to choose products wisely. If a product does not have an ingredient list, or it lists stuff you can't identify, avoid it in favor of one that fully discloses ingredients you know are not harmful.

- If there is no ingredient list, you can bet the product includes a slew of chemicals that you probably don't want to have much to do with. Find another product.
- Vague references to ingredients generally mean the ingredients are questionable. For instance, when a soap or detergent lists *surfactant* but does not disclose what it is made of, it most likely contains a synthetic surfactant and therefore is not readily biodegradable. *Fragrance* is another nebulous term to look out for. If the type of fragrance or its source is not explained, it could be made from anything and may contain phthalates and other petrochemical nasties. (See page 122 for more information on phthalates.)

Instead of products with questionable ingredients, choose naturally nontoxic, biodegradable products that will do the job and keep you and the planet green.

---

useless by-product, and string it together with benzene (which happens to be carcinogenic[1]). The result is a compound that can be made into soap and detergent. It sounds like a nifty science project, but one you would want to wear gloves for, and certainly nothing anyone would want to wash down the drain or find in their drinking water.

Natural dish soaps and detergents use the power of plants to create suds, and some contain oxygen bleach for nontoxic, deep-cleaning results. No mess, no fuss. They're made with renewable resources (plants) and are biodegradable. Everybody wins.

## The Deal with Dyes

Bright colors can be a beautiful thing, especially in flowers, sunsets, and crayons. But the colorants that make many a liquid dish soap colorful do not make soap work better.

## Levels of Impact

Synthetic dish soap and detergent ingredients have an impact on humans and the environment throughout their life cycle—during their manufacture, use, and disposal.

**Manufacture.** Manufacturing surfactants used in dishwashing soaps is not a pretty process. Petroleum-based ingredients take a heavy toll on the environment beginning with the pollution involved with its extraction from the earth, and they are likely to create more pollution during processing—a double whammy for the environment. During processing, synthetic surfactants like ethoxylated alcohol can become contaminated with 1,4-dioxane, a nasty by-product of manufacturing. This compound is known to cause cancer in animals and thought to do so in humans as well,[2][3] and it ends up in the final product.[4] Chlorine bleaches, which are often included in detergents for automatic dishwashers, leave behind a mess of toxic impurities that must be disposed of or incinerated after processing.

**Use.** Synthetic surfactants are just plain irritating to the skin. Ethanol, a widely used ingredient, dries out delicate skin, causing "dishpan hands." Synthetic colors and dyes and contaminants like 1,4-dioxane are readily absorbed through the skin and may leave residue on dishes even as they are being swept down the drain and ultimately into the water table. In automatic dish detergents, chlorine compounds yield noxious fumes during dishwasher cycles that use hot water. Those fumes can escape even when the dishwasher door is closed, and they are in no way good to breathe.

Furthermore, although the mothers of sassy children will always threaten to "wash your mouth out with soap," we all know it's not advisable to eat dish soap. But the likelihood of synthetic residue being left on dishes washed with synthetic soaps or detergents is pretty strong. Chlorine compounds included in automatic dishwasher powders and the fragrances that cover them up are especially likely to leave residues. Some freshly washed and dried dishes smell like a chemical garden. It's not natural and can't be tasty or good to eat.

**Disposal.** It's easy to subscribe to an out-of-sight-out-of-mind complacency when washing suds down the drain. But synthetic detergent that takes a long time to biodegrade isn't going anywhere anytime soon. It'll stick around to contaminate water systems,[5][6][7] soil fed by those waters,[8] and critters that live there.[9] The thing about water is that there is a finite amount of it on the planet. It cycles between the earth and the sky, but they're not making any more of it, so it's up to us to be conscientious stewards of what we've got.

## Rinse Aids

As their name implies, rinse aids prevent spotting from droplets of water drying on dishes, especially clear glass and shiny flatware. They can be helpful if you have really hard water that leaves mineral deposits, making glasses and silverware look grimy. Rinse aids are really just a bunch of special surfactants that lower the surface tension of water so much that it can't form into droplets, but instead drains off dishes, glasses, and flatware in thin sheets. Unless specified as doing so,

*(continued on page 84)*

### LIQUID DISH SOAPS

I investigated 24 brand-name liquid dish soaps. They will remain nameless, but the findings were consistently concerning. Here's what I discovered.

All contain unspecified "surfactants," which strongly suggests that they are nonbiodegradable. They also contain ethanol/SD alcohol 40, which is harsh, drying, and possibly irritating to the hands (I like to call them *paws*).

A good number of them contain more irritants, like dodecylbenzene sulfonate (of either the ammonium or sodium variety). Some contain ethoxylated alcohol, which is especially toxic to aquatic critters[10] and which during processing is commonly contaminated with 1,4-dioxane (a carcinogen in animals and possibly also in humans).[11] [12]

Diethanolamine (DEA) is yet another irritating detergent used in liquid dish soap, and it also has contamination problems. DEA can react with nitrites (which may be added as undisclosed preservatives or present as processing contaminants)[13] to form carcinogenic nitrosamines.

The vague ingredients *fragrance* and *color* are also popular. They may make soap look and smell more enticing, but they don't do a thing for its performance and may be unnecessarily harmful to humans and the environment.

### AUTOMATIC DISH DETERGENTS

Automatic dishwashing powders and gels contain the usual synthetic surfactant suspects plus a few more eco-brutes.

Conventional automatic dish detergents are generally riddled with chlorine bleach in one form or another, as well as a host of chemical fragrances. The trouble with chlorine being in dish detergents isn't so much that you'll come in direct contact with it (you're unlikely to sift through the detergent with your bare hands), but that you'll breathe in the fumes generated during the wash cycle and ingest the residue that's left on the dishes.

Another concern with dish detergents is the phosphates they include. Phosphates are minerals that soften the water to boost the detergent's action, just as they do in laundry detergent. Though fairly nontoxic for humans, phosphates wreak havoc in the ecosystem, especially for fish and other water beings. Phosphates in wastewater cause blooms of algae, which in turn eat up all the oxygen and kill off all the fish. While major laundry detergent makers are phasing out phosphates, dishwashing detergent makers haven't gotten on the bandwagon quite yet.

*Look to these dish soaps, detergents, and rinse aids for clean, green spotless results.*

## LIQUID DISH SOAPS

### BIOKLEEN

#### Hand Moisturizing Dishwash Liquid

**Ingredients:** This liquid is biodegradable and contains plant-based surfactants but no phosphates. The Lemon Thyme variety is scented with natural plant extracts. Free and Clear is unscented and without dyes.

**Available:** at natural markets and online

www.biokleenhome.com

### CALDREA

#### Dish Soap Liquid

**Ingredients:** This biodegradable liquid contains plant-derived surfactants. In Basil Blue Sage, Ginger Pomelo and Green Tea Patchouli (and others!), it's derived from natural sources and some well-researched, biodegradable, human-safe synthetic sources.

**Available:** in select home stores such as Sur la Table, Smith & Hawkin, and online

www.caldrea.com

### CITRA-SOLV

#### Citra-Dish Liquid

**Ingredients:** This liquid dish soap is biodegradable, contains plant-based surfactants, and includes no phosphates or artificial dyes. It has natural citrus and essential oils.

**Available:** at natural markets and online

www.citra-solv.com

### EARTH FRIENDLY PRODUCTS

#### Ultra Dishmate
**Ingredients:** This product is biodegradable, contains plant-based surfactants, and has no phosphates or artificial dyes. Its natural almond, apricot, grapefruit, lavender, and pear fragrances are derived from plant oils.

#### Natural Spa Dish Soap

**Ingredients:** This dish soap is biodegradable, contains plant-based surfactants, and has no phosphates or artificial dyes. Its thoughtfully blended varieties include Apricot, Black Currant, Grapefruit, Lemongrass, Pear, Pomegranate, and Rosemary.

**Available:** at natural markets and online

www.ecos.com

### METHOD

#### Dish Soap

**Ingredients:** It's biodegradable and contains naturally derived surfactants and no phosphates. Lavender, Cucumber, Peppermint Vanilla, and Pink Grapefruit get their fragrances from essential oils.

**Available:** at many markets and grocery stores and online

www.methodhome.com

### MOUNTAIN GREEN

#### Dishwashing Liquid

**Ingredients:** It's biodegradable and contains plant-based surfactants, but no phosphates or artificial dyes. The two natural fragrances are Fresh Green Apple and Orange Burst.

**Available:** at natural markets and online

www.mountaingreen.biz

### MRS. MEYER'S CLEAN DAY

#### Dish Soap

**Ingredients:** Biodegradable and containing plant-based surfactants, this dish soap uses natural colors and natural preservatives. Lavender, Lemon Verbena, and Geranium use essential oils fragrances.

**Available:** at natural markets and specialty markets and online

www.mrsmeyers.com

*(continued)*

## PLANET

### Ultra Dishwashing Liquid

*Ingredients:* This product is biodegradable with plant-based surfactants and natural fragrances, but no phosphates or artificial dyes.

*Available:* at grocery stores and natural markets and online

www.planetinc.com

## SEVENTH GENERATION

### Dishwashing Liquid

*Ingredients:* This biodegradable liquid contains plant-based surfactants, but no phosphates or artificial dyes. It comes in two plant-oil fragrances, Lavender Floral and Mint and Lemongrass and Clementine Zest, and in unscented Free and Clear.

*Available:* at grocery stores and natural markets and online

www.seventhgeneration.com

## STONEWALL KITCHEN

### Dish Soap

*Ingredients:* A biodegradable dish soap containing plant-based surfactants and natural colorants, and no phosphates. It's available in Lavender Mint, Lemon Parsley, Grapefruit Thyme, and Rosemary Lime.

*Available:* at kitchen and home stores and online

www.stonewallkitchen.com

# AUTOMATIC DISHWASHING DETERGENTS

## BIOKLEEN

### Automatic Dish Powder

*Ingredients:* It's biodegradable, nontoxic, dye free, chlorine free, and phosphate free, and instead uses plant-based surfactants and oxygen bleach for naturally tough stain removal. The regular variety contains natural fragrances; Free and Clear is unscented.

### Automatic Dish Gel

*Ingredients:* This gel is biodegradable, nontoxic, dye free, chlorine free, and phosphate free. It contains plant-based surfactants and natural fragrances, and it cleans using the power of grapefruit seed extract and orange peel extract.

*Available:* at natural markets and online

www.biokleenhome.com

## CALDREA

### Dishwashing Powder

*Ingredients:* This biodegradable powder leaves dishes sparkling clean. Free of phosphates and chlorine bleach. It's available in Ginger Pomelo, Basil Blue Sage and Lavender Pine, derived from natural and some well-researched, biodegradable, human-safe synthetic sources.

*Available:* in select home stores such as Sur la Table, Smith & Hawkin, and online

www.caldrea.com

## CITRA-SOLV

### Citra-Dish Automatic Dishwashing Detergent

*Ingredients:* This powder is biodegradable and nontoxic. It cleans using the power of oxygen bleach and citrus extracts. Free of chlorine, phosphates, and artificial dyes, its fragrance comes from lavender oil.

*Available:* at natural markets and online

www.citra-solv.com

## EARTH FRIENDLY PRODUCTS

### Wave Machine Dish Wash Powder HP

*Ingredients:* This powder is biodegradable, nontoxic, and free of chlorine, phosphates, and artificial dyes. It contains plant-based surfactants and gets its fragrance from lavender oil.

### Wave Machine Dish Wash Gel

*Ingredients:* It has plant-based surfactants and is biodegradable, nontoxic, chlorine free, phosphate free, and artificial dye free. Its fragrance comes from lavender oil.

*Available:* at natural markets and online

www.ecos.com

## ECOVER

### Automatic Dishwashing Powder

*Ingredients:* This powder is biodegradable, nontoxic, plant and mineral based, chlorine free, and phosphate free. It includes enzymes, a sugar-based bleach activator, and a plant-based fragrance. The box is made of 95 percent recycled cardboard.

### Dishwasher Tablets

*Ingredients:* These tablets are biodegradable, nontoxic, chlorine free, and phosphate free. They have plant-based surfactants, oxygen bleach, and a plant-based lemon fragrance. The box is made of 95 percent recycled cardboard.

*Available:* at natural markets and online

www.ecover.com

## METHOD

### Dish Cubes Dishwasher Detergent

*Ingredients:* These cubes come in a pouch that dissolves in the dishwasher. The detergent inside is biodegradable, nontoxic, chlorine free, and phosphate free. It uses naturally derived surfactants. The Cucumber-Lemon, French Lavender, and Pink Grapefruit fragrances come from essential oils.

*Available:* at many markets and grocery stores and online

www.methodhome.com

## MRS. MEYER'S CLEAN DAY

### Dishwashing Powder

*Ingredients:* Made with biodegradable, nontoxic, plant-based surfactants, this powder uses oxygen bleach for stain removal. It's free of chlorine, phosphates, and artificial dyes. The Lavender, Lemon Verbena, and Geranium varieties get their fragrances from plants and essential oils.

### Automatic Dishwashing Liquid

*Ingredients:* It's biodegradable, nontoxic, and free of chlorine, phosphates, and artificial dyes, but it does contain plant-based surfactants as well as minerals. The natural Lavender, Lemon Verbena, and Geranium fragrances come from plants and essential oils.

*Available:* at natural markets and specialty markets and online

www.mrsmeyers.com

## SEVENTH GENERATION

### Free and Clear Automatic Dishwasher Powder

*Ingredients:* This unscented powder is biodegradable, nontoxic, and free of chlorine, phosphates, and dyes.

### Automatic Dishwasher Gel

*Ingredients:* Biodegradable and nontoxic, this gel has no chlorine, phosphates, or artificial dyes. It's available with a gentle green apple or lemon fragrance.

*Available:* at grocery stores and natural markets and online

www.seventhgeneration.com

# RINSE AIDS

## EARTH FRIENDLY PRODUCTS

### Wave Jet Rinse Aid

*Ingredients:* Wave Jet is biodegradable and contains plant-based surfactants, not chemicals. No harmful residues or fumes are produced.

*Available:* at natural markets and online

www.ecos.com

## ECOVER

### Rinse Aid

*Ingredients:* This product uses biodegradable, plant-based surfactants. It has no chemicals, generates no fumes, and leaves no harmful residues.

*Available:* at natural markets and online

www.ecover.com

the surfactants don't biodegrade. Typically, some sort of alcohol is included to improve drying because it evaporates quickly. Most rinse aids also contain chemical fragrances. After all, where would we be without china that smells of synthetic ingredients?

If you are determined to have sparkly, streak-free glasses and flatware but don't want to contaminate the water supply or breathe in conventional rinse aids' synthetic fragrances, then natural rinse aids are for you. One of the most effective is white distilled vinegar. It really does the trick. It's cheap and nontoxic, and it dissolves the grimy buildup and mineral spots caused by hard water better than spit and a shirtsleeve will. Simply fill the rinse-aid compartment of your dishwasher with white vinegar. The machine will do the rest.

There are also a few naturally great consumer products that will make your dinner knives so spotless you'll be able to use them to check your reflection for spinach in your teeth.

## Hand Washing versus Automatic Washing

There is debate over whether hand washing or automatic dishwashing is more water and energy efficient. The verdict hinges on two main considerations: how stingily water is used during hand washing and how full the dishwasher is. Here are some tips to help you get the most out of both methods.

### Hand Washing

- Scrape the dishes before washing them to get the most out of clean, soapy water. Compost plant-based food scraps for the greenest disposal.

- Suds all the dishes up first, then rinse them all at once. Instead of washing items under running water, fill a bowl with hot water and a squirt of soap to wash.

- Wash lightly soiled and less greasy items—like glasses and flatware—first to keep the wash water fresher. Save the pots and pans for last. Stack the messier dishes in the sink to give them a few minutes to soak while you're working on the other dishes.

- Soak dishes, pots, and pans that are caked with food residue before washing them. For tips on dealing with tough stuff, see "Pots and Pans" on page 86.

- Wash plastic and wooden dishes and flatware by hand. Washing plastic items by hand will prevent wearing and scratching, which increase the likelihood of plastic leaching into food. Dry wooden items immediately after washing them to prevent damage and warping.

### Automatic Washing

- Less is more in terms of detergent. Contrary to popular belief, using more detergent doesn't wash the dishes better, it just makes them dingy with residue. Most of us fill the detergent

# How to Clean and Deodorize a Dishwasher

If your dishwasher is looking or smelling funky, first clean the filter according to the manufacturer's directions. Then, use white distilled vinegar to deodorize the inside and dissolve water spots. Pour 2 cups white vinegar into a bowl and sit it upright in the bottom rack. Run the machine through a short wash cycle and it will be clean, deodorized, and ready to run!

compartment so full that it's hard to close it or the gel squishes out, but that's unnecessary and wasteful, and it undermines cleaning. And using that second detergent compartment is overkill. One tablespoon of detergent is enough to clean a full load in an efficient dishwasher, and use 2 tablespoons maximum in older models. If you use powdered detergent, try mixing 1 teaspoon of baking soda with your detergent to boost its action (but don't wash aluminum pans when you've mixed in baking soda because it may discolor them).

- Use white distilled vinegar as a rinse aid. If your dishes suffer from hard-water spotting, pour white vinegar into the rinse compartment for shiny, spotless glasses, flatware, and china.

- Resist running partial loads in the dishwasher. Wash full loads only! If only a few dishes need washing, do them by hand to save water, energy, and detergent. Wash oversize platters and bowls by hand to maximize the available space in the dishwasher.

- Don't wash plastic or wooden items in the dishwasher. Hot water and deter-gent will wear out plastic and may increase the leaching of plastic into food.[14] Wooden items washed in a dishwasher will age and deteriorate more quickly than when washed by hand.

- Choose the right wash cycle. Many machines have a few different wash cycles. Options usually include something like "normal wash," "light china" or "quick rinse" for less intensive cycles, and "pot and pans" for heavy-duty jobs. A lot of the newer energy-efficient machines even have an "energy saver" button for smart cycles, which should always be used if you have it!

- Turn off the "heat dry" option. A machine full of dishes will dry more quickly with heat, but it won't sterilize the dishes and is a big energy hog. If you run the dishwasher at night, most loads will have air dried by morning with no problem. When the wash cycle is complete, open the door and pull out the top rack to keep it propped open. For quicker drying, check over-turned cups and bowls for puddles and drain them.

## Pots and Pans

Washing pots and pans is generally low on the totem pole of fun domestic chores. I would rather cook a six-course meal for a dozen people than scrub cookware. However, if you're forced to the chore, a few tips and tools can make it easier without resorting to harsh detergents.

**Baking soda is your friend.** Baking soda is a great ally for cleaning pots and pans that have a caked-on, baked-on crust. And, it's cheaper than beans. Here are some great ways to use it for maximum results.

- **General Baking Soda Scrub.** Sprinkle 2 tablespoons baking soda on the bottom of a mucky pot or pan. Add 2 inches or so of hot water and a little squirt of dish soap. Let it stand for 10 to 15 minutes before scrubbing. For pots that have grease and grime built up on the sides, add 1 additional tablespoon of baking soda for every 2 inches of water needed to cover the gunk.
- **Extra-Strength Baking Soda Scrub.** Sprinkle 2 tablespoons baking soda in the bottom of a really mucky pot or pan and add ¼ cup white distilled vinegar. It will foam like mad. Push the mixture around with a wooden spoon to coat the food that's caked on the bottom and sides of the pot. Add 2 inches or so of hot water and a little squirt of dish soap. Let it stand for 10 to 15 minutes before scrubbing.
- **Oxy-Tough Baking Soda Porcelain Scrub.** Powdered oxygen bleach will put some muscle into cleaning stains on porcelain casserole dishes. Sprinkle 1 tea-spoon each of oxygen bleach powder and baking soda in the dish (use 2 teaspoons each for larger dishes or really tough jobs). Fill the dish with hot water and swirl to dissolve the powders. Let it stand for 10 to 15 minutes before scrubbing.
- **Burned Food-Off.** For stubborn, burned-on food, mix 2 tablespoons of baking soda with 1 quart of water in the dirty pot or pan and bring it to a boil. Remove the pan from the heat and let the solution cool to a temperature that can be handled, then scrub. For dishes, such as casserole dishes, that can't be put on the stove top, mix 2 tablespoons of baking soda with each quart of water needed to cover the stuck-on food and put the dish in an oven preheated to 350°F for 5 to 10 minutes. Let the dish cool, then scrub.

*BIG NOTE:* Do not use baking soda solutions with nonstick pots and pans because they may scratch the coating, which may then leach into food (see page 107 for details about nonstick cookware and why it may be harmful). Do not use these solutions with aluminum pots and pans either, because they may discolor them.

## Washing Produce

Washing fruits and veggies is generally a good idea. With organic produce, it's a matter of washing off human paw prints and residual dirt and compost. With conventional produce, washing can reduce pesticide residue, but it can't eliminate it. Peeling conventional fruits and veggies also can reduce the chemical pesticides, sprays, and waxes that are concentrated in the skin (though healthy, happy minerals and nutrients are also concentrated in skins). However, the reality is that conventional produce is laden with pesticides inside and out, especially soft-skinned specimens like tomatoes, grapes, berries, peaches, and lettuces, so going organic is a smart green priority.

To be honest, I am not big on heavy-duty produce washing because I choose organically grown produce whenever possible and think that a wee bit of organic dirt helps to keep the immune system robust. Not all soilborne organisms and bacteria are bad; in fact, the human digestive tract depends on microorganisms by the trillions. Helpful bacteria found in foods like yogurt and miso are key elements in maintaining a healthy balance of microorganisms in our guts, which is essential for robust digestion and assimilation of food and nutrients. But some kinds of bacteria, on the other hand, are not so good. Produce can be contaminated by bacteria growing in a festering fridge or picked up from hands or surfaces when animal products like meat, poultry, and fish are handled in an unsanitary way, causing major stomach upset or worse. Washing fruits and veggies with nontoxic formulas is the ecological and healthy way to be safe.

A few naturally nontoxic produce-washing products are available commercially (see the "Green Thumb Guide"), but blending your own homemade tonics is cheap, easy, and no-nonsense. Some good ones to try are on the following pages.

*To help remove unwanted chemical residues and bacteria from food, try these nontoxic, biodegradable produce washes.*

## BIOKLEEN

### Concentrated Produce Wash

This concentrated formula effectively removes pesticides, herbicides, fungicides, waxes, and soil by using the power of grapefruit seed extract and lime peel extract. It contains no synthetic preservatives and leaves no residue. It can also be used to clean cutting boards, appliances, and counters.

*Available:* at natural markets and online www.biokleenhome.com

## EARTH FRIENDLY PRODUCTS

### Fruit and Veggie Wash

This wash helps remove pesticides, chemicals, heavy metals, dirt, wax, and bacteria from fruits and veggies. It contains plant-based surfactants and citric acid and leaves no residue or taste on produce.

*Available:* at natural markets and online www.ecos.com

## ENVIRONNÉ

### Fruit and Vegetable Wash

Designed to remove residues from pesticides, fungicides, and herbicides as well as waxes and oils, this wash uses nontoxic, biodegradable surfactants. It's available in screw-top and spray bottles or as individually packaged wipes.

*Available:* at natural markets and grocery stores and online www.vegiwash.com

# Fruit and Veggie Washing Tonic

*Diluted vinegar is the backbone of this tonic. A touch of baking soda adds a little abrasiveness, but be sure to rinse the produce thoroughly so no baking soda taste lingers on the food. Double or triple the recipe for bigger jobs.*
Note: *Don't use this tonic on mushrooms because they will absorb the flavor, which is not so tasty.*

3 cups filtered water*
3 tablespoons white distilled or apple cider vinegar
2 tablespoons baking soda

Mix the water, vinegar, and baking soda together in a spray bottle or bowl, depending on how you will use it.

*\*You can find information about filtering water in my last book,* The Balanced Plate *(Rodale, 2006).*

**Spray Tonic.** Spray it on fruits and veggies. Scrub firm fruits and veggies like cucumbers, apples, and potatoes, especially if you plan to eat the skin (which generally contains bountiful nutrients). Rinse well and carry on.

**Dunk Tonic.** Dunk, swish, and scrub the produce as desired. Put veggies in a colander or strainer that fits inside the bowl for easy draining and to allow you to use the same batch of tonic multiple times.

# Extra-Strength Homemade Lemon Peel Produce Wash

*If you would like to bump it up a notch to make a more powerful wash, add some of the ingredients that are in the Fruit and Veggie Washing Tonic, above.*

**YIELD: ABOUT 1 QUART**

4 cups filtered water
3 tablespoons white vinegar
2 tablespoons Homemade Lemon Peel Concentrate (see page 89)
2 teaspoons baking soda
4 drops grapefruit seed extract (available at most natural markets)

Mix all the ingredients together thoroughly until the baking soda has dissolved.

Pour it in a spray bottle for spritzing on fruits and veggies or in a bowl for dunking. Rinse the produce before carrying on.

# Homemade Lemon Peel Concentrate and Produce Wash

*This potent formula is made to be diluted—use 2 tablespoons per quart (32 ounces) of water. Dilute it in a spray bottle to spritz fruits and veggies or in a bowl so you can dunk leafy greens to more easily clean inside their folds. It will stay fresh for about a year in a cool, dark pantry.*

**YIELD: 1 CUP, ENOUGH FOR 1 GALLON DILUTED**

4 organic* lemons
1 cup vodka

Scrub the lemons with water. Peel away the yellow part of the skin (which cooks call *zest*) and chop it finely. Try not to include any of the white pith because it's bitter (especially if you plan to bake with the extract). Place the chopped peel in a freshly washed glass jar and cover it with the vodka. Cap the jar tightly and let it stand for 2 weeks. Strain out the solids before using the concentrate.

*\*Using organic lemons is highly recommended.*

To make the produce wash, dilute 2 tablespoons of concentrate in each quart of water. Put it in a spray bottle for spritzing or a bowl for dunking. Rinse the produce after using the wash.

If you would like to make a pretty gift of the strained concentrate, add curly fresh lemon peels made with a zest tool.

Store the concentrate in a tightly capped jar, away from direct light and at room temperature.

# Fruit and Veggie Oxygen Wash

*Diluted hydrogen peroxide—yup, the same stuff you use to clean cuts—works brilliantly for washing produce. Simply spray or dunk the produce for clean, fresh results.*

3 cups filtered water
1 cup 3 percent hydrogen peroxide

Mix the water and hydrogen peroxide together in a spray bottle or bowl, depending on how you want to use it.

**Spray Tonic.** Spray it on fruits and veggies. Scrub if appropriate (cucumbers, apples, potatoes, and the like). Rinse well and carry on.

**Dunk Tonic.** Dunk, swish, and scrub the produce as desired. Place veggies in a colander or strainer that fits inside the bowl for easy draining and to allow you to use the same batch of tonic multiple times.

## Cutting Boards

Cutting boards are kitchen essentials. Brilliantly low-tech, they can last a lifetime if they're cared for wisely. There's a huge variety of sizes, shapes, and thicknesses to meet your personal preference, and these days cutting boards are made of some fabulously sustainable materials.

Bamboo is one of the most durable and sustainable materials for cutting boards. It's brilliantly strong, looks good, and grows like a weed. Bamboo is a giant grass that grows impressively quickly, and when used for a cutting board, it's as sturdy and long lasting as wood. Bamboo cutting boards come in a wide selection of dimensions, grain patterns, and shades. My favorite has been with me for about a dozen years, and it will likely last a lifetime. A bamboo cutting board should be treated like one made of wood: Don't submerge it in water, and massage it with vegetable oil from time to time.

## *Clean Those Cutting Boards*

In many kitchens, cutting boards play an important role in preparing every meal. In my kitchen, I have a 3- by 4-foot built-in wooden cutting board kitty-corner to the stove. It is where I spend some of the most enjoyable time ever. I take cutting-board hygiene personally. We have an industrial-strength kitchen that gets serious traffic: a 12-burner stove; a stainless steel, double-door commercial fridge; a wok station; and a salamander finishing oven. It's great fun and the heart of our home. I tend to that built-in board like it's an altar, using homemade formulas like the one below to keep it as clean as a whistle and always ready for action. Though my wooden cutting board will last a lifetime, if I were to build it from scratch, I would choose bamboo, hands down.

# Homemade Cutting Board Sanitizer

¼ cup 3 percent hydrogen peroxide

¼ cup white distilled vinegar

4 drops grapefruit seed extract (optional; available at most natural markets)

4 drops essential oil of oregano (optional; available at most natural markets)

1 tablespoon baking soda

Mix the hydrogen peroxide, vinegar, grapefruit seed extract, and essential oil of oregano in a spray bottle or bowl.

Sprinkle the baking soda on the cutting board. Spray the board with or dunk a clean sponge in the mixture and scrub the board. It should fizz up a storm.

Wipe the board thoroughly with fresh water before using it.

*In your search for an über-green cutting board, consider any of these bamboo beauties that will likely last a lifetime.*

## CRATE AND BARREL

The selection of bamboo products varies by store and may include cutting boards, serving boards, and trays.

www.crateandbarrel.com

## MIU FRANCE

MIU France is a renowned maker of world-class kitchen tools that are elegant in both form and function. Their beautiful line of products now includes sustainable materials, including a selection of solid bamboo butcher blocks, chopping blocks, cutting boards, butcher boards, and an exquisite oval serving board with a stainless steel band and handles. High-end form, function, and durability meet at MIU France.

www.miufrance.com

## SEATTLE LUXE

Seattle Luxe offers smart-looking striped bamboo cutting boards in both oval and rectangular shapes. They are solid, heavy, and mighty good-looking with dark and light variegation.

www.seattleluxe.com

## SUR LA TABLE

The selection of bamboo products varies by store and may include cutting boards, a cutting block with a knife drawer, a prep board, bowls, serving dishes, utensils, mixing spoons, disposable veneerware plates, placemats, and food covers.

www.surlatable.com

## TOTALLY BAMBOO

Totally Bamboo pioneered the trend. They carry a fantastic selection of cutting board styles, shapes, and dimensions. Among the more than 230 products on offer are durable bowls, plates, serving platters and other dishes, kitchen accessories, utensils, even countertops, rolling butcher blocks, and director's chairs (perfect for the kitchen supervisor). Totally Bamboo is a go-to site for sustainable bamboo kitchen accoutrements.

www.totallybamboo.com

## WHOLE FOODS

The selection of bamboo products varies by store and may include cutting boards, cheese boards, bowls, utensils, mixing spoons, and serving ware. Many of the products are made by Totally Bamboo.

www.wholefoodsmarket.com

## WILLIAMS AND SONOMA

The selection of bamboo products varies by store and may include cutting boards, a bamboo board and mezzaluna, and an oval serving tray made by MIU France.

www.williams-sonoma.com

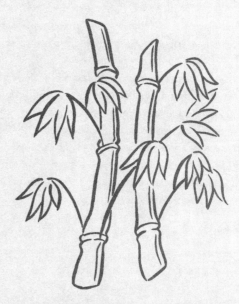

## Plastic Cutting Board Questions

If you like a touch of plastic in your food, then plastic cutting boards are for you. It's safe to say that plastic is not healthy to eat. If you look at a plastic cutting board that's been well used, you will see that it's nicked, cut, and scratched. Guess where all the plastic shards end up? And those nicks and cuts harbor the same bacteria that we have all been warned about. But it's not just the plastic; the additives and plasticizers used to make the plastic hard and durable are also worth worrying about. Hard plastics can contain insidious bisphenol A, which makes plastic strong but also damages the reproductive system,[15] disrupts hormones,[16] mimics estrogen,[17] and is linked to breast and prostate cancer[18] and even to obesity. Scratched and worn plastic cutting boards leach this and other nasty chemicals into food.[19] Hungry?

Yes, yes, I have considered the argument that plastic is more sanitary than wood for cutting boards, and I beg to differ strongly. Proponents claim that plastic can be put in the dishwasher to sterilize it. First, household dishwashers don't get hot enough to sterilize—sorry, folks. (Dishwashers typically reach temperatures of 120°F to 140°F, but solid surfaces need to be at a temperature of 250°F for 15 minutes to be properly sterilized.). Second, washing plastic cutting boards with hot water and detergent wears them down, which may make more plastic leach into foods, especially fatty and oily foods. If I sound very opinionated, it is because I am. I really care, and I hope you do, too.

## Dioxin-Free Cup o' Joe: Unbleached Coffee Filters to the Rescue!

A cup of fresh-brewed java is a brisk delight that seduces all our senses. Opting for unbleached coffee filters is a healthy green detail that's better for you, the planet, and your treasured cup of perky pleasure. As do all chlorine-bleached paper products, conventional coffee filters harbor dioxins, carcinogenic chlorinated hydrocarbons[20] that accumulate in our bodies and persist in the environment. None too friendly, especially in your cup of joe. Dioxins are classified by scientists and the US Environmental Protection Agency (EPA) as persistent organic pollutants, which means that they are able to migrate not just within the ecosystem, but also from, for example, coffee filters to coffee. Up to 24 percent of the residual dioxins in bleached coffee filters can leach and migrate into the brewed java[21] for us to ingest.[22] Since dioxins bioaccumulate, drinking even small amounts on a regular basis adds up to dangerous levels. According to studies performed by the EPA, the exposure you get to dioxins via bleached coffee filters alone is enough to exceed the lifetime limit for an "acceptable level." In fact, there is no "safe" level, period.[23]

Unbleached coffee filters are a simple way to get a delicious cup of dioxin-free coffee, with no strings attached. They're available at any old grocery store for the same cost as the snowy white kind. Be green, go unbleached!

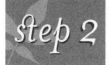

Depending on how you use your oven, cleaning its inside may be no more than a once-in-a-while chore. The best measure is a preventive one: Wipe up overflows and spills when they're fresh to prevent the crusty, caked-on crud that will later season foods with the distinctive taste of burned toast. But if, alas, grease and grime build up and get the best of you, choosing a chemical-free, nontoxic oven cleaner is the healthy way to go.

While conventional oven cleaners provide elbow-grease-free action, they are loaded with terribly toxic and caustic chemicals. The chemicals do the work so you don't have to. Heavy-duty solvents are favored, along with super-caustic chemicals. They work, but they are wickedly dangerous to touch or breathe, and they're prone to causing highly unpleasant side effects.

Some solvents that popular oven-cleaning formulas lean on include glycol ethers, which are severe irritants of the eyes, skin, and lungs;[24] extremely dangerous to inhale;[25] and prone to causing reproductive problems.[26] There's also 2-butoxyethanol, which is also a severe irritant of the eyes, skin, and lungs;[27] seriously dangerous to inhale;[28] and easily absorbed through the skin,[29] and it may damage the liver, kidneys, lymph- and blood-forming organs,[30] and nervous system.[31]

For caustic action strong enough to cut through tough oven gunk, many conventional oven cleaners contain severe corrosives like sodium hydroxide, which can be extremely dangerous to inhale or touch;[32] can burn the eyes, skin, and lungs;[33] and can cause chronic damage to tissues.[34]

You can also find in them such nefarious propellants as propane, butane, and isobutene, which are harmful to inhale. Considering the chemicals that are in these aerosols, it would be wise to wear a respirator when using them.

Basically, you don't want to touch or inhale conventional oven cleaners. That can be tough, because cleaning the inside of an oven requires you to be in pretty close quarters. Also, the residues left by these toxic oven cleaners aren't what you want seasoning your roasted or baked foods, let alone being distributed throughout the house as fumes. Nontoxic options sound like the smart, safe way to get your oven spic-and-span.

## Safer Oven Cleaners

Unfortunately, there aren't many nontoxic commercial oven-cleaning products on the market. Arm and Hammer Oven Cleaner has been deemed nontoxic by Consumers Union, and Restore makes a nontoxic oven-cleaner (www.restoreproducts.com), but I have found good old baking soda to be the best thing around.

## Self-Cleaning Ovens Are Naturally Nontoxic

Many ovens are *self-cleaning*, which means that they have a high temperature cycle that will burn off crusty, caked-on spills without using chemical cleaners. It's a good way to go to avoid having to use elbow grease or solvent-heavy caustic cleaners to cut through tough grease and grime. I suggest you let the self-cleaning cycle rip when the room is well ventilated: Open windows and doors and maybe get a fan spinning for good measure.

## Heavy-Duty Homemade Oven Cleaner

*Citra-Solv is a concentrated citrus cleaner that can cut through and clean just about anything in its path. When mixed with water and baking soda, it makes an industrial-strength, nontoxic oven cleaner. This formula works with very little elbow grease if it's allowed to sit on the oven's bottom for a few hours. Be sure to wipe it away with a damp cloth or sponge and then rinse the surface thoroughly to avoid leaving any residue.*

16 ounces baking soda

4 tablespoons Citra-Solv Cleaner and Degreaser concentrate

water

Place the baking soda in a bowl. Add the Citra-Solv concentrate and mix well. Add water a little at a time to form a paste that is thick enough to spread (a thin paste won't work as well). Spread it evenly over the bottom of the oven. Let it stand for a minimum of 1 hour and as long as 3 hours. Use a scrubber sponge to wipe and scoop away the loosened gunk (wearing rubber gloves is advised because Citra-Solv is very potent). For really stubborn spots, take a piece of steel wool and show 'em who's boss. Wipe and rinse very thoroughly with a damp cloth.

# Sunday Oven Cleaner

*This formula offers elbow-grease-free action if allowed to sit for a good 12 hours. If you slather it on your oven on Saturday afternoon, by Sunday the cooked-on grime will slip right off with a scrubber sponge and warm water (ergo, the name). It's hard to believe plain old baking soda can have so much might, but I tell you, its quiet alkaline action really works!*

16 ounces baking soda
   water

**Spray method.** Sprinkle the baking soda evenly over the bottom of the oven. Spray with water from a spray bottle until the soda is very damp, but not running wet. Let it stand for 12 hours (check it and spritz again if necessary to keep it moist). Then, simply wipe and scoop the remains with a scrubber sponge—all of the grime will be as loose as a goose and easy to wipe away. Wipe the oven thoroughly with a damp cloth to remove all of the baking soda (this is the most elbow grease you'll need for this method; it takes a few minutes, but it's worth the nontoxic effort).

**Paste method.** Place the baking soda in a bowl. Add water a little at a time to form a spreadable paste (be careful not to add too much water at first—a runny paste won't work as well). Spread the paste evenly over the bottom of the oven and let it sit for 12 hours. Wipe using the procedure described for the spray method to finish.

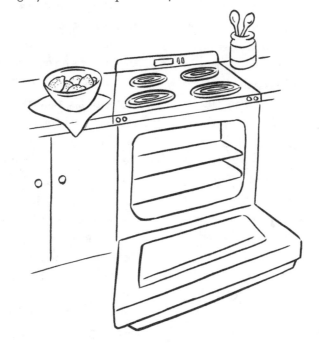

Here are some smart green tips for getting the most out of your oven and stove. They will save you time, energy, and money.

- **PUT A LID ON IT.** Save time and energy by covering pots when warming food or boiling water. Containing heat with a lid is a simple way to speed up heating and save energy in the process.

- **USE THE RIGHT-SIZE POT ON THE RIGHT-SIZE BURNER.** Placing a small pot on a big burner is a silly waste of energy. Choose the right-size pot to save energy and money.

- **KEEP STOVE-TOP REFLECTORS CLEAN.** Reflector pans under stove-top burners reflect and amplify the heat. The cleaner they are, the more efficient the burners will be.

- **LET LEFTOVERS COOL.** Before stashing leftovers in the fridge, let them cool to room temperature. It will keep the fridge from working overtime to chill them out.

- **DON'T PEEK.** Opening the oven door to check on what's cooking can reduce the temperature inside the oven by 25°F or more per peek. It's a hemorrhaging of energy that also causes distress to happily roasting or baking foods. Either wait until you think the food has cooked or flip on the oven light and peer through the oven's window.

- **KEEP THE SEAL CLEAN AND TIGHT.** A tight, clean oven seal will retain the heat with maximum efficiency and keep the oven's temperature even, which means foods will cook better and more quickly.

- **USE GLASS OR CERAMIC BAKING DISHES.** They retain heat better than metal pans do, allowing you to set your oven temperature 25°F lower for the same great results.

- **THAW FOODS IN THE FRIDGE.** Cooking frozen foods takes longer than cooking thawed foods, whether on the stove top or in the oven. In addition, thawing foods, especially animal products, in the fridge will help prevent bacterial buildup.

- **SKIP OR ABBREVIATE PREHEATING.** Roasting savory dishes in the oven doesn't require extensive preheating. To simply warm up goodies, skip preheating the oven altogether—just pop 'em in and turn it on to use less energy. Baking things like cookies, cakes, and bread does require a stable starting temperature, so get to know how many minutes it takes your oven to reach full temperature; there's no need to let the oven preheat for longer than it needs to.

- **CONSIDER A TOASTER OVEN.** For small jobs, a toaster oven will perform as well as a big oven. They require less time to heat up and less energy to stay hot. Some are pretty cute, too.

- **TRY A CONVECTION OR MICROWAVE OVEN.** According to the American Council for an Energy-Efficient Economy, "convection ovens are usually more energy efficient than conventional ovens because the heated air is continuously circulated around the food being cooked, reducing [the] required temperature and cooking times. On average, you'll cut energy use by about 20 percent. Microwaves use a lot of energy when operating, but because cooking times are so drastically reduced, using a microwave to prepare a meal will reduce energy use by about two-thirds compared to a conventional oven. . . . New 'rapid-cook' ovens combining microwaves with other cooking technologies—notably halogen lights or convection—are designed to cut cooking time and improve the quality of foods compared to standard microwave preparation."

## Green Stainless Steel Care

Many ovens, oven doors, and oven hoods are made of stainless steel, which is a durable, rustproof material that doesn't corrode, but does require the right formulas for steak-free cleaning and polishing. Keeping stainless steel surfaces buffed and twinkly with nontoxic products is a bright idea for a green, clean home and planet.

Conventional stainless steel cleaners rely on heavy-duty solvents to get the job done. Solvents do the job, but possibly at the expense of your health and the ecosystem's well-being. I researched the formulas of nine conventional stainless steel cleaners to see what powerful chemicals are the norm. All of them contain really nasty, heavy-duty solvents derived from petrochemicals, like the highly toxic naphtha compounds and petroleum distillates, all of which are extremely harmful to

*If your oven won't clean itself and you aren't keen on homemade solutions, check out some of the nontoxic products designed for cleaning barbecue grills. They're formulated to take off heavy grease and grime and will make cleaning the oven as easy as a walk in the park. Here are two to try.*

## SOYCLEAN

### BBQ Grill Cleaner

*Ingredients:* This all-natural soy-based formula is biodegradable, nontoxic, and nonflammable and will create no caustic fumes.

www.soyclean.biz

## SUNBRITE

### Grill and Oven Cleaner

*Ingredients:* This industrial-strength cleaner is biodegradable, nontoxic, nonabrasive, and water soluble.

www.sunbrite.biz

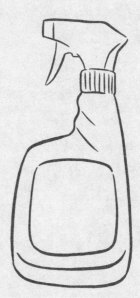

*For naturally buff, streak-free stainless steel cleaning, look for these nontoxic products.*

## CALDREA

### Stainless Steel Spray

*Ingredients:* This nontoxic spray is formulated from an ancient remedy that does not use chemical solvents. Its fragrances are derived from natural sources and some well-researched, biodegradable, human-safe synthetic sources.

*Available:* in select home stores such as Sur la Table, Smith & Hawkin, and online

www.caldrea.com

## METHOD

### Stainless Steel Cleaner Plus Polish

*Ingredients:* This nontoxic cleaner's label is a little vague, but says it contains "biodegradable ingredients" and natural and synthetic fragrances.

*Available:* at most grocery stores and retail chain stores and online

www.methodhome.com

## MRS. MEYER'S CLEAN DAY

### Stainless Steel Spray

*Ingredients:* It's biodegradable and nontoxic, and it has plant-based surfactants, but no solvents. Its natural lavender, lemon verbena, and geranium fragrances come from plants and essential oils.

*Available:* at most natural markets and online

www.mrsmeyers.com

## SIMPLE GREEN

### Stainless Steel One-Step Cleaner and Polish

*Ingredients:* They're biodegradable and nontoxic.

*Available:* at natural markets and online

www.simplegreen.com

inhale[35] [36] and damage the skin, with repeated exposure defatting skin and causing cracking, irritation, and dermatitis.[37] [38] Furthermore, naphtha is a possible carcinogen because it may contain benzene[39] and petroleum distillates that can damage the nervous system with repeated exposure.[40] Another solvent that's widely used in stainless steel cleaners is 2-butoxyethanol, a toxic irritant that's both harmful to inhale[41] and easily absorbed through the skin—repeated exposure can damage the liver, kidneys, lymphatic system, and blood.[42] None of these solvents sound like a very good deal, even for spiffy, shiny results.

Using an aerosol cleaner on your stainless steel surfaces is like adding insult to injury. Along with the hazardous hydrocarbon propellants aerosols contain, the chemical solvents are sprayed in a fine, misty vapor that is easy to inhale. This is not a good thing, especially because those solvents are seriously dangerous to breathe in.

The good news is that there is a brood of nontoxic, eco-friendly cleaning products designed specifically for stainless steel surfaces. They harness the power of plant-based surfactants, natural solvents, and essential oils, and I guarantee that you will step back to admire the fine job they do. No harm, no foul. There's no need to sacrifice health, happiness, or the planet to bust smudges. You can get exceptionally reflective results with products like these. See the "Green Thumb Guide" at left for recommendations.

Here are some all-natural ways to clean stainless steel surfaces.

- Don't use abrasive cleaners or sponges to clean stainless steel. They can scratch the surface irreparably. Baking soda is one abrasive that won't scratch stainless steel.
- Club soda removes streaks and heat stains from stainless steel. Pour club soda into a spray bottle to spray and wipe dry or simply dampen a clean towel with it and wipe dry.
- For streak-free results, first clean the surface with a damp sponge or cloth, then shine it up with a dry cloth. If a grain is visible in the stainless steel surface, rub in that direction.
- Less is more. Natural stainless steel cleaning products usually contain plant oils for shiny results. A little goes a long way, and too much may leave streaks.
- Undiluted white distilled vinegar is a great tonic for cutting grease and grime and polishing stainless steel. Pour vinegar into a spray bottle to spray and wipe dry, or simply dampen a clean towel with it, swipe, and then wipe dry. No need to rinse afterward.

## Homemade Stainless Steel Cleaners

Dedicated do-it-yourselfers may want to mix up a batch of homemade stainless steel cleaner. Here are two formulas for shiny surfaces.

## All-Purpose Stainless Steel Cleaner

*Baking soda is brilliant once again—it's gently abrasive but won't scratch, leaving only clean, shiny results. Club soda is full of alkaline minerals that produce a streak-free finish.*

½ cup baking soda

1 cup club soda

Combine the ingredients in a bowl. Use a damp cloth or sponge (not the scrubber side) to rub the mixture on the steel surface. Wipe it clean and follow with a dry cloth (no need to rinse).

## Creamed Stainless Steel Buff Formula

*Cream of tartar is a great natural bleaching agent. Mixing it with gently abrasive baking soda and hydrogen peroxide produces a formula that will make any stainless steel sink or surface shine.*

2 tablespoons cream of tartar

2 tablespoons baking soda

2 tablespoons 3 percent hydrogen peroxide

Combine all the ingredients in a bowl. Use a damp cloth to massage the mixture into the surface. Let it dry completely and then wipe with a damp cloth (no need to rinse).

# Cleaning Fixtures with Club Soda

Club soda is indispensable not only for certain cocktails, it can also clean kitchen fixtures to a brilliant shine. Club soda is chock-full of alkaline minerals, which eat away stains and hard-water buildup. It doesn't get easier than this.

Simply pour club soda over grungy, greasy, or mineral-stained metal fixtures and wipe with a rag. Alternatively, pour club soda into a bowl, moisten a clean rag with it, and rub the fixtures until they gleam.

## Naturally Fresh Fridge

The refrigerator is home to culinary desires, as well as lingering aromas that can get quite funky over time. With a few green tricks and tools, keeping a fridge smelling naturally fresh is simple. To be green, choose nontoxic products that can be replaced without a lot of wasted packaging, such as baking soda or zeolite. Air filters for the fridge can be helpful for keeping things fresh and clean, but avoid bulky, disposable plastic units that can only be used once.

Baking soda is a time-tested material that absorbs odors and moisture. It's cheap and pretty effective when used properly and changed from time to time. You can simply pop open a box and stash it on a shelf in the fridge, though the more baking soda that is exposed, the more action it provides. Try filling a shallow container 1 inch deep for better odor absorption. A good trick is to use a disposable deli container (finally, something useful to do with those things!) and punch holes in the lid to let the baking soda breathe while decreasing the chance of a messy mishap if the container gets knocked over. Replenish it every 2 to 3 months, because once the baking soda becomes saturated, it's inactive and should be refreshed.

Zeolite is another highly absorbent material that works wonders for keeping a fridge fresh. A naturally occurring mineral found in lava rock, it munches, absorbs, and neutralizes odors with a vengeance. Zeolite, which comes in granules or chunks, is also useful for deodorizing closets, cars, and garbage cans.

Zeolite also absorbs moisture and is said to prolong food life, curb staleness and freezer burn, and actually save electricity. One of the brilliant properties of pure zeolite is that it's rechargeable! That means that, once it has soaked up funky odors and moisture for about a year, it can be laid out in the sun to dry and recharge for using again and again. There are a few products on the market designed with this purpose in mind. Check out the green options for keeping a naturally fresh, nontoxic fridge in the "Green Thumb Guide" on the opposite page.

*If you'd like to keep your fridge fresh and eodorized, check out these products to neutralize odors naturally.*

## CYCLETROL DIVERSIFIED INDUSTRIES

### Omni-Zorb Odor, Moisture, and Mold Eliminator

These granules are made from high-grade zeolite and amino acids for ultimate odor control. It recharges in the sun, so it can be used again and again! If you live in a dry climate, spread the granules in the sun for a day to dry them. If you live in a damper climate, dry the granules on a sunny windowsill. It's brilliant and reduces waste like a champ.

### ZeoFresh Refrigerator Packet

These handy packets keep fridges and freezers fresh by controlling odor and preventing odor cross-contamination.

*Available:* at natural markets and online

www.omni-zorb.com

## IMTEK ENVIRONMENTAL

### Smelleze Refrigerator Deodorizer Pouch

IMTEK has a wide range of environmentally friendly odor-control products, including the Smelleze Refrigerator Deodorizer Pouch in small and medium sizes. Each pouch contains a granulated odor absorber that neutralizes and eliminates odors.

*Available:* at select markets and online

www.no-odor.com

## NATURE'S ODOR AND GERM CONTROL

### Odor and Germ Control Refrigerator and Freezer Packets

Stash these convenient zeolite packets in the fridge or freezer to soak up odors for up to a year.

*Available:* at select markets and online

www.nogc.com

## PURIFIERS

Refrigerator air purifiers are another way to go to both deodorize a fridge and snuff out bacteria, though they are typically made of plastic and require batteries. However, they should last a long time, and if you use rechargeable batteries, you can stay in the green.

## NEOTEC

### Refrigerator Odor Remover, XJ-100 Refrigerator Air Purifier

Both refrigerator deodorizers employ ozone to purify air, neutralize odors, and snuff out the bacteria that lurk inside refrigerators. They're compact, effective, and battery operated.

www.neotecstore.com

## ULTRA-PURE

### Refrigerator Deodorizer and Freshener

This friendly looking unit resembles a squared 5½-inch-high egg and generates activated oxygen and ozone to ward off odors, bacteria, and mold. It's available in white or orange. It takes four C batteries, which are widely available and will last for 4 months of continuous use. A 1-year warranty is included.

www.ultra-pureair.com

# Unstoppable Sinks

Sinks tend to clog and back up at the most inconvenient times. There are a few ways to free them up that don't require the caustic ingredients (like sodium hydroxide and sodium hypochlorite) and ecologically injurious acids found in conventional drain cleaners, which can permanently and seriously damage skin and eyes. *Note:* Conventional drain cleaners, with their extremely harsh chemicals, should never be used if you have polyvinyl chloride (PVC) pipes because they will literally eat them away.

## PREVENTING CLOGS

Prevention, of course, is the best way to keep drains flowing freely. Consider any of these options for preventing clogs.

*Mesh sink drain screen.* While a standard drain basket that sits in a kitchen sink helps to prevent major debris from being sucked down the drain, it has its limits, and smaller dregs will slip right by it. A mesh drain screen that sits in the drain, flush with the sink, is a fantastic low-tech tool for catching all sizes of particles that are attempting to escape down the drain. It costs just a few bucks and will last for years. Avoid plastic models in favor of stainless steel. They're available at many grocery, home, hardware, and plumbing stores and online (www.plumbingsupply.com/stainlessscreenstrainers.html).

*Baking soda and boiling water.* Another preventive for keeping drains from backing up is to pour 1 cup of baking soda down the drain followed by 2 quarts of boiling water. Some say this will unclog drains, but I haven't found that to be the case. It works well as a preventive measure though, and can be done every few weeks, once a month, or whenever you think of it. Here's a thought: After cleaning your teakettle with vinegar and water (see page 104), dump ½ cup baking soda down the drain before pouring out the liquid. You will get double-duty action with the added vinegar. Presto, multitasking action!

*Natural enzyme drain products.* A few natural products contain active enzymes that munch on and clear food debris to free up drains. They are highly effective when used as a preventive on a monthly or bimonthly basis. See the opposite page for a guide to these products.

## FREEING CLOGGED SINKS

Sinks that have become hopelessly clogged can be approached in a few ways: You can bust out your handy plumber's snake and ream the pipe, you can use a natural drain cleaner, or you can call a plumber to do these things for you.

A plumber's drain snake is an invaluable tool that can be used to manually clear a pipe. A flexible rod or tube, it's the single most effective tool for nontoxic, autonomous drain cleaning. They're available at just about any plumbing supply store or in the plumbing section of hardware stores.

Natural drain cleaners have active enzymes that literally eat away organic material that lodges in pipes. Look to the muscle of any of these products for unstoppable drain help.

## BIO-CLEAN

Bio-Clean's granulated powder is a concentrated blend of natural bacteria and enzymes (not genetically modified) that digest the waste that accumulates in pipes and drains in no time. I have a personal stash for preventive use.

*Available:* from plumbers and online www.statewidesupply.com

## CITRA-SOLV CITRA-DRAIN

Made with natural enzymes, bacterial cultures, and a biodegradable surfactant, this liquid drain cleaner is a nontoxic way to keep drains and pipes flowing freely without damaging the plumbing.

*Available:* at most natural markets and online www.citra-solv.com

## EARTH FRIENDLY PRODUCTS EARTH ENZYMES DRAIN OPENER

Earth Enzymes is a granulated powder that effectively digests clogged debris with natural enzymatic action for clearing and maintaining free-flowing pipes.

*Available:* at most natural markets and online www.ecos.com

Calling a plumber will likely be unnecessary if you have these savvy skills. After all, a hired plumber will simply use a snake to free the clog and possibly follow that with a heavy-duty, poisonous drain cleaner.

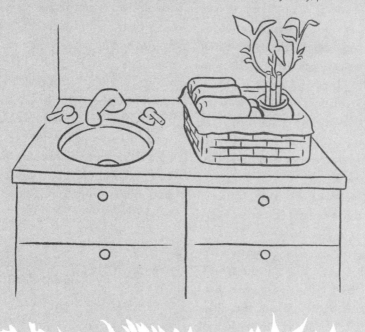

# Sterling Silver Care (for Jewelry, Too!)

Sterling silverware and candleholders are indulgences of yesteryear that are largely out of vogue. Though impressively beautiful, their being passé is a relief, really, because silver tarnishes easily and requires a lot of upkeep to maintain its high, lustrous shine. If you don't have a chest filled with solid silver flatware to polish for special occasions, this homemade solution can be used to buff up jewelry instead. The secret ingredient is a creamy toothpaste (don't use a gel; see "Green Thumb Guide: Toothpastes" on page 208 for eco-friendly toothpastes for the task).

Dab a little toothpaste on a cloth and rub the silver item. Then polish the piece with a clean, soft cloth (an old T-shirt works beautifully). Ta-da!

## Squeaky Clean Coffee Makers

Coffee is a beloved morning brew that deserves to run through a clean machine. Over time, coffee makers suffer from the grungy stains that build up from all the luscious oils that impart coffee's delicious aroma and flavor. That buildup isn't just unsightly—it can make even freshly brewed coffee taste stale. Of course, if your coffee maker is black, you won't see it, but it's still there. To remedy the situation, here are two green cleaning practices for freshening and deodorizing a coffee maker to squeaky-clean status.

**Vinegar Cycle Freshener.** Pour 1 cup white distilled vinegar into the water reservoir. Add 6 cups cold water. (For 4-cup coffee makers, use ½ cup white vinegar and 3 cups water.) Flip on the switch and let it run through a cycle, just like you do when you brew coffee, but sans coffee and filter. Empty the pot. Refill the water reservoir with just water and run the cycle again to remove the vinegar residue. Repeat if it still smells. Then it's good to go!

**Oxygen Bleach Stain Remover.** Oxygen bleach is a brilliantly effective alternative to chlorine for removing stains, especially on light-colored coffee makers. Remove the coffee filter basket from the machine. Place 2 tablespoons powdered oxygen bleach in a bowl large enough to submerge the filter basket in and fill the bowl with warm water. Swish the solution around to dissolve the powder and then submerge the filter basket. Let it soak for 20 minutes before taking a scrub brush or scrubber sponge to it. Rinse it, dry it, and carry on.

## Spiffy Clean Teakettles

Teakettles are companions that will last for years when given due diligence. With loving care, a good kettle can and should last a lifetime, though the inside may get encrusted with the minerals deposited by hard water and then deposit sediment in your piping-hot cup'a. Floating debris does not go hand in hand with properly brewed tea, and the mineral deposits that cause them are tough to get off with even serious elbow grease.

I am deeply attached to the stainless steel teakettle that perennially perches on our stove. This beloved kettle was procured as a gift from a chaotic open-air market in India by Roger Verge (an extraordinary chef and man), and it survives daily use and the constant demands of being shuffled among a dozen burners, finally resting there with contentment when all else has been cleared away. It's a little battered, but I wouldn't trade it for anything—even the most über state-of-the-art model. The inside does suffer from white mineral deposits, which I deal with from time to

time by using a simple, effective method, and you can too. Here's how.

Fill the kettle two-thirds full with a solution of half white distilled vinegar and half water.

Bring the solution to a rolling boil for 3 minutes. It will smell strongly of vinegar, which will deodorize the kitchen and dissipate quickly, though you may want to open the windows and turn on the exhaust fan.

Empty and rinse the kettle. (To keep your drain clear, pour 1/2 cup baking soda down the drain before pouring off the hot water and vinegar—together, they will eat away debris in the pipes. See page 102 for more "Unstoppable Sinks" tips.)

Fill the kettle two-thirds full with water and again bring it to a boil for 3 minutes to remove any lingering vinegar residue. Empty and rinse the kettle, then repeat once more if necessary.

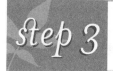

# step 3 — Green and Safe Cookware

Good cookware is the cornerstone of the kitchen. Whether your finesse in the kitchen is limited to basic pasta or extends to five-course meals paired with the perfect wine, choosing the right pots, pans, and ovenware is not only essential for consistent results, it's a key influence on personal and planetary health.

Heat tends to make materials more reactive. That can be very delicious (espe-

cially when it involves good olive oil and shallots). The duty of good cookware, such as pots and pans, is to conduct heat without reacting with or destructively leaching into the food cooked in them. For example, stainless steel, glass, and enameled cast iron conduct heat brilliantly and remain inert no matter how high the temperature climbs. On the other hand, aluminum and Teflon-coated or other nonstick pots and pans are not benign and can leach substances into the food and cause toxic fumes, respectively. Although aluminum conducts heat excellently, it is reactive when heated. With an inside coating of stainless steel, however, aluminum can do its job safely without coming into contact with food. Copper is another material that is better used when coated with stainless steel because it is also highly conductive but reactive and can leach into food. Though a little bit of copper isn't bad for you, too much can be poisonous. Cast iron, on the other hand, offers you a little iron that is actually good for your body and blood.

## Materials to Avoid (at All Costs!)

To run a greener kitchen and household, some cookware materials are better than others. Whether you simply dabble in the kitchen or cook up a storm, here are some kinds of cookware to steer clear of when buying pots and pans.

### Aluminum

Aluminum conducts heat brilliantly, but it's really dangerous to allow it to come in direct contact with food. It's a soft, highly reactive (especially with acidic foods) metal that can leach into food. It's toxic,[43] genotoxic (can cause genetic mutation),[44] and may disrupt hormones.[45] The most serious danger is that aluminum is neurotoxic;[46][47][48] it can cross the blood–brain barrier[49][50] and may be linked to Alzheimer's disease.[51][52][53] Proponents of aluminum cookware say it's debatable how many aluminum molecules get into food, but many scientists and doctors say it's a serious health risk. I won't use aluminum cookware and avoid allowing aluminum foil to come in contact with cooking food at all costs. Aluminum cookware that is coated with stainless steel is safer—in fact, some of the best heavy-bottomed stainless steel pots and pans have aluminum in their bases to better conduct heat. However, I would advise you to avoid nonstick-coated aluminum pots and pans at all costs because I believe that both materials are really bad for you.

### Teflon-Coated and Other Nonstick Pots and Pans

The chemicals used to make pots and pans nonstick are toxic and hazardous to humans, wildlife, and the environment. They're widely believed to be carcinogenic,[54][55][56] bioaccumulate in tissues over time,[57] and persist in perpetuity in the environment[58] because there is no known mechanism that can break them down.[59][60] Nonstick chemicals have consistently been linked with developmental disorders, birth defects, and cancer[61][62] and have been shown to be highly toxic to the liver, kidneys, and blood.[63][64] Companies that manufacture nonstick products insist that they're safe and they won't break down or emit fumes under normal cooking conditions. But it doesn't take a doctoral degree to contest that pots and pans can get very hot very fast and that they scratch easily, which means flecks of the coating can end up in food. Manufacturers say chemical fumes from cooking with nonstick cookware have little to no effect on humans, but they also acknowledge that those same fumes might kill a pet bird in the kitchen.[65] Hmmm. I say just don't use 'em, because they're really dangerous. The original manufacturers of nonstick chemicals, 3M, even stopped making them, citing "principles of responsible environmental management,"[66] but one company (ahem, DuPont) keeps up production despite the EPA's campaign to reduce and eliminate the use of these dastardly chemicals for the sake of all beings on the planet. The bottom line is, don't buy them. If you have them, don't use them for cooking.

Unfortunately, there is no way to recycle nonstick pots and pans, but a good idea might be to send them back to the manufacturer with a little note saying, "Enough is enough, stop with nonstick chemicals already. Quit harming humans and the world at large."

## Nonstick Wonder (Just Mind the Fumes)

Nonstick pots and pans might seem like an ingenious invention for no-fuss cleanup, but be mindful of the acute and chronic human and ecological hazards that may come along with them. An EPA advisory panel voted unanimously to recommend that a chemical used in nonstick coatings, perfluorooctanoic acid (PFOA),

be considered a likely carcinogen,[67] [68] [69] and the compound is wickedly persistent in the environment.[70]

The components of nonstick coatings on pots and pans, like PFOA, might not stick to food, but they stick to humans and the environment. They're found in the blood of nearly all Americans and also at low levels throughout the environment worldwide,[71] and they endure in both places for a very long time.[72] A number of studies have shown that nonstick chemicals like PFOA are likely to cause developmental problems like birth defects and cancer.[73] [74]

### Nonstick Profiles

There are a few nonstick siblings that are closely related in chemical makeup and behavior. They all have nonstick properties, and they can also have stain-resisting, water-repelling, and fire-retarding characteristics according to their application. They're all considered by the EPA to be persistent, bioaccumulative, and toxic. Like a bad houseguest, once invited in, they just won't leave.

PFOA has gotten the most press of this bunch of perilous nonstick chemicals, and rightly so. It's really nasty in its own right and is also a key player in manufacturing other favored nonstick chemicals like polytetrafluoroethylene (PTFE), which is used in Teflon, and perfluorooctyl sulfonate (PFOS), which was once used in Scotchgard and is still used in stain-resisting treatments for textiles and in polishes, waxes, varnishes, and firefighting foams.

## NONSTICK CHEMICALS PROFILE

| FLUOROPOLYMERS | COMMON USES | HUMAN EFFECTS | ECOLOGICAL EFFECTS |
|---|---|---|---|
| Perfluorooctanoic acid (PFOA), perfluorooctane sulfonate, polytetrafluoroethylene (PTFE) | • Nonstick cookware<br><br>• Stain-, soil-, and grease-resistant coatings on textiles, carpets, upholstery, furnishings, bedsheets, and clothing<br><br>• Waterproofing of fabrics, clothing, and upholstery<br><br>• Personal care and cosmetic products (those with *fluoro-*, *perfluoro-*, or PFTE ingredients, such as face and body moisturizers and makeup<br><br>• Coating on microwave popcorn bags<br><br>• Coating on fast-food packaging and candy wrappers<br><br>• Weatherproof waxes, varnishes, and polishes<br><br>• Surfactant in cleaning products and firefighting foams | • Virtually indestructible [75][76] and highly toxic<br><br>• Suspected carcinogen[77]<br><br>• Accumulates and remains in the body for a very long time[78] because it is not metabolized[79][80]<br><br>• Widely found in the blood of the the world's population[81] and 95% of Americans[82]<br><br>• Distributed to the liver, kidneys, and blood[83][84]<br><br>• Linked to developmental toxicity[85][86][87]<br><br>• Linked to cancer of the liver, kidneys, testes, and pancreas[88] | • Very persistent in the environment;[89] virtually indestructible,[90][91] and there is "no known environmental breakdown mechanism for PFOA"[92][93]<br><br>• Contaminates wildlife around the globe, from whales, tuna, and dolphins in the Mediterranean Sea; to seals, sea eagles, and Atlantic salmon; to dolphins in the Ganges River in India; to polar bears and turtles in the Arctic; to albatross in the Pacific; to harbor seals in the San Francisco Bay; and other wildlife[94] |

Other nonstick chemicals that aren't made with PFOA tend to release PFOA when they break down. It's no good at all. None of these substances breaks down in the environment or bloodstream. It's fair to say that every nonstick molecule produced since 1938 is still circulating somewhere on the planet, showing up in the far corners of the globe and even in the blood of Arctic polar bears.[95] Holy smokes!

## Teflon

Teflon is the household name when it comes to nonstick cookware, but those wickedly slick chemicals are a virtually indestructible hazard to humans, wildlife, and the environment. They're toxic, and they persistently accumulate in the tissues of humans and wildlife, and in the environment.[96][97] They might not stick to food, but they sure do stick around and have been linked with some very ugly health effects.

DuPont has been making Teflon for the past half century, and the company stands by its safety. It claims that Teflon coatings just don't release toxic or hazardous chemicals under conditions of normal use. According to DuPont, "At high temperatures, the quality of the coating may begin to deteriorate. . . . This can begin to occur at temperatures above 500°F (260°C). If heated to an extremely high temperature, the coating may begin to decompose and give off fumes."[98] Further,

# It's in Our Blood!

According to samples 3M, the original manufacturer of PFOA, collected from blood banks, that chemical is present in the blood of 90 percent of Americans.[99] Other independent studies, commissioned by the Environmental Working Group, a Washington, DC-based environmental research organization, registered the chemical pollutant in more than 95 percent of Americans' blood.[100] Because PFOA never degrades or breaks down in the environment,[101, 102] every molecule of it produced in the last 60 years will be forever present on the planet—circulating in the water, the air, and our bodies. Therefore, it's advisable for the health of all humans and the planet at large that we reduce our direct exposure to nonstick cookware and food containers and stain-resistant fabrics.

if an "empty non-stick cookware pan is accidentally heated above 660°F (348°C), a temperature that far exceeds what food preparation calls for, the non-stick coating may begin to deteriorate."[103] Hmmm.

Well, if you've ever fired up a pan on high heat, you may beg to differ about just how fast it will get very hot, and empirical studies will back you up. University food safety scientists measured that very relationship by placing a generic nonstick frying pan on a regular old electric burner preheated on high. In just 3 minutes and 20 seconds, the pan reached a whopping 736°F![104] The same test performed by the same cats with a Teflon-coated pan showed that it reached 721°F in a mere 5 minutes,[105] with the temperature still climbing when the test was stopped. I hope they were wearing gas masks. While empty pans on the stove get hotter more quickly than pans with food in them, it seems worth considering that fumes may still be an issue when you are cooking up a storm.

DuPont also says that "in rare instances, a person may accidentally ingest a flake of non-stick coating from an aged pan. The coating flake is non-toxic and would pass through the body without being absorbed. Based on the inert characteristics of the coating, data indicate that there are no health effects from the incidental ingestion of pieces of non-stick coating."[106] Based on the nature of these nasty chemicals, none of us should take ingesting them lightly. I say that to be safe, it's best to avoid them altogether.

## Safer Cookware: Pots, Pans, and Ovenware

If you are looking for cookware materials that are better for you, your family, and the environment, the first step is knowing the features and benefits of the different materials that are available. Here's an introduction to some of the best of what's around for all of your cooking needs.

(continued on page 112)

# Greener Kitchen Papers

Opting for unbleached kitchen papers is an eco-savvy move for a greener kitchen.

Parchment paper, a friend to cooks and chefs everywhere, is a naturally nonstick alternative to greasing up roasting pans, cake pans, and cookie sheets. It makes cleanup a cinch and is extra-handy as a lining for cookie sheets when you're pumping out multiple batches. Unbleached parchment paper can be used several times before tossing it, and it can serve as a protective barrier between questionable bakeware materials (like aluminum and nonstick coatings) and food. I use it to line my two commercial aluminum baking sheets to prevent baked, roasted, and toasted goods from coming in direct contact with the aluminum. Instead of tossing your baking sheets into the landfill, with a lining of parchment paper, they can serve safely for years to come!

The parchment sheets are disposable, yes, and therefore somewhat wasteful, but they're a whole lot better than using nonstick cookware. When in need, unbleached parchment products are the green way to go. Most white paper products (including parchment paper) are bleached with chlorine, which creates dioxins during its manufacture and leaves residues in finished products. Most parchment paper is also coated with Quilon, a chemical that may contain chromium (a heavy metal), which is toxic when incinerated and may leach into foods. To avoid contributing to the dioxin pollution of the planet and inviting these undesirable chemicals into your sumptuous food as some heavy metal seasoning, be green and opt for unbleached parchment paper. And with mindful management, parchment paper can be used more than once—I wipe it with a damp sponge, let it dry, fold it, and stash it for the next time I need it.

For other baking needs, unbleached cupcake or muffin liners are a wise green pick. You can grease stainless steel muffin pans to prevent sticking, but if you use aluminum or nonstick-coated pans, unbleached baking cups put a layer of nonstick protection between those materials and your baked goods.

Unbleached waxed paper is also worth looking into. It's dioxin free, you don't risk low-grade exposure to toxins when you use it, and you don't have to worry about the contaminants in bleached paper ending up in landfills. Handy unbleached waxed bags are a fantastic alternative to plastic bags for packed lunches and on-the-go goodies. Life is good.

The same considerations apply to cheesecloth. Unbleached cheesecloth is a safer, greener option compared to the bleached kind.

There are a few companies that produce fantastic unbleached paper baking products, as well as unbleached waxed paper, cheesecloth, and coffee filters. It just makes good, green sense. Here are some products to look for.

## BEYOND GOURMET

Unbleached parchment paper, baking cups, coffee filters, and cheesecloth. No chlorine used in any products.

*Available:* at most natural markets and online www.avolsson.com/beyondgourmet.com

## IF YOU CARE

Unbleached parchment paper, baking paper (parchment in a roll of precut sheets), baking cups, and coffee filters. All paper products are unbleached. The parchment paper is coated with silicone for safe use. The company also makes 100 percent recycled aluminum foil, which can be recycled again after use.

*Available:* at most natural markets and online www.ifyoucare.com

## NATURAL VALUE

Unbleached natural parchment paper, natural waxed paper, and natural waxed paper bags. All of Natural Value's paper products are made with unbleached fibers.

*Available:* at most natural markets and online www.naturalvalue.com

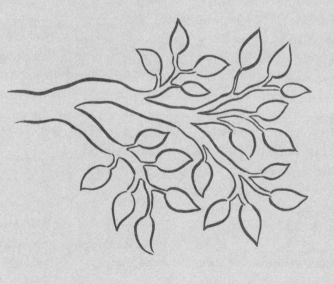

# Tips for Avoiding Nonstick Chemicals

- Replace Teflon- and nonstick-coated pots and pans, including rice cookers and hot air popcorn makers. Send them back to the manufacturer or dispose of them properly as hazardous waste.
- Opt out of stain treatments for new furnishings like carpets and upholstery.
- Avoid clothing and fabrics treated to be stain, dirt, and grease resistant.
- Avoid fast-food containers, especially coated french fry containers, burger boxes, and wrappers.
- Avoid microwave popcorn. The bags are usually coated with nonstick chemicals. Instead, make your own microwave popcorn using a brown paper lunch sack, with or without a little olive oil and/or salt. Or, go for stove-top-popped corn—it tastes better anyway!
- Avoid cosmetics with ingredients that contain the words *fluoro-*, *perfluoro-*, or *PFTE* (which is Teflon). They are usually found in face and body moisturizers and cosmetics.

## Stainless Steel

Stainless steel is favored by cooks for a host of positive features. It's durable: Stainless steel resists scratches and dings, doesn't corrode, and can last a lifetime. It's versatile: It doesn't react to acidic or alkaline foods, and it can be used for just about anything.

To make the most of stainless steel cookware, heat the pan first before adding oil to coat it. Food can stick to stainless steel pretty stubbornly, but using a little oil will make food cook better and stick less, and cleanup will be easier. Soaking the pan before washing or scrubbing it will also help with the chore. Stainless steel is dishwasher safe.

The best stainless steel pots and pans have a heavy bottom of copper or aluminum for optimal heat conductivity. The thicker the bottom, the better. Other metals like chromium and nickel are typ-

ically mixed into the steel alloy. Most pots and pans have a number imprinted on the base indicating the mixture—look for a minimum of 18/8 or 18/10 ("18" indicates the amount of chromium, whereas "8" and "10" are the amount of nickel). There are murmurs from the peanut gallery that other metals mixed with steel, like nickel, chromium, and molybdenum, can leach into food, but unless your cookware is severely battered and dinged, it's a negligible concern.

## Enameled Cast Iron

Enameled cast iron is one of the most durable, versatile, and long-lasting cookware materials. The best Dutch ovens (heavy, steep-sided pots with two handles) are made of enameled cast iron, though enameled cast iron pots and pans are available in a wide variety of shapes and sizes. These pots and pans are made with heavy cast iron that is covered with smooth enamel, and they typically have tight-fitting lids. They can be used on the stove top or in the oven and are highly prized by chefs and home cooks for a multitude of uses.

Enameled cast iron is impervious, stable, and dependable, and cookware made of it will probably outlive you. With its very heavy, thick construction, this kind of pot is a superior conductor of heat. Cast iron absorbs and distributes heat evenly, so less heat is required for optimal results.

Enameled cast iron cookware is versatile, too. You can use it on the stove top, in the oven, under the broiler, on the grill, or even on an open fire. It's excellent for slowly cooking soups, casseroles, and stews; quickly searing or sautéing just about anything; and even baking bread or cakes. The lids can also be inverted for use as frying pans. Brilliant.

Enameled cast iron cookware that has been seasoned is by nature nonstick (no chemicals included). It's important to season new cast iron cookware to create the nonstick surface and prevent rusting. It takes a little time, but it's easy and only needs to be done once to last a lifetime. First, wash and scrub the pot with warm, soapy water to remove any oil or wax used to protect the cookware prior to purchase. Second, preheat the oven to 300°F. Dry and coat the pot inside and out, including the lid, with a heavy fat like coconut oil or a vegetable oil with a high smoke point, such as grape seed oil. Next, place the pot

upside down (yes, upside down) in the oven for at least 1 hour (line the bottom of the oven with foil to protect it from drips). Let it cool, then repeat the process by coating it with oil and baking it for an hour again. Ta-da! You're ready to sear for the rest of your life.

Enameled cast iron pots (including Dutch ovens) come in many different shapes, sizes, and colors. They aren't cheap, but they will last forever and are truly phenomenal (I can't endorse them enough!). A few companies manufacture them, but the two most respected are old-school manufacturers Le Creuset and Staub (both from France). See the "Green Thumb Guide" on page 116 for some recommendations.

## Cast Iron Cookware

Cast iron cookware is an old-school, durable choice that's a supreme heat conductor and naturally nonstick. It's heavy and heats up more slowly than stainless steel, but it retains heat brilliantly. Cast iron gets better with time—its performance is legendary. It releases a small amount of iron into foods, which is good for the body, especially for red blood cell production.

Cast iron is durable: It's an enduring material that, once seasoned, can last a lifetime if it is well cared for.

Cast iron cookware is versatile, too. Its optimal heat conductivity makes it ideal for high-temperature cooking, like searing and pan-frying, and for mid-range heat, like sautéing. It's also good for slowly toasting seeds and nuts. Cast iron is heavy and retains heat like a champ, so using lower temperatures can yield the same results as higher temperatures with other materials like stainless steel, coated aluminum, anodized aluminum, and even copper. It must be seasoned to acquire a permanent, natural nonstick surface and to seal and protect it from rust.

Some manufacturers sell factory-seasoned pieces, but it's easy to do yourself and only needs to be done once to last a lifetime. First, wash and scrub the pan with warm water and soap to remove any factory-applied protective coatings and dry it thoroughly (you can put it in the oven for a brief time to dry). Second, preheat the oven to 300°F and line the bottom with foil to prevent drips. Third, rub and coat the pan, inside and out, with a rich fat like coconut oil or a vegetable oil with a high smoke point, such as grape seed oil. Next, place the pan upside down in the oven for about an hour—placing it right side up will make the oil collect in the bottom of the pan, which defeats the purpose. Then remove it from the oven and let it cool. For the best results, repeat the process by coating it with oil again and baking it for another hour.

Once seasoned, cast iron will retain a permanent nonstick surface as long as it is not washed with soap. Instead, scour it with super-hot water and coarse salt. Always dry it thoroughly and completely after washing to prevent rusting and corrosion.

There are a few manufacturers of cast iron cookware today, but Lodge Manufacturing is one of the oldest and most respected, and Iittala Hackman is fabulously stylish. Beware of brands of cast iron cookware that have a nonstick coating, which should be avoided at all costs (see "Nonstick Wonder [Just Mind the Fumes]" on page 107 for more information).

## Glass and Ceramic Cookware

Glass and ceramics are both nonreactive and conduct and retain heat quite well, and they have a nonporous surface that won't stain. They won't warp, dent, or ding, but they are breakable. Glass and ceramics are considered fantastic choices for ovenware, but there's also glass and ceramic cookware designed to withstand the direct heat of stove-top cooking. This kind of cookware is versatile—it's great for cooking, serving, and storing food in one shot. It won't scratch, and can be used safely in the microwave and dishwasher. Clear glass cookware can even be recycled if it breaks. Glass and ceramics conduct and retain heat so superbly that when you bake with them, you can reduce the oven temperature by 25°F. One caveat: Be sure the glazes on your ceramic cookware are lead free.

Glass and ceramic cookware can go from fridge to oven and back again, but pieces designed for the stove top shouldn't be taken directly from the fridge to the rangetop. Extreme temperature changes can cause them to break, so let them reach room temperature before heating. As for cooling, heat-resistant glass should be cooled a bit before cold water hits it, though ceramics are generally impervious to thermal shock. Yee-ha!

## Copper

Copper is a superlative conductor of heat, evenly distributing and retaining heat for superior results. Because it's a reactive metal, it must be lined with stainless steel to prevent the production of toxic salts when in contact with some foods, especially acidic foods like tomatoes, lemons, wine, and vinegar. Copper is prized by top chefs as the ultimate cookware material, though it is quite expensive and can dent and tarnish easily. Look for copper cookware with a heavy bottom and an inside lined with stainless steel. Avoid aluminum linings and nonstick coatings.

## Anodized Aluminum

Anodized aluminum, a new-generation material, is treated with an electrolytic passivation process to develop an extremely hard and nonreactive coating on its surface. These pots and pans are dark in color and look much like nonstick cookware. For all intents and purposes, anodized aluminum is sealed, which supposedly prevents it from reacting with or leaching into food (even really acidic stuff like lemons, rhubarb, and wine) and makes it relatively nonstick. It's received good marks on the green, safe culinary front, though it is less conductive than regular old aluminum. Calphalon and Cuisinart are both big proponents of anodized aluminum. If you are in the market for anodized aluminum cookware, be sure to avoid those with nonstick coatings. Personally, I'll stick to stainless steel and enameled cast iron, which have both been around long enough for a clear verdict to be declared.

## Silicone

Silicone bakeware is strangely rubbery and needs no chemical coating to make it nonstick. It's hard to believe it doesn't melt in the oven or give off gases like mad, but so far the verdict is that the stuff is safe. Silicone is made basically from sand. It's inert and doesn't react with food or heat. It looks very futuristic, like something I imagine the Jetsons would use. It may be hard for more traditional chefs and home cooks to accept these rubbery muffin and Bundt pans. But silicone has some attractive properties: It's nonstick and nonreactive, it doesn't retain odors or flavors, it's stain resistant, it distributes heat evenly, and it's dishwasher safe. Silicone is impervious to extreme thermal changes—it can go from freezer to piping hot oven and back again. It's pretty nifty and pretty indestructible stuff—I mean, you could throw it on the floor and it would bounce.

Here's another tip: Silicone rubber spatulas are fantastically long lasting, heat resistant, and a safe, green alternative to plastic ones. They come in fun colors, too.

*If you are in the market for cookware that is better for you, your family, and the environment, check out the best of what's around.*

# ENAMELED CAST IRON

## CHANTAL

United States-based German makers of fine enamel-on-steel cookware, Chantal offers a wide variety of pots, pans, bakeware, and serveware in vibrant colors and shapes. The company's pots and pans have tight-fitting tempered glass lids made in Japan. The pots and pans are shaped like traditional cookware and have a carbon steel core and handles that stay cool to the touch, and all their products are expertly enameled for classic nonreactive, nonstick performance. Basic and specialty bakeware is also available in many shapes and sizes, including square, rectangular, and round baking dishes, ramekins, casseroles, quiche dishes, and pie plates, as well as festively shaped pieces. Chantal also manufactures copper fusion and stainless steel pots and pans.

*Available:* at culinary and home stores and online

www.chantal.com

## KINETIC

Kinetic offers a respectable selection of enameled cast iron cookware (and great stainless steel goods too!). The products are available in several shapes, sizes, and colors, including Dutch ovens, saucepans, grill pans, casseroles, and roasting dishes.

*Available:* at culinary and home stores and online

www.innova-inc.com

## LE CREUSET

Le Creuset has been crafting the finest enameled cast iron cookware since 1925. Prized by French chefs, each piece of cookware is one of a kind, cast and molded from molten steel and skillfully enameled to yield magnificent results by distributing the heat evenly to brown and caramelize food to perfection.

The cookware comes in a wide range of shapes, sizes, and colors—round and oval pots, pans, ovens, and casserole dishes; rectangular and round roasting pans; skillets and griddles; tagine ovens; and even oven dishes shaped like apples, bell peppers, and pumpkins. The company also makes enamel-on-steel tea-kettles and traditional enameled stoneware dishes for baking. There's also a line of bakeware: Bijou by Le Creuset. All are top-shelf products.

*Available:* at culinary, home, and department stores, Whole Foods, and online

www.lecreuset.com

## STAUB

Staub is synonymous with quality and style when it comes to enameled cast iron cookware. Its most famous model is a round casserole with brass knobs and rounded metal buds on the underside of the enameled cast iron lid that cause steam from the cooking food to condense and drip down, producing sublimely moist food.

Available in a wide range of shapes, sizes, and colors, there are round and oval pots, pans, ovens, and casserole dishes; rectangular and round roasting pans; skillets and griddles; woks; tagine ovens and stoneware; and La Théière teapots and other signature specialty items.

*Available:* at culinary, home, and department stores and online

www.staubusa.com

# CAST IRON

## IITTALA HACKMAN

Iittala Hackman is where form and function meet. The company offers pots and pans of the highest quality and great style, created by a handful of award-winning Finnish designers in collaboration with world-class chefs and materials specialists. With its signature thick base, this cookware has superb heat retention. And here's a bonus: It's preseasoned! Pots, pans, and skillets are available in a few versatile sizes. One classic piece in the Iittala collection is the Sarpaneva cast iron pot, designed in 1960, which has an ingenious detachable wooden handle and is lined with enamel. It's fantastic looking—when you see it, you'll get what I mean. This company also produces a fabulous line of other kitchen goods that shouldn't be missed.

*Available:* at fine culinary and home stores and online

www.iittala.com

## LODGE MANUFACTURING

Lodge Manufacturing has been producing the finest cast iron cookware in a little town in Tennessee since the early 1800s. Family owned and operated, Lodge offers the most extensive selection of cast iron cookware on the market—skillets, grill pans, griddles, Dutch ovens, fryers, and bakeware as well as enameled cast iron cookware, pots, and casserole dishes in great colors. Its products are durable and long lasting—the company claims some of its pieces are still in use after 100 years.

*Available:* at culinary, home, and department stores and online

www.lodgemfg.com

# GLASS AND CERAMIC

## CORNINGWARE

Perfectly blending style and function, CorningWare cookware and bakeware is the one-stop shop for cooking, serving, and storing, all in one dish. CorningWare has been an all-time best seller since 1958. Available in a wide variety of shapes, styles, and sizes for stove-top and oven use, this opaque ceramic stoneware is nonporous, nonreactive, and durable—it won't crack or chip easily. Most pieces have fitted glass lids and some have tight-sealing plastic covers to make storing foods a cinch.

*Available:* at culinary, home, and department stores and online

www.corningware.com

## KITCHENAID

KitchenAid is a solid source for many kitchen appliances, tools, cookware pieces, and accessories, including an ample selection of fine, heavyweight ceramic bakeware. Promoting even baking and superb heat retention, KitchenAid ceramic bakeware can travel between the oven, broiler, microwave, fridge, and freezer like a champ. All the pieces are double-fired so they won't scratch or stain and, of course, they're dishwasher safe. Many even have handy, snazzy removable silicone grips on the handles for slip-proof control. KitchenAid bakeware is available in a wide selection of shapes and sizes, including square, rectangular, and oval baking dishes (with silicone grips), loaf pans, round quiche and pie dishes, deep-dish pie pans, and ramekins. Only one round 3½-quart dish has a cover.

*Available:* at most culinary and home stores and online

www.kitchenaid.com

*(continued)*

## LUMINARC

Made from glass and ceramic, Luminarc cookware for the stove top and oven is versatile and resists breaking and chipping. A wide variety of opaque glass–ceramic stove-top cookware is available in a diverse selection of shapes and sizes, including saucepans with removable handles for easy storage. The company's clear glass ovenware is also a great pick, with roasting pans and casserole dishes with domed covers, baking dishes (with or without storage covers), quiche and pie pans, and custard cups to choose from. Luminarc cookware is nonporous, nonreactive, and safe for the dishwasher and microwave.

*Available:* at culinary and home stores and online

www.luminarc.us

## PYREX

Pyrex bakeware is transparent and durable, and it provides good heat conduction for even, consistent baking. Pyrex glassware can go directly from the fridge or freezer to a preheated oven and back again safely. Made of nonporous glass, it won't absorb flavors, odors, or stains. This bakeware is nonreactive to even acidic foods and is microwave and dishwasher safe. It's available in a wide selection of shapes and sizes—square and rectangular baking dishes, loaf pans, pie plates, round casserole dishes with covers, and roasting dishes. Some even have snazzy, tight-fitting plastic lids that allow you to store leftovers right in the baking dish. Pyrex also makes fantastic glass storage containers in many shapes and sizes with lids that seal tightly. They can't be beat for safely keeping food and leftovers.

*Available:* at most grocery and home stores and online

www.pyrexware.com

## VISIONS

Made from translucent glass–ceramic, Visions cookware is wonderfully versatile. It's safe for the stove top, oven, broiler, and microwave. It's nonreactive and nonporous, so it won't absorb flavors, stain, or react with acidic foods. The fitted lids make Visions cookware ideal for oven and stove-top cooking that requires covering, and make storing leftovers in the fridge or freezer a convenience (they can be heated again without transferring them to another dish!). Visions products won't scratch, and they're dishwasher safe. Several shapes of pots and pans, all with fitted lids, are available.

*Available:* at culinary and home stores and online

www.visions-cookware.com

# SILICONE

## CALPHALON

Purveyors of fine culinary pots, pans, and accoutrements, Calphalon stocks a great supply of silicone bakeware—muffin pans, Bundt pans, loaf pans, round and square cake pans, and nifty baking mats.

*Available:* at culinary and home stores and online

www.calphalon.com

## KITCHENAID

KitchenAid is a go-to brand for solid kitchenware across the board, including silicone bakeware. With an extensive selection of shapes and sizes, KitchenAid is a one-stop shop for silicone splendor—muffin pans in several sizes, fluted cake pans, rose-mold pans, an assortment of mini-bakeware, loaf pans, round cake pans, heart-shaped pans, mini-animal shaped pans, square and Bundt pans, madeleine pans, and handy baking mats.

*Available:* at most kitchen and home stores and online

www.kitchenaid.com

## LÉKUÉ BAKEWARE

Ooh-la-la, it's French silicone! Lékué makes two lines of silicone bakeware, Classic and Gourmet, both having an outstanding array of choices. The Classic line includes muffin and popover pans, Bundt and deeply fluted Bundt pans, and loaf and heart-shaped pans. The Gourmet line includes mini-loaf, cake, and pyramid pans and mini-muffin-top pans. They're worth looking into.

**Available:** at culinary stores and online www.amazon.com, www.kitchen-universe.com

## step 4 — Safer Plastics

Plastics are ubiquitous elements of our daily lives. They're everywhere—holding the food we eat and the water we drink, constructing the toys our kids play with, the bottles they nurse from, and the sippy cups they graduate to. Plastics house the computers we work on and the remotes that control our entertainment systems. They make up the interiors of the cars we drive. They're cheap, versatile, and convenient. What's not to love? Plenty. Plastics are taking a serious toll on our health and environment. Plastics are made with petroleum, a nonrenewable resource with a host of human and ecological concerns at every stage of its life cycle, from extraction, through processing and use, to disposal in landfills and by way of incineration. Manufacturing plastics involves a mess of petrochemicals that spew into the air and water toxic by-products that stick around for a very long time and creep up the food chain. Though seemingly über-convenient for holding food and drink, plastics have been found to leach chemicals into that food and drink. Plastics are usually disposed of by incineration, which releases some of the most toxic chemicals known to man, like dioxins and furans.[107] They are also disposed of in landfills, where they occupy at least 20 percent of the space by volume[108] and break down at a glacial pace, leaving behind more toxic junk.

Let's face it, using plastics is up there with death and taxes in inevitability. But that doesn't mean we have to sit back and take what's being fed to us on a polyethylene spork (that strange hybrid spoon—fork utensil). There are simple skills you can learn to help you pick plastic products more wisely.

# DECODING PLASTICS: THE NUMBERS

Most plastic products are neatly stamped with a number (1 through 7, usually on the bottom of the container) that says just what kind of plastic it is and determines whether it can be recycled. Different kinds of plastic are used for different purposes (though all are used for food and drinks). Some are less harmful than others that are truly terrible and should be avoided with a ten-foot pole. In reality, plastics are unavoidable, so knowing which ones to lean toward and which ones to steer clear of is a smart, green, healthy agenda.

Not all containers are labeled, and not all containers marked with a number with the recycling arrows are readily recyclable (where were the recycling police when all of this was decided?). For example, #1 and #2 plastics with narrow necks are recyclable in most areas, whereas other #1 and #2 plastics may not be. Different municipalities accept different plastics for recycling, so check what your recycling program accepts.

This table is a simple guide to the plastics that are populating our world.

| PLASTIC TYPE | RELATIVE RISK | DETAILS |
|---|---|---|
| **1** **PETE** | **SAFER** ☑ | Polyethylene terephthalate ethylene<br><br>*Used for:* Water, soda pop, juice, and shampoo bottles; detergent and peanut butter containers<br><br>*Profile:* Contains stabilizers and flame retardants, but fewer additives that leach into foods, drinks, and the ground under landfills than other plastics<br><br>*Widely recyclable |
| **2** **HDPE** | **SAFER** ☑ | High-density polyethylene<br><br>*Used for:* Opaque milk and water jugs , bleach bottles, detergent and cleaning product containers, plastic bags<br><br>*Profile:* Safer for food than many other plastics (doesn't leach as much) and not quite as toxic to produce<br><br>*Widely recyclable |
| **3** **PVC** | **DANGER!** ⊠ | Polyvinyl chloride (PVC) or vinyl chloride<br><br>*Used for:* Plastic cling wrap; cooking oil, cleaning product, and some plastic squeeze bottles; toys (this use has been banned in many countries); phonograph records; water pipes<br><br>*Profile:* Avoid these plastics at all costs. Vinyl chloride is a human carcinogen.[109] Persistent toxic dioxins are produced during manufacture and incineration of these plastics. Common additives that leach into food include plasticizers (softeners) like phthalates and di-(2-ethylhexyl)adipate (DEHA), both considered carcinogenic.[110] Phthalates are known hormone disrupters,[111] and DEHA is linked to deleterious effects on the liver, kidneys, spleen, and bone formation.[112]<br><br>*Not recycled |

| PLASTIC TYPE | RELATIVE RISK | DETAILS |
|---|---|---|
| 4 LDPE | SAFER ☑ | Low-density polyethylene<br><br>*Used for:* Plastic wrap, grocery store bags, some baby bottles<br><br>*Profile:* Like its high-density cousin, LDPE is safer for food (it doesn't leach as much) and less toxic to produce than other plastics are.<br><br>*Not commonly recycled |
| 5 PP | SAFER ☑ | Polypropylene<br><br>*Used for:* Food containers and tubs and some plastic squeeze bottles, like those for ketchup and syrup<br><br>*Profile:* Safer than many other plastics (it doesn't leach as much) and can withstand higher temperatures than other plastics without melting.<br><br>*Not commonly recycled |
| 6 PS | DANGER! ⊠ | Polystyrene<br><br>*Used for:* Styrofoam containers, opaque plastic cutlery<br><br>*Profile:* Styrene, used to make polystyrene, is highly toxic to the brain and nervous system[113] [114] and is a suspected carcinogen[115] that can leach from this stuff. It may also have adverse effects on red blood cells and the liver, kidneys, and stomach.[116] [117] Manufacture involves the carcinogen benzene, which is notorious for sticking around for eons. Steer clear of this stuff at all costs.<br><br>*Not recycled |
| 7 OTHER | DANGER! ⊠ | Other (usually polycarbonate)<br><br>*Used for:* Hard plastic baby bottles, "sippy" cups, 5-gallon water bottles, sport water bottles, metal food can liners<br><br>*Profile:* This classification is for any plastic other than #1 through #6, but usually it's polycarbonate. Bisphenol A (BPA) leaches from polycarbonate plastic and mimics and disrupts estrogen, which may alter the normal functioning of the endocrine system;[118] affect growth, puberty,[119] and the size of reproductive organs;[120] and decrease sperm production.[121] It has been found to spark prostate and breast cancer.[122] [123] Studies show that early-life exposure may cause genetic damage. Almost all government-funded studies clearly link BPA with adverse effects, including changes in hormone levels; early puberty; changes in gender-specific behavior; prostate enlargement; decreased sperm production; altered immune function; and behavioral effects including hyperactivity, increased aggression, and impaired learning.[124] Industry-funded studies say it's safe. Be your own judge, but steering clear is likely safer.<br><br>*Not recycled |
| 7* PLA | SAFER ☑ | Polylactic acid and other bio-based plastics (biodegradable plastics made from corn, potatoes, soy, and/or wheat)<br><br>*Used for:* Deli and take-out food containers, cold cups, straws, cutlery, food wraps, bags<br><br>*Profile:* These are the great hope for our future health and that of the environment. Nontoxic, biodegradable, and made with renewable resources, bioplastics need 65% less energy to produce and generate 68% fewer greenhouse gases.[125] |

# COMMON INGREDIENT HAZARDS: PLASTIC

The process of turning petroleum into plastic resin for making the oodles of products we depend on is where things get really nasty. Plastic resin is pretty rigid, so plasticizers and chemical softeners are added to create an endless profile of qualities. Manufacturers can make the resin flexible, strong, pliable, stretchy—you name it, plastic can be molded for the job. The trouble is, plasticizers and softeners inflict dire harm on humans and drift into foods and drinks with remarkable ease. Fortunately, not all plastics include these additives, so knowing what's what is essential for choosing plastics wisely.

Here are the most common additives lurking in everyday plastics, and especially those bearing the numbers 3 and 7.

| ADDITIVE | THE STORY | USES | HUMAN HAZARDS |
|---|---|---|---|
| **BISPHENOL A (BPA)** | BPA was first synthesized at the turn of the 20th century, investigated in the 1930s as a synthetic estrogen, and added to plastics in 1953. Today it's used to bind plastics, making them malleable and strong. The problem is that it leaches into food and drink—95% of people tested by the US Centers for Disease Control and Prevention have BPA in their bodies.[126] | Hard, clear polycarbonate (#7); baby bottles; sippy cups; sports water bottles; 5-gallon water bottles; metal food can liners | Has toxic developmental, neural, and reproductive effects;[127] is a hormone disrupter (mimics estrogen);[128] linked to breast and prostate cancers;[129] promotes early puberty;[130] damages sperm and reverses normal gender differences in the brain;[131] linked to obesity, diabetes, hyperactivity, and impaired immune function[132] |
| **PHTHALATES** | Phthalates make plastics more flexible. They are cheap and about 800 million pounds a year are produced for use in a wide variety of products. Phthalates are added to soften plastics, to help paints and solvents work better, and even to enhance the penetration of cosmetics and personal care products into the skin and to "fix" fragrances to make them stick round longer. According to the US Centers for Disease Control and Prevention, more than 75% of Americans have measurable amounts of phthalates in their bodies.[133] See "Phthalates" on page 170 for more details. | Vinyl and polyvinyl chloride (#3); plastic cling wrap; cooking oil bottles; plastic squeeze bottles; cleaning products; shower curtains; toys; phonograph records; water pipes; nail polish; adhesives; paint and caulk | Probable human carcinogens;[134] hormone disrupters;[135] teratogens of genital development in boys;[136] cause testicular atrophy;[137] linked to kidney and liver damage and lesions[138] |

To use plastic wisely and more safely in the kitchen, follow these tips.

1. **DON'T MIX HOT FOODS AND PLASTIC.** Putting hot foods or drinks in plastic containers is never a good idea. The chemicals and additives in plastics are not especially stable. They are released when the plastic is heated and then can leach into the food or drink. That's not good for anyone. Fatty foods and plastics are the worst combination of all because the chemicals in plastics are more soluble in fat, so they leach greater amounts of those chemicals into fatty foods.

   - *Microwaving.* Putting plastics in the microwave is a no-no unless you wish to season your food or drink with chemicals. Plastics labeled "microwave safe" are supposed to be safer, but that doesn't mean there isn't any leaching going on. Glass and ceramic containers (without metallic paint or glaze) are the best for use in the microwave.

   - *Serving.* Serving hot foods and drinks in plastic is a prescription for chemical ingestion. Harder plastics are safer, but all plastics leach, especially into fatty food. Glass, ceramic, and stainless steel serving dishes are the most functional, food-friendly choices. And they look nice, too.

   - *Storing.* When storing leftovers in plastic containers, wait for the food to cool to room temperature before putting it in the container. That way, you'll avoid heating up the plastic and minimize the leaching.

2. **USE LESS PLASTIC CLING WRAP.** Plastic wrap is a mainstay in kitchens everywhere, though its clingy convenience comes at quite a cost. Most plastic wraps are made with the worst kind of plastics (PVC and its cousins), which are laden with softening chemicals like phthalates and plasticizers that are believed to readily migrate into foods. Reusable glass containers with lids and unbleached waxed paper are great, greener alternatives for storing food. Aluminum foil can also be used and then recycled, though it should not come in direct contact with hot foods because it is a soft metal that can leach into the food and cross the blood–brain barrier[139][140] and is linked to neurotoxicity,[141][142][143] hormone disruption,[144] and Alzheimer's disease.[145][146][147]

   Curbing your use of plastic cling wrap is not rocket science, and choosing and using it wisely is worthy of a noble prize: a long, healthy life.

   - Choose PVC-free plastic wrap. See "Plastic Cling Wraps and Bags" on page 125 for a guide to better products.

   - Don't let plastic wrap come in direct contact with food, especially fatty foods. Use a plate to cover dishes of food instead. Or snazzy glass containers with lids or PVC-free plastic containers will do the trick. If plastic wrap is too convenient to give up entirely, first cover the food with something safe, like a cloth napkin or towel, unbleached waxed paper, parchment paper, or a chlorine-free paper towel, then cover that with plastic.

   - Do not put plastic wrap in the microwave, period. If you must use it, never let it touch the food directly. Try covering the food with a glass or ceramic lid or plate, unbleached wax paper, parchment paper, or a chlorine-free paper towel instead. I don't care what it says on the box, I avoid it altogether.

- For deli foods that are wrapped in plastic (like cheese), slice off a thin layer where the food came in contact with the plastic, then wrap the rest in waxed or parchment paper and place it in a container or PVC-free plastic wrap.

3. **TOSS OUT OLD, SCRATCHED PLASTIC CONTAINERS.** Plastic containers that are scratched and cracked leach more unwanted chemicals into foods and drinks than new containers do.[148] Any plastic that is the worse for wear should not be used for foods. As plastic containers wear out, replace them with glass containers for long-lasting, safe food storage. Unfortunately, many plastic containers can't be recycled, but they can be repurposed for organizing stuff in drawers, closets, and offices or used as gardening tools.

4. **DODGE THE DISHWASHER.** Hand wash plastic items instead. It's simple—don't put plastics in the dishwasher, wash them by hand. Hot water and the detergents used in automatic dishwashers break down plastics and increase chemical leaching. Wash plastic items by hand, using a sponge that won't scratch them.

5. **GO FOR GLASS CONTAINERS.** Even "safer" plastics, like #1, #2, #4, and #5 (see page 120 for information), leach malicious chemicals into foods. We all wish they didn't, but they do. For food storage, glass containers are the way to go. They come in all shapes and sizes, and with tight-fitting lids for all the convenience and none of the concern. A green bonus is that glass containers can last for decades, and even if they suffer an untimely demise, they can be recycled with the glass bottles.

Stainless steel containers are another great option. Some sets of stainless steel mixing bowls come with fitted lids. Beautiful.

6. **RETHINK PLASTIC WATER BOTTLES.** Plastic water bottles are the bane of eco-green living, and they're pretty impossible to avoid. The reality is that we require fluids to live, and we need something to carry them in. Plastic bottles are the ubiquitous standard, but glass and stainless steel water bottles are great green options that let you avoid ingesting the chemicals that migrate from plastic and contributing to the piles of waste created by thirsty people everywhere. Glass bottles are an ideal substitute that can be used many times before recycling, but of course they are also breakable. Stainless steel is not only impervious to breaking, it's long lasting and safe to tote around everywhere.

Glass water bottles can be refilled again and again with filtered water—just be sure to wash the inside with hot water or hydrogen peroxide to sterilize it as needed. Reuse empty glass juice bottles as water bottles—they're perfect for chilling water in the fridge.

Stainless steel water bottles are practically indestructible and can last a lifetime. They are sturdy enough to take anywhere—the car, the gym, all kinds of urban and rural terrain—and they are a great, green stand-in for plastic sports bottles.

If you do use plastic water bottles, try reusing them. Water bottles made with #1 and #2 plastic are intended for a single use, but they can be used again and again. I try to avoid plastics, but I regularly clean the plastic bottles I do use by swishing the inside with hydrogen peroxide rather than washing them with hot water and/or harsh detergents, because they break down the plastic and increase the chemical leaching. To get the most life out of a plastic water bottle, avoid letting it heat up in indirect sunlight, especially in the car.

## Plastic Cling Wraps and Bags

The modern marvel of plastic has given us ultra-clingy wrap and sealing bags, but not all are made alike. Many one-use disposable plastic goods are laden with chemical additives that can leach into food. When we eat foods stored in this stuff, the chemicals migrate into our bodies and do no good. The good news is that there are plenty of convenient plastic products that don't have all the extra chemicals. While abstaining from plastics is a high ideal, it's so difficult to achieve that choosing safer products that don't have the toxic additives is the better bet. Check out the PVC-free wraps listed in the next column. They don't contain any plasticizers or chlorine and they're noncarcinogenic.

Here are some guidelines for choosing safer plastic wraps, bags, and containers.

### Plastic Cling Wraps

Avoid at all costs plastic wraps that are made with #3 PVC. The safer choice is plastic wraps made with #4 LDPE, including Best Yet Clear Plastic Wrap, Diamant Food Wrap, Glad Cling Wrap, and Saran Cling Plus Premium Wrap.

### Plastic Bags

Avoid at all costs bags that are made with #3 PVC or vinyl chloride. The safer choice is bags made with #4 LDPE, including Glad Storage, Freezer, and Sandwich bags; Hefty Baggies and One-Zip Slides; and Ziploc bags and Double Guard Freezer bags.

### Plastic Containers

Avoid at all costs #6 PS and #7 polycarbonate containers, including all Styrofoam goods. Safer choices include containers made with #4 LDPE, which includes all Tupperware containers except Rock 'n Serve containers, and #5 PP containers, including all Gladware containers, all Rubbermaid containers except Stain Shield, the Container Store's Tellfresh containers, and all Ziploc containers.

## Baby Bottles and Sippy Cups

Graduating to using baby bottles and then sippy cups are rites of passage for young kids that should be safe and carefree. It's deplorable that products mar-

# Bioplastic Cling Wrap! Welcome to the Future

The idea of wrapping food in corn-based cling wrap may seem like a futuristic sci-fi fantasy, but it's not. Imagine convenient, stretchy plastic wrap that's made from plants, contains no plasticizers, and is biodegradable. It clings to dishes and foods, but not to the planet. It's real—check it out! Here are two brands.

Garden Bio-Film (made by BioBag USA) looks and acts just like a plastic wrap should. Made from corn for covering seedlings, it's 100 percent biodegradable and comes in a roll like conventional wraps, though you may have to cut its 3-foot width for use with food. You can find it at www.biobagusa.com.

Eco Film (made by Cortec) is stretchy and versatile, 100 percent biodegradable, and available in three stock sizes. You can find it at www.ecofilm.com.

keted for use by infants and children are laden with toxic chemicals that may negatively affect their health and growth, but parents who choose wisely can minimize the risks from these bottles and cups.

Here's the trouble with baby bottles: bisphenol A (BPA) is a standard chemical used to make clear #7 (polycarbonate) plastic products, including most baby bottles. After as few as 50 washings, substantial amounts of bisphenol A may leach into the milk or formula the bottles contain.[149] It's amazing that it's legal to use BPA in baby bottles because it migrates from plastic to food readily and is known to cause developmental, neural, and reproductive problems.[150]

When you're in the market for kid-friendly goods, avoid shiny polycarbonate (#7) plastics at all costs. Go for tempered glass baby bottles—they have

been around forever and, despite the claims of the plastic industry, they are extremely durable and safe and can withstand a terrific amount of washing. Or, choose bottles made of "safer" plastics—polyethylene and polypropylene (#1, #2, and #5)—which usually are opaque or less shiny.

Consider Born Free vented glass and BPA-free plastic bottles; Evenflo glass, opaque plastic, and pastel plastic bottles; Gerber opaque polyethylene bottles; the Klean Kanteen stainless steel bottle (which converts to a sippy cup); and Medela plastic bottles, feeders, and breast milk storage bottles. Plastic bottle inserts that are considered safer include Playtex Nurser and Playtex Drop-Ins. Note that some companies' brands include both safer products and products made with materials you should avoid. Read the labels carefully!

# PAPER OR PLASTIC?

You are checking out at the grocery store when the cashier asks, "Paper or plastic?"

The jury is out on which is greener. Of course, using fewer of both is the first step in being greener, but there are a few things to consider in the debate over which is better. I can count on my fingers and toes how many bags I use in a year because I bring a bag with me pretty much all the time. However, if I must, I choose paper over plastic because it is made from a renewable resource, can hold more items, can be recycled, and, at the end of the day, is biodegradable.

Here are some facts that might help you weigh the options the next time you are asked, "Paper or plastic?"

| VARIABLE | PAPER | PLASTIC |
|---|---|---|
| Raw material | Trees | Polyethylene plastic (petroleum or natural gas) |
| Renewable resource? | Yes | No |
| Manufacturing process | Includes harvesting the timber, pulping, and making the paper and bag | Includes drilling and extracting petroleum, making ethylene plastic, polymerizing the ethylene, and making the bag |
| Quantity used in the United States | 10 billion, requiring 14 million trees[151] [152] | 100 billion, requiring 12 million barrels of oil[153] |
| Energy required to produce (including transportation, electricity, fuel extraction, and processing) | 1 paper bag = 1,680 kilojoules (kJ)<br><br>*As the rate of recycling increases, the feedstock energy of wood to produce paper can be reduced to zero[154] | 1 plastic bag = 735 kJ<br><br>*As the rate of recycling increases, the feedstock energy of natural gas can be reduced by only half and of petroleum by a quarter[155] |
| Production waste | Paper production creates 72% more solid waste, 35% more air pollution, and 50% more water pollution than plastic[156] | Plastic produces less solid waste and air pollution than paper, though the pollution caused by petroleum drilling, extraction, and spills may not be accounted for |
| Weight | 2,000 paper bags weigh 280 pounds | 2,000 plastic bags weigh 30 pounds |
| Carrying capacity | Can hold more and heavier items than a plastic bag | Less than a paper bag |
| Reusability | Reusable several times as a grocery bag and then as wrapping paper | Reusable depending on strength of the plastic |
| Compostable? | Yes | No |
| Recyclable? | Yes, mixed with newspaper or cardboard | In most places |
| Biodegradable? | Yes | No; photodegrades into smaller toxic bits, contaminating the soil and water and entering the food chain[157] |
| Time required to break down | 1 month | 1,000 years, by releasing toxic materials into the soil and water[158] |
| Other environmental impacts | None | Hundreds of thousands of sea turtles, sea birds, whales, and other marine life die from eating discarded plastic bags mistaken for food[159] |

Bringing a reusable bag on shopping excursions is the greenest choice of all. To make a habit of it, here are a few tips to make it easy to remember to have reusable bags on hand.

- Keep cloth bags in the trunk of your car. After unloading your purchases, put the bags back in the car immediately, before you forget!

- Get an ultra-compact bag with an integrated pouch (nylon or mesh), one of those bags that folds up into a pouch that's attached to the bag. This kind of bag comes complete with a nifty elastic string to cinch it up and a handy clip to attach it to something so it won't get lost. These bags are no bigger than half your fist and they're brilliant for stashing in your computer case, attaché case, tote bag, or purse for on-the-fly purchases. Three to look for are:
  - ACME Workhorse Style 1501 (black mesh), available at www.reusablebags.com
  - ChicoBag (nylon), available at www.reusablebags.com
  - Small Nylon Shopping Bag (nylon), available at www.thecontainerstore.com

## Greener Garbage Bags

Greener trash bags made from recycled, degradable, and/or biodegradable plastic just make sense. Why create more trash when you're taking out the trash? Choosing trash bags and garbage bags might seem like a small detail, but our collective use of them is impressively large. According to the EPA's figures on municipal solid waste, trash bags make up 4 percent of discarded disposable plastic goods—to the tune of 2.2 billion pounds annually![160] That's a serious heap that doesn't include what was stuffed into the bags.

There are several ways you can be green with trash bags.

**Use recycled plastic trash and garbage bags,** made from recycled and especially postconsumer-recycled plastic. *Recycled* plastic is generally made from scraps recovered from manufacturing new plastic. It's called "recycled," but it's more accurately described as plastic that has been saved from being discarded and is reprocessed into new products. *Postconsumer* recycled plastic is manufactured from materials recovered from finished products that were used and recovered to make new products. Postconsumer plastic is the greener of the two.

These bags save energy and resources and reduce waste and pollution. Plastics manufactured from recycled materials require 40 percent less energy to produce.[161] Processing virgin plastics involves massive amounts of dangerous

# San Francisco Earns Green Stripes
## by Banning Plastic Bags

After much lobbying on both sides from environmentalists and supermarket trade grocers, in 2007 San Francisco city leaders, in a landslide 10–1 vote, approved a groundbreaking law banning plastic grocery bags. The estimated 200 million petroleum-derived plastic bags consumed annually in the city[162] are the source of widespread pollution, littering streets and parks and choking marine life in the Bay Area. Under the law, markets and drugstores with retail sales of more than $2 million a year can only offer customers paper bags that can be recycled or biodegradable plastic bags that break down easily enough to be composted. The citywide move will save 450,000 gallons of oil a year and prevent 1,400 tons of waste from entering landfills annually.[163] "Hopefully other cities and other states will follow suit," said Ross Mirkarimi of the city's Board of Supervisors. In 2005, the board considered instituting a 17-cent-per-bag tax, but reached an agreement with retailers to reduce bag use instead.[164]

chemicals and toxic air pollution. Making plastics from recycled materials curbs that pollution and reduces the amount of waste that ends up in landfills. Seventh Generation is one brand to look for in stores.

**Use degradable plastic trash and garbage bags,** which are made from plastic that contains additives that accelerate the breakdown and degradation of plastic. It looks, feels, and functions just like standard plastic. Degradable bags reduce waste because they disintegrate in 12 to 24 months.[165] Most degradable plastic trash bags contain recycled and postconsumer recycled plastic, which also saves energy and resources and reduces the waste and pollution generated during manufacturing. Look for Natural Value brand bags in natural markets.

**Use biodegradable plastic trash and garbage bags** made with plant-based polymers manufactured from renewable resources like corn and potatoes. According to the American Society for Testing and Materials (ASTM), biodegradable,

> *Worldwide consumption of plastic bags is 500 billion a year.*[166]

compostable plastic is "capable of undergoing biological decomposition . . . such that the plastic is not visually distinguishable and breaks down to carbon dioxide, water, inorganic compounds, and biomass,

# Irish Tax Cleans Up 90 Percent
## of Plastic Bag Use

In 2002, the Republic of Ireland introduced a 15-cent-per-bag tax on disposable plastic shopping bags in a move to curb litter. The program has been an outstanding success and had immediate results. More than 100 million of the estimated 1.2 billion free plastic bags that were being handed out every year have been removed from circulation,[167] and the millions of euros raised by the tax will be directed toward environmentally friendly initiatives. Shoppers are urged to use reusable bags and, according to environment minister Martin Cullen, "It is clear that the levy has not only changed consumer behaviour in relation to disposable plastic bags, it has also raised national consciousness about the role each one of us can, and must play if we are to tackle collectively the problems of litter and waste management." The United Kingdom is watching the move's outcome closely, as are countries like Taiwan, as they consider similar "plastaxes." Let's hope it's contagious.

at a rate consistent with known compostable materials (e.g., cellulose) and leaves no toxic residue."[168]

The bags are 100 percent biodegradable, breaking down in 3 to 6 months in commercial composting conditions.[169] In a home composting situation, they break down in 4 to 5 months. The jury is out on how long it will take for them to break down in a landfill, but it is likely to be much quicker than for petroleum plastic (which never *entirely* breaks down, but rather breaks up into smaller and smaller fragments).

Although the bags are biodegradable, they do not fall apart while in use. The plastic is stable until it is subjected to heat or the microorganisms that initiate biologic breakdown. The bags can be stored in their package for 1 to 2 years with no problem.

These bags are a renewable resource. Their manufacture uses about 68 percent less fossil fuel[170] and creates 80 to 90 percent less greenhouse gas pollution.[171]

Biodegradable plastic does not produce toxic materials; on the contrary, composted bioplastics can support plant growth.[172]

Using biodegradable bags is the greenest option! See the "Green Thumb Guide: Trash and Garbage Bags and Liners" on page 132 for brands to look for.

Here are some ways to be greener with trash disposal.

- **REDUCE WASTE.** Buy products with less packaging or packaging that can be recycled. Recycle everything you possibly can—paper, plastics, glass, cardboard, and metal—and compost plant-based food scraps to make a great soil conditioner for your garden.
- **REUSE PLASTIC GROCERY AND SHOPPING BAGS.** They make great liners for smaller wastebaskets.
- **EMPTY SMALLER WASTEBASKETS INTO A LARGER TRASH CAN.** That way you don't have to throw away the bag used to line the smaller basket.
- **CHOOSE THE RIGHT-SIZE BAG.** Using bags that are larger than you need is simply a waste of resources and money.
- **COMPACT YOUR TRASH BY HAND.** Reduce the volume of bulky items like milk jugs and soy milk cartons by pressing or stepping on them.
- **CONSIDER INVESTING IN A TRASH COMPACTOR.** It will reduce the volume of trash and the number and size of the bags you use.
- **BUY GREENER TRASH BAGS.** Get those made with recycled materials, degradable plastic, or biodegradable plastic.

## SAVING THE PLANET
## ONE GARBAGE BAG AT A TIME

According to the Seventh Generation company, if every household in America replaced just 20 tall kitchen drawstring trash bags made with virgin plastic with 20 bags made with 65 percent recycled bags (like the company's Tall Kitchen Bags), we would save 39,000 barrels of oil, enough to heat and cool 2,200 US homes for a year, and 720,000 cubic feet of landfill space—that's 1,100 full garbage trucks' worth. We'd also have 30 million fewer pounds of air pollution.[173]

If every American household replaced a 20-count package of trash bags made from virgin plastic with 80 percent recycled ones (like Seventh Generation's Large Trash Bags), we would save 81,000 barrels of oil, enough to heat and cool 4,700 US homes for a year, and 1.48 million cubic feet of landfill space—that's 2,200 full garbage trucks' worth. We'd have 60 million fewer pounds of air pollution, too.[174]

*To create less trash, look for these garbage bags made from recycled, degradable, and biodegradable plastic.*

# RECYCLED AND DEGRADABLE

## NATURAL VALUE

### Degradable Trash Bags

Natural Value's EcoSafe degradable trash bags are engineered to perform like ordinary plastic trash bags, but they degrade much more quickly. They contain a proprietary additive called DCP (which stands for *degradable compostable plastic*) that accelerates their breakdown. They're available as 13-gallon tall kitchen bags and 33-gallon large trash bags.

***Available:*** at most natural markets and online

www.naturalvalue.com

## NATURE SAVER

### Recycled Trash Liners

These liners are made of 100 percent recycled plastic (30 percent postconsumer plastic). Sizes are 7–10 gallons, 16 gallons, 31–33 gallons, 40–45 gallons, 56 gallons, and 55–60 gallons.

***Available:*** at select grocery, hardware, and custodial supply stores and online at www.buyonlinenow.com

## SEVENTH GENERATION

### Tall Kitchen Bags
### Large Trash Bags

Seventh Generation is devoted to manufacturing ecologically sound products across the board. Its trash bags are made with recycled and postconsumer recycled plastic. The 13-gallon tall kitchen bags contain 65 percent recycled material (45 percent postconsumer), whereas the 30- and 33-gallon large trash bags contain 100 percent recycled plastic (70 percent postconsumer).

***Available:*** at most natural markets and grocery stores and online

www.seventhgeneration.com

## WEBSTER INDUSTRIES

### EarthSense Recycled Plastic Trash Bags

These liners are 100 percent recycled and heavy duty, but they contain no postconsumer plastic. They come in 13-, 30-, 33-, and 39-gallon sizes.

***Available:*** at grocery and hardware stores and online at www.greenlinepaper.com

### ReClaim Trash Bags

These heavy-duty liners are 80 percent recycled (10 percent postconsumer plastic). Sizes are 7–10 gallons, 13 gallons, 16 gallons, 31–33 gallons, 33 gallons, 40–45 gallons, 55–60 gallons, and 56 gallons.

***Available:*** online at www.amazon.com, www.buyonlinenow.com

# BIODEGRADABLE AND COMPOSTABLE

Products marked with an asterisk (*) are certified by the Biodegradable Products Institute as meeting the standards for biodegradable or compostable plastic set by ASTM.

## AL-PACK

### Compostable Bags*

These bags are made with 100 percent biodegradable and compostable plastic. Sizes are 3½ gallons, 14 gallons, 39 gallons, and 63 gallons.

***Available:*** at select hardware stores and markets and online

www.mycompost.com

## ALTE-REGO

### Compost-a-Bags*

These trash and waste bags come in a variety of home and commercial sizes. They're made with 100 percent biodegradable and compostable plastic.

**Available:** at select markets and online

www.compost-a-bag.com

## BIOBAG USA

### Bags*

BioBag makes 100 percent biodegradable and compostable kitchen and yard waste bags for home and commercial use. They're available as food waste bags (3 gallons), tall kitchen bags (13 gallons), and lawn and leaf bags (33 gallons). The company also makes dog waste bags, (8 by 12 inches) and cat pan liners (31.1 by 15.3 inches), as well as Garden Bio-Film, a biodegradable plastic for garden use that can also be used for wrapping food.

**Available:** at select markets and online

www.biobagusa.com

## CORTEC

### Eco Works Bags*

Cortec makes 100 percent biodegradable and compostable plastic bags that are available in custom shapes, sizes, elasticities, and thicknesses for home and commercial use. It also makes Eco Film, a certified 100 percent biodegradable and compostable plastic stretch wrap.

**Available:** at select markets and online

www.ecofilm.com

## FORTUNE PLASTICS

### Comp-Lete Bags

Fortune Plastics makes trash and garbage bags for home and commercial use. The 33-by-39-inch lawn and leaf bags hold 33 gallons, but custom sizes are available. They're 100 percent biodegradable and compostable plastic.

**Available:** at select hardware stores and markets and online

www.fortuneplastics.com

## HERITAGE BAG

### BioTuf Compostable Bags*

These bags are for home and commercial use. The sizes available hold 30, 32, 48, and 64 gallons. They're 100 percent biodegradable and compostable plastic.

**Available:** at select hardware stores and markets and online

www.heritage-bag.com

## INDACO MANUFACTURING

### Bio-Solo Bags*

This company makes trash and waste bags for home and commercial use. Its kitchen bags are available in mini (17 by 16 inches, 4 gallons) and jumbo (24 by 30 inches, 13 gallons) sizes. Its garbage bags are 26 by 36 inches, or approximately 33 gallons. The leaf and yard bags are 30 by 48 inches (approximately 39 gallons), whereas the heavy-duty industrial bags are 35 by 50 inches (approximately 55 gallons) and the cart liners hold 64 or 94 gallons. All are made with 100 percent biodegradable and compostable plastic.

**Available:** at select markets and online

www.biosolo.com

*(continued)*

# NATURE FRIENDLY PRODUCTS

### Biodegradable Trash Bags*

These 100 percent biodegradable and compostable plastic trash and garbage bags are intended for home and commercial use. The food waste bags hold 4 gallons; the tall kitchen bags, 13 gallons; the lawn and leaf bags, 33 gallons; and the trash bags, 39, 45, 55, and 69 gallons. Dog waste bags and cat pan liners are also available.

*Available:* at select markets and online

www.nfpco.com

# PLASTIC SOLUTIONS CANADA

### EcoBio Compostable Bags*

The company makes 100 percent biodegradable and compostable plastic kitchen bags (24 by 30 inches, 13 gallons); regular organics bags (30 by 36 inches, 33 gallons); lawn and leaf bags (33 by 44 inches, 39 gallons); and bin liners (33 by 48 inches, 39 gallons; 42 by 48 inches, 55 gallons; and 48 by 60 inches, 69 gallons).

*Available:* at select markets and online

www.ecosafeplastics.com

# POLY-AMERICA

### Husky EcoGuard Compostable Lawn and Leaf Bags*

These 100 percent biodegradable and compostable plastic lawn and leaf bags hold 33 gallons.

*Available:* at select hardware stores and markets and online

www.poly-america.com

# TRELLIS EARTH PRODUCTS

### Bioplastic Bags*

Trellis Earth Products makes 100 percent biodegradable and compostable plastic trash and garbage bags for home and commercial use as well as produce and retail bags. The tall kitchen bags hold 13 gallons and the commercial trash bags, 33 gallons. Produce and retail bags come in 9½ by 10½ inches, 12½ by 15 inches, and 12½ by 20 inches.

*Available:* at select markets and online

www.trellisearth.com

# US COMPO SOLUTIONS

### Bags and Liners*

These 100 percent biodegradable and compostable plastic trash bags and liners for food, kitchen, yard, and compost waste come in a wide variety of sizes.

*Available:* at select hardware stores and markets and online

www.uscompo.com

# W. RALSTON

### Biosak Compostable Brown Bags*

These trash and waste bags are available in several sizes: kitchen bags (16.75 by 17.5 inches, approximately 3 gallons); bin liners (25 by 30 inches, approximately 13 gallons; and 29 by 30 inches, approximately 20 gallons); leaf and yard bags (30 by 33 inches, approximately 33 gallons); and cart liners (48 by 60 inches, approximately 69 gallons). They're made with 100 percent biodegradable and compostable plastic.

*Available:* at select hardware stores and markets and online

www.cttgroup.com

# LINERS WITH RECYCLED CONTENT

If you are in the market for greener garbage bags for heavy-duty home use or for commercial, retail, or industrial use, check out some of the products these companies offer.

## APCO EXTRUDERS

### Trash Liners

These heavy-duty trash liners are made with 100 percent recycled LDPE (76 to 100 percent postconsumer content).

*Available:* at Apco Extruders, 732-287-3000 (no Web site)

## DYNA PAK

### Full Circle Trash Bags

Dyna Pak makes trash bags, liners, bags on a roll, box liners, ice bags, and more. The company's Full Circle trash bags are made with 80 percent recycled plastics (11 percent postconsumer content).

www.dynapak.com

## NATURE SAVER

### Bags and Liners

These trash bags and liners are made with 100 percent recycled content (10 percent postconsumer content).

www.buyonlinenow.com

## POLY-AMERICA

### Bags and Liners

Husky garbage can liners and lawn and landscaping bags contain 50 to 100 percent recycled content (10 percent postconsumer content).

www.poly-america.com

## POLYETHICS INDUSTRIES

### Bags and Liners

Polyethics offers retail and industrial bags and liners that are flat, gusseted, tear-off, zip-lock, or custom printed and contain 100 percent recycled content (10 percent postconsumer content).

www.polyethics.com

## RESOURCEFUL BAG AND TAG

### Bags, Liners, Carts, and Bins

This company makes trash and recycling bags, liner and drawstring bags, yard waste bags, and carts and bins. All are made with 75 percent recycled content (25 percent postconsumer content).

www.bagandtag.com

## WEBSTER INDUSTRIES

### Bags

Webster's heavy-duty trash and garbage bags are made with 100 percent recycled content (10 percent postconsumer content). They're sold under the brand names Sure-Tuff, Good'n Tuff, and ReClaim.

www.websterindustries.com

To find more recycled commercial, retail, custom, and industrial bags and packaging products, check out these directories.

*Recycled Content Products Directory*, from the California Integrated Waste Management Board: www.ciwmb.ca.gov/rcp

*Recycled Plastic Products Directory*, from the American Chemistry Council and the Environment and Plastics industry Council of Canada: www.recycledproducts.plasticsresource.com

## Step 5 — Recycled Paper Towels and Napkins

Americans love paper and we use tons of it—literally. The general MO for being green with paper products is less is more, so be green and choose wisely.

### Less Is More

The green mission of "reduce, reuse, recycle" gets nipped in the bud with disposable paper goods like paper towels and napkins. Reusing them is prohibitive and recycling services are not readily available. According to the EPA's figures on municipal solid waste, we send about 6.8 billion pounds of disposable tissue products to landfills annually.[175] It's hard to say just how much of the mound is paper towels and napkins because the total includes toilet paper and tissues, but you can bet your bottom dollar that they're a hunk of it, and less than 0.5 percent of all disposable tissue products get recycled.[176] Hence, using fewer is better. Paper towels can be handy for quick wiping and paper napkins are useful when you're on the go, but curbing your use of both in favor of cloth is a smart green move overall.

### Be Greener: Choose Cloth over Paper

Choosing reusable cloth over disposable paper is a positive step toward a greener kitchen. Cloth dish towels and rags go a lot farther than single-use paper towels. Wiping hands and drying dishes with cloth does the planet good. Dish towels that become the worse for wear can be recycled into rags for dirty tasks like cleaning up food spills and floor mishaps. Old T-shirts are also perfect for repurposing as rags for cleaning up.

Buying a nice set of cloth napkins is a small investment that makes for feel-good eco-style. They're economical, and you can even fold them into napkin origami shapes for special occasions. Seriously, though, they save resources, and save you a small wad of cash over the years as you do your small part to prevent paper-manufacturing pollution. When I was growing up, we had only cloth napkins in our house, so for me it's simply a reflex to use them. If you are new to the idea, I guarantee that once you get in the habit, you won't want to go back to using flimsy, crumply paper napkins. However, if and when paper towels and napkins are called for, go for the good stuff and buy recycled ones.

### Choose Wisely: Recycled and Chlorine Free

When disposable paper products are called for, opt for eco-friendly products with recycled content and chlorine-free bleaching.

Go for *postconsumer recycled* products for eco-heroic status. With paper, the word *recycled* by its lonesome doesn't mean that the napkin or towel is actually made from recycled paper. The recycled paper can also be leftovers from virgin-paper runs. It's better than virgin paper, but products with postconsumer content are the über-green choice—and the higher the percentage, the better. Postconsumer recycled paper is made from the pulp of paper that has already been used, so it doesn't require pillaging more trees to manufacture a new product. And not only do postconsumer recycled paper towels and napkins not consume virgin trees, they require a lot less energy and water to produce and thus generate less pollution.

If the thought of recycled paper towels and napkins brings to mind rustic brown burlap, things are looking up. More good news comes with snowy white paper goods that are bleached with chlorine-free processes. Chlorine-free oxygen bleaching has hit the big time as an economical eco-option for whitening all kinds of paper products without leaving an environmentally disastrous wake. Manufacturing chlorine-bleached paper products is a notorious source of dioxin pollution, which brings with it a wicked spectrum of ecological and human health effects. Dioxins are highly toxic persistent organic pollutants (POPs) that have a nasty habit of migrating and traveling up the food chain.[177] They are carcinogenic[178] and have been found to mess with estrogen receptors[179] and growth regulators,[180] among other things. Since dioxins accumulate in tissues,[181] even exposure to small amounts adds up to dangerous levels over a lifetime. (See "Dioxins" on page 42 and "Persistent Organic Pollutants" on page 43 for details). By flexing our consumer muscles and choosing paper products that are processed without chlorine, we can curb this impending mess one paper towel and napkin at a time. Go green with postconsumer recycled, chlorine-free goods!

## SAVING THE PLANET
## ONE PAPER TOWEL AT A TIME

According to the Seventh Generation company, if every household in America replaced just one 70-sheet roll of virgin paper towels with a roll of 100 percent recycled ones, we would save:

- 575,000 trees
- 1.5 million cubic feet of landfill space—that's 2,200 full garbage trucks' worth
- 207 million gallons of water—a year's supply for 6,400 people
- 35,000 pounds of pollution [182]

*When you are scouting the store for greener paper towels, look for these recycled products that are whitened without chlorine.*

## ATLANTIC PACKAGING PRODUCTS

### Atlantic Paper Towels

These 100 percent recycled towels (80 percent post-consumer content) undergo chlorine-free processing.

### Fiesta Paper Towels

Buy these for chlorine-free processing and 100 percent recycled content (80 percent postconsumer content).

*Available:* at most markets

## CASCADES TISSUE GROUP

### Paper Towels

Cascades paper towels are processed without chlorine and made with 100 percent recycled content, though less than 40 percent is postconsumer content.

*Available:* at most markets

## MARCAL PAPER MILLS

### Paper Towels

Processed without chlorine, these towels are 100 percent recycled, with more than 60 percent of that postconsumer content.

*Available:* at most markets

## NATURAL VALUE

### Paper Towels

These towels are processed chlorine free and made with 100 percent recycled content (more than 25 percent postconsumer content).

*Available:* at most natural markets

## PLANET

### Green Forest Paper Towels

These 100 percent recycled paper towels are processed without chlorine and contain more than 40 percent postconsumer content.

### Planet Paper Towels

Planet towels are processed without chlorine and made with 100 percent recycled content (80 percent postconsumer content).

*Available:* at most natural markets

## ROYAL PAPER

### Earth First Paper Towels

Processed free of chlorine, these 100 percent recycled towels have 80 percent postconsumer content.

*Available:* at most markets

## SEVENTH GENERATION

### Paper Towels

Processed without chlorine, these towels are made with 100 percent recycled content, with 80 percent of that postconsumer content.

*Available:* at most markets

## TRADER JOE'S

### Paper Towels

These towels are processed without chlorine and are 100 percent recycled, 35 percent of which is postconsumer content.

*Available:* at Trader Joe's markets

## WHOLE FOODS

### 365 Everyday Value Paper Towels

These paper towels undergo chlorine-free processing and are made with 100 percent recycled content (80 to 95 percent postconsumer content).

*Available:* at Whole Foods markets

*Curbing the use of disposable napkins is the greenest choice! But if you are in need of paper napkins, go for these chlorine-free products made from recycled content to save trees, energy, and water and prevent more pollution.*

## MARCAL PAPER MILLS

### Bella Dinner Napkins

Processed chlorine free, they contain 100 percent recycled content (40 percent postconsumer content).

### Marcal Napkins

Processed without chlorine, they are made with 100 percent recycled content (more than 60 percent of which is postconsumer content).

*Available:* at most markets

## NATURAL VALUE

### Napkins

Processed without chlorine, these napkins are 100 percent recycled (more than 25 percent postconsumer content).

*Available:* at most natural markets

## PLANET

### Green Forest Napkins

These napkins are processed without chlorine and made with 100 percent recycled content, more than 40 percent of which is postconsumer content.

*Available:* at most natural markets

## ROYAL PAPER

### Earth First Napkins

Processed chlorine free, Earth First napkins contain 100 percent recycled content, 80 percent of that postconsumer.

*Available:* at most markets

## SEVENTH GENERATION

### Napkins

These 100 percent recycled napkins (80 percent postconsumer content) are processed without chlorine.

*Available:* at most markets

## WHOLE FOODS

### 365 Everyday Value Napkins

These napkins are processed without chlorine and made with 100 percent recycled content (80 to 95 percent postconsumer content).

*Available:* at Whole Foods markets

## SAVING THE PLANET ONE NAPKIN AT A TIME

The Seventh Generation company has compiled figures showing that if every household in America replaced just one 500-count package of virgin fiber napkins with 100 percent recycled ones, we would save:

- 2.4 million trees
- 6.3 million cubic feet of landfill space—that's more than 9,400 full garbage trucks' worth
- 887 million gallons of water—that's a year's supply for 27,600 people[183]

# 4 Steps to a Spic-and-Span Green Bathroom

**Eco-**

**combining form—etymology:** late Latin oeco, household;
Greek oik-, oiko-, house
**2.** ecological or environmental (*Merriam-Webster's Collegiate Dictionary*)

**Home** *noun*

**1.** A place where one lives; **3.** A place where something
flourishes (*Oxford English Dictionary*)

am hard-pressed to think of anyone who *enjoys* cleaning the bathroom. It's a frequent chore involving plenty of gross corners and crannies. But I'd bet most everyone is happy to groom, shower, and shave in spic-and-span quarters. After all, the bathroom is where *we* get clean. So having a clean bathroom is important, and having a clean, *green* bathroom is essential.

It makes sense to clean such intimate quarters with products that are kind to your body and the planet. Years ago, my buddy Woody Harrelson summed it up clearly. He said, "I can't think of anything more absurd than cleaning something disgusting with toxic chemicals." Woody is one of the most au naturel cats around, and though I can't exactly picture him cleaning a bathroom, he frowns upon chemical cleaners, and with good reason.

The bathroom is home to a lot of surfaces that take a lot of abuse, beginning with all of the activities that go on there. You don't want harsh chemical cleaners on the surfaces that your—or your children's—precious skin touches. Tackling the task with the right product might not exactly be everyone's choice for fun, but the results are rewarding.

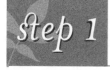

## step 1 — Hand Soap: Be Kind to Your Paws and the Planet

Two roads diverge in the world of hand soaps: natural (plant based) and synthetic (petroleum based). The first is a kind choice for your paws and the planet, the latter is worth opting out of because of the effects they can have on water ecosystems by taking a long time to biodegrade and on your skin by being petrochemicals.

Natural hand soaps use effective but gentle plant-based surfactants to work up cleansing suds with sumptuous smells derived from plant-based fragrances and essential oils. They give you delectable, au naturel paws all around. Synthetic soaps, on the other hand, are formulated with petrochemicals that are harsh and drying to the skin and that also cause a mess in the ecosystem. Sodium lauryl sulfate (SLS) is a foaming agent very commonly used in conventional soaps. It's very irritating to the skin, and it increases the absorption through the skin[1] of other syn-

thetic ingredients, delivering them to the bloodstream more readily than products without it. That's not good news, especially if the soap gets its scent from synthetic perfumes or fragrances that may contain undisclosed compounds such as phthalates, which bioaccumulate,[2] disrupt hormones,[3][4] and are linked to cancer[5][6] and developmental and reproductive toxicity.[7][8] SLS may also be contaminated with unpleasant impurities[9] like 1,4-dioxane, a persistent pollutant in the environment[10] that can bioaccumulate and travel up the food chain and is a probable carcinogen[11] associated with developmental effects.[12] Other possible contaminants are nitrosamines, which are, reasonably, believed to cause cancer in humans because they do so in animals.[13][14]

Many conventional hand soaps include other synthetic ingredients, like synthetic moisturizers, to counter the drying action of petroleum-based surfactants, giving you a double whammy of chemicals. Synthetic moisturizers just don't nourish and moisturize skin. Petroleum-based moisturizers may seem to moisturize, but they're only drawing moisture from the deeper layers of the skin to make the top layer feel smoother temporarily, they aren't truly moisturizing the skin in the long run. They also tend to sit on the skin, creating a synthetic seal that doesn't allow the skin to breathe.

Most natural soaps are available in a bouquet of scents that are derived from plant-based sources like essential oils and plant botanicals. Synthetic soaps, on the other hand, typically obtain their aromas from artificial perfumes and fragrances that may contain phthalates and other menacing chemicals. Phthalates are a nasty group of chemicals that cause scents to "stick" and last a long time, but they are associated with some very bad health effects (see page 170 for more details about phthalates).

## Antibacterial Soaps and Hand Sanitizers: Helpful or Harmful?

Antibacterial soaps and hand sanitizers have become all the rage. There are no more germs and bacteria at large today than there were, say, 20 years ago, but we seem to be way more paranoid about them now.

More than 700 antibacterial products are currently on the market. That's a lot.

And while it's true that there are incalculable amounts of bacteria everywhere, antibacterial soaps and hand sanitizers are not always the answer for confronting them for a few good reasons.

1. Not all bacteria are bad. A lot of bacteria are benign and some of them are truly helpful. For instance, the bacteria in our guts are absolutely essential for digesting and absorbing food, and they are an important part of our immune system.[15] Antibacterial soaps kill bacteria indifferently, wiping out the good and the bad with broad strokes.

2. Overusing antibacterial cleaners messes with our immune system.[16] Bacteria and germs are everywhere, but they have a tough time infiltrating our bodies because we have many levels of defense. We are designed to fight off mild bacteria and germs. Your body is quietly, heroically doing it right now. However, the immune system gets lazy and weak when all the day-to-day defense work is done for it. This becomes a big issue when really nasty stuff comes along. A strong immune system is one that's in fighting form.

3. Casual, regular use of antibacterial products promotes the growth of resistant strains of bacteria and germs. This spells trouble for antibiotics in the big picture. Over time, our most effective antibiotics will be rendered useless. We need antibiotics and antibacterials for the really nasty bacteria and pathogens like *Staphylococcus*

(continued on page 146)

*Whether you favor liquid soap, foaming soap, or bar soap, this will point you toward some smart choices for happy hands and a healthy planet.*

## LIQUID HAND SOAPS

### AVALON ORGANICS

**Glycerin Hand Soap**
12-ounce hand-pump dispenser

*Ingredients:* Delightfully clean and enriched with vegetable glycerin to impart hydrating moisture even with frequent washing, these soaps are infused with organic essential oils and pure botanicals: Lavender, Lemon, Peppermint, Rosemary, and Chamomile (in an extra-gentle baby soap).

*Available:* at most natural markets and online

www.avalonorganics.com

### BURT'S BEES

**Hand Soap**
7.5-ounce hand-pump dispenser

*Ingredients:* This soap's ingredients are naturally derived. It contains cleansing, softening moisturizers, fragrances from plant and essential oils (Citrus and Ginger Root, Green Tea, and Lemongrass), and natural preservatives.

*Available:* at most grocery stores, drugstores, and natural markets and online

www.burtsbees.com

### EARTH FRIENDLY PRODUCTS

**Natural Spa Hand Soap**
17-ounce hand-pump dispenser

*Ingredients:* These pure, plant-based hand soaps contain 100 percent biodegradable earth salts, glycerin, natural preservatives, and pure essential oils for their crisp, clear scents: Black Currant, Cucumber Mint, Grapefruit, Lavender, Lemongrass, Meyer Lemon, Pear, Pomegranate, and Rosemary.

*Available:* at natural markets and online

www.ecos.com

## KISS MY FACE

**Obsessively Organic Self Foaming Liquid Soap**
8.75-ounce foaming hand-pump dispenser and 17.5-ounce refill bottle

I would walk to the end of the earth for this self-foaming hand soap.

*Ingredients:* These certified organic soaps have no synthetics, chemicals, SLS, or artificial preservatives. You can choose from scents like Grapefruit and Bergamot, Rosemary and Melon, Lemon and Ginger, and Lavender and Chamomile, all derived from essential oils. Author's pick!

**Sudz Organic Foaming Soap**
8.75-ounce foaming hand-pump dispenser

*Ingredients:* These natural soaps have no synthetics, chemicals, SLS, or artificial preservatives. You can choose from scent blends with fun names like In the Pink and Sports Complex.

*Available:* at natural markets and online

www.kissmyface.com

## METHOD

**Foaming Hand Wash**
12-ounce foaming hand-pump dispenser

*Ingredients:* This biodegradable soap is nonaerosol and contains all-natural fragrances—Eucalyptus Mint, Green Tea, Sea Minerals, and Sweet Water. *Note:* I spoke with Method about some of their soaps' fragrances and colors that don't smell or look natural. The company admitted that some are synthetic, but says it has thoroughly researched all the ingredients and that all are plant based and biodegradable. If this concerns you, try Method's Go Naked varieties, which have no dyes or perfumes.

*Available:* at most grocery stores and online

www.methodhome.com

*(continued)*

# HAND AND BODY BAR SOAPS

Bar soaps are a long-lasting way to lather hands and body without a lot of packaging. Look for soaps made with plant-based oils and natural fragrances. For clean, green suds, steer clear of bar soaps with synthetic ingredients like petroleum-derived oils, SLS, and artificial preservatives, colors, and fragrances.

A plethora of natural bar soaps can be found in every natural market and a growing number of grocery stores. Here are a few of my favorite bar soaps for lustrously cleansing hands and bodies in the sink, shower, and bath.

## AUBREY ORGANICS

**Bar Soap**
3.6-ounce bar

*Ingredients:* Made with pure plant ingredients, botanicals, and essential oils, these soaps lather up beautifully without drying out skin. Choose from nine varieties, including scents like Evening Primrose and Lavender, Honeysuckle Rose Vegetal, Sea Buckthorn with Sandalwood, and Men's Stock.

*Available:* at most natural markets and online

www.aubrey-organics.com

## DR. BRONNER'S MAGIC SOAPS

**Bar Soap**
2- and 5-ounce bars

*Ingredients:* These soaps contain only pure organic plant oils, essential oils, and vitamin E. The available varieties include Almond, Eucalyptus, Lavender, Lemon, Peppermint, Tea Tree, Rose, and unscented Baby Mild.

*Available:* at most natural markets and online

www.drbronner.com

## DRUIDE

**Bar Soap**
3.2-ounce bar

*Ingredients:* Handmade with exquisite vegetable oils, then cold-pressed and air-dried for 2 months for softness, these soaps are 100 percent pure, with no synthetic ingredients whatsoever. Different formulations are available for several types of skin, whether on the body or face.

Choose from 13 varieties, including inviting formulas like Honey and Glycerin, Purified Clay, Ginseng and Rose, Hibiscus Flower/Shea Butter, Mango Butter and Chamomile, and Unscented.

*Available:* at select markets and online

www.druide.ca

## JUNIPER RIDGE

**Bar Soap**
3.5-ounce bar

*Ingredients:* Made with moisturizing pure olive oil and shea butter, and scented with pure plant extracts. Choose from six scents like White Sage, California Bay Laurel, and Western Juniper.

*Available:* at select markets and online

www.juniperridge.com

## KISS MY FACE

**Big Kiss Organic Bar Soap**
10-ounce bar

*Ingredients:* These soaps are made with pure palm oil, olive oil, herbal extracts, and natural fragrances including Lavender and Tangerine, Eucalyptus and Grapefruit, and Sweet Orange and Lime.

**Organic Sudz**
8-ounce bar

*Ingredients:* These soaps are made with pure palm oil, plant extracts, and natural fragrances like grapefruit and lemongrass, sweet orange and lime, jojoba and eucalyptus, and lemon and verbena.

**Olive Oil Bar Soap**

4-ounce bar

*Ingredients:* These soaps are made with olive oil, plant extracts, and natural fragrances like Olive and Green Tea, Olive and Lavender, Olive and Honey, Olive and Aloe, and Olive and Chamomile, as well as Pure Olive Oil (unscented).

*Available:* at most natural markets and some grocery stores and online

www.kissmyface.com

## PANGEA ORGANICS

**Bar Soap**

3.75-ounce bar

*Ingredients:* These cleansing and moisturizing soaps contain fine organic plant oils like extra-virgin olive oil, soybean oil, and coconut oil, along with pure organic essential oils and herbal extracts. They're packaged in 100 percent recycled cardboard.

Choose from nine varieties, including scents like Indian Green Tea with Mint and Rose Petals, Pyrenees Lavender with Cardamom, and Tunisian Olive Oil and Coconut.

*Available:* at most natural markets and online

www.pangeaorganics.com

## CASTILE SOAPS

Castile soap is as pure as it gets. Made exclusively with vegetable oils—typically olive, coconut, almond, hemp, and/or jojoba—it was called *seafarer's soap* once upon a time for its broad range of uses. Castile soap dates back to the 15th century, and today it is still made with the same simple, no-fuss process. With a pH of 9, it's highly alkaline and terrifically good for cleaning hands, and almost anything else. It's a great all-purpose cleaner and an essential ingredient in many homemade cleaning formulas. Though quite thin, castile soap is very concentrated and a little goes a long way. When I travel, I always bring along a small bottle so I can avoid busting into a bar of some questionable hotel soap, which I never use up and feel it is wasteful to throw away.

## DR. BRONNER'S MAGIC SOAPS

**Pure Castile Soap**

2-, 4-, 8-, 16-, and 32-ounce and 0.5-, 1-, and 5-gallon bottles

*Ingredients:* A family I babysat for as a kid used this stuff and I thought it was very strange—all the sayings on the bottle weirded me out. Now I get it: It's the pure end-all and be-all of castile soaps. It's made with only organic vegetable oils and organic plant extract fragrances: almond, peppermint, eucalyptus, lavender, and the unscented Baby Mild. Dr. Bronner's castile soap is a must-have in every green household for scores of uses.

*Available:* at most natural markets and online

www.drbronner.com

## MOUNTAIN ROSE HERBS

**Liquid Castile Soap**

8- and 16-ounce hand-pump dispensers and 1- and 5-gallon refill bottles

*Ingredients:* This perfectly pure soap is made with organic coconut and olive oils, aloe vera, and rosemary extract.

*Available:* at select natural markets and online

www.mountainroseherbs.com

## OMEGA NUTRITION

**Face and Body Liquid Soap**

*Ingredients:* This pure and perfect soap, made from organic, food-grade oils, contains essential fatty acids that are ideal for conditioning and moisturizing skin. It's available in orange and peppermint scents (made with essential oils), as well as unscented.

*Available:* at natural markets and online

www.omeganutrition.com

# 2 Effective Words: Soap and Water

The largest study done on hand hygiene shows that nothing works better to get rid of disease-causing bacteria and viruses than good ol' soap and water,[17] period. The best way to protect yourself against everyday germs is to wash your hands several times a day. It's as simple as that. (I really do think this works. We get very few colds and stuff in our house, and our cuts and scrapes don't get infected.)

and *Escherichia coli*, but not for common bacteria and germs that mill around in the bathroom.

4. Research is linking too stringent hygiene with an increase in allergies, especially in kids, and notable increases in asthma and eczema to boot.[18 19 20]

## Triclosan: The Antibacterial with Hazardous Side Effects

Triclosan is one of the most common ingredients found in synthetic antibacterial products. It's a broad-spectrum biocide that kills everything in its path, but its hazards to human health and the environment are not trivial. Triclosan is a type of phenol that, though it has antiseptic properties, is a chemical pollutant that persists in the environment and bioaccumulates in humans and animals.[21] It's acutely toxic to aquatic life[22] and causes serious havoc in water ecosystems. One of the big concerns with triclosan is that it's highly reactive with compounds like chlorine,[23] both in the environment at large and possibly at home when mixed with chlorine-based cleaners. The interaction creates carcinogenic compounds like chlorinated dioxins[24] and chloroform.[25] This is not a good picture to be in. Choosing nontoxic, biodegradable products that use the naturally antiseptic powers of plants and essential oils instead of products containing triclosan is clearly the green way to go.

## Make Liquid Soap Naturally Antibacterial with Essential Oils

The essential oils of some plants have natural antibacterial properties, and they smell good, too! Add a dozen drops to your favorite (plant-based, biodegradable) liquid hand soap and shake it up for a fine way to improve the natural antibacterial action of good ol' soap and water. Mix and match fragrances for a bouquet of aroma and healthy hygiene.

Essential oils with natural antibacterial properties include cinnamon, clove, lavender, lemon, lemongrass, oregano, rosemary, sweet orange, tea tree, and thyme.

Naturally occurring compounds in these oils have antibacterial, antifungal, antiviral, and antiparasitic effects, and they support the immune system.

See "Essential Oils for Cleaning" on page 64 for descriptions of essential oils' properties and Aroma Combo Blends.

## Natural—and Portable— Antibacterial Protection

Warding off bacteria naturally is a great idea, especially in public places. Ever think about what is crawling on the handrail in a subway car or the doorknob of a restaurant or office? How about the grime on a dollar bill? Walking around with surgical gloves is pretty much a social and fashion faux pas, but a few natural hygiene tricks can offer you protection without undermining how effective antibiotics are against more dangerous strains of bacteria, germs, and viruses.

There are a few excellent sanitizing hand wipes that contain effective, natural ingredients like essential oils and organic alcohol for on-the-go action. I have them stashed all over—in my purse, my computer bag, my gym bag, and my car. I don't leave home without them!

### Homemade Formulas

If you prefer to mix up your own hand sanitizer, try a few of my favorite effective blends on page 148.

*For safe, sanitized hands on the go, try these naturally effective, nontoxic products.*

## DESERT ESSENCE

### Aroma Essence Towelettes
Plastic canister of 25 towelettes

*Ingredients:* Palmarosa, lavender, tea tree oil, and essential oils

### Tea Tree Moist Towelettes
Individually packaged towelettes

*Ingredients:* Purified water, organic tea tree oil, organic lavender oil, organic orange, and wild-crafted rosewood go into these towelettes.

*Available:* at most natural markets and online

www.desertessence.com

## EO

### All-Purpose Sanitizing Wipes
Box of 24 singly-packed towelettes

*Ingredients:* Made with organic, non-GMO alcohol, purified water, and vegetable glycerin, it also contains organic lavender essential oil, organic flower extracts of chamomile and calendula, safflower oil and aloe vera extracts, and dimethicone (a silica-derived moisturizer). It's also available as a sanitizing gel in a squeeze bottle or hand-pump dispenser.

*Available:* at most natural markets and online

www.eoproducts.com

## PERX ORGANIX

### Natural Wipes
Box of 20 singly-packed towelettes and plastic canister of 90 towelettes

*Ingredients:* These towelettes include the essential oils of chamomile, lavender, sage, rosemary, peppermint, spearmint, lemon, and tea tree.

*Available:* at natural markets and online

www.perxorganix.com

# Clean Hands Spritz (Homemade Formula)

**YIELD: 1 OUNCE**

2 tablespoons + 1 teaspoon plain, aloe vera, or lemon witch hazel

⅛ teaspoon tea tree oil

24 drops essential oils of lavender, lemon, cinnamon, peppermint, and/or thyme (use two or more for good action and a balanced aroma, and also because these oils are potent)

4 drops grapefruit seed extract

Mix all the ingredients in a I-ounce glass spray bottle (available at natural food stores and online, or reuse a bottle that something else came in).

Shake well before using.

Spray two or three times on grimy paws and rub them together.

Note: *Use this to sanitize hands on the go. It has an indefinite shelf life. Add a handwritten label for a nice touch—use an address label or simply tape one on with clear shipping tape. I give bottles of this spritz as gifts during the winter holidays, when colds and the flu are rampant (and I receive thanks-yous all year long!).*

# Lovely Lavender Antiseptic Deodorizing Spray

*This lovely-smelling spray can be used on any surface, and there's no need to wipe it after. Alcohol deodorizes and lavender has powerful natural antiseptic properties,[26] leaving a fresh, lingering aroma. For a bouquet of custom scents, choose from other essential oils with antiseptic properties like cinnamon, clove, lemon, lemongrass, rosemary, sweet orange, and thyme. (See "Essential Oils for Cleaning" on page 64 for details about their properties and Aroma Combo blending ideas.)*

¾ cup filtered water

¾ cup vodka

16 drops essential oil of lavender

Mix all the ingredients in a spray bottle. Spray four to six times to freshen any area. It may be stored for 6 months if kept out of direct sunlight.

# Organic Towels

A fluffy towel is a heavenly thing to behold and dry off with. And when it's organic, it's a feel-good proposition with effects that reach well beyond a quick towel-off. Pure cotton is the obvious choice for absorbency and luxurious softness when it comes to towels, and choosing organically grown cotton towels instead of those made with conventionally grown threads is a champion green option.

The difference between conventionally and organically grown cotton is significant. Cotton is one of the most versatile natural fibers, but conventional methods of growing it are highly toxic to the environment. Cotton is grown on less that 3 percent of farmland worldwide, but it uses about 25 percent of the insecticides applied.[27] If it takes a quarter of a pound of pesticides to grow enough cotton to make a T-shirt,[28] can you imagine how much it takes for a big, thick towel? A lot.

The good news is that those pesticides can't be applied to plants producing certified organic cotton. I have to say, the cotton doesn't suffer in quality—organic cotton is just as fluffy, soft, and absorbent as its conventional counterparts. In fact, it tends to be more absorbent than conventionally grown cotton, because a lot of organic cotton producers do not finish their cotton with formaldehyde products for sizing and stain resistance, as is the norm in commercial textile production. If you've ever tried to dry off with a brand-new towel that hasn't yet been washed and it just won't mop up the water, then you know what I'm talking about. It makes no sense to make towels slick, but it's a standard practice in conventional production to make fabrics easy to care for and stain resistant. The result isn't just frustratingly nonabsorbent towels, it's low-grade formaldehyde fumes too.

I'd say it's a fair bet that most companies that go to the trouble of using organic cotton opt out of chemical finishing, but it's always worth investigating before making a purchase. If you are in a store selecting towels, the best thing to do is to feel them for slickness and, if you're still not sure, ask someone who works there whether the fabric was finished. If you are shopping online, look for companies that talk about how they finish their products. If all else fails, e-mail or call the company. It's worth the effort because towels that aren't finished with formaldehyde feel and absorb much better.

Bright white and colorfully dyed towels are another consideration when choosing towels. With conventionally dyed products, anything goes, which typically includes scouring with chemicals and chlorine before subjecting the cotton to ecologically devastating dye baths that may include heavy metals and chemical fixers. Bright white conventional towels undoubtedly took loads of chlorine to get that way, and you know about the toxic dioxin by-products of chlorine. Most white organic towels are bleached with oxygen, and colorful pieces are dyed with low-impact vegetable dyes. Some organic cotton towels are even made with "color grown" fiber, meaning that they're made from plants that naturally have cotton colored in earth tones like sage and a variety of brown hues, with no dye added. That's one smart plant.

Lastly, while you're at it, consider seeking out US-grown or fair-trade cotton. Both are good for the economy and good for humans.

There are more than a handful of organic cotton towel options these days, though if you ask me, Coyuchi makes some of the best of all time. I've had some of their sets for years and they are still divine. Check out some of the sources on pages 150 and 151 for eco-friendly towels and other fine products.

*(continued)*

## ANNA SOVA LUXURY ORGANICS

Bath towels, bath sheets, hand towels, wash-cloths, and bath mats

Colors: white, cream, espresso, raspberry

Anna Sova stocks an incredible assortment of luxury goods, including spa-quality, thick, plush organic cotton Turkish towels. They contain no rayon, polyester, or viscose and are processed without dioxin bleaches, heavy metals, azo dyes, or formaldehyde fin-ishing. The company will even embroider your towels with a monogram for you and yours. If you're in the market for luxurious sheets (or other products such as soy can-dles or zero-volatile-organic-compound paint with essential oil aromatherapy—see Chapter 9 for information), this is the place to peruse.

*Available:* online at www.annasova.com

## COYUCHI

Bath towels, bath sheets, hand towels, wash-cloths, bath mitts, tub mats, bathrobes

Colors: ivory, white, blue, taupe

Coyuchi is my favorite of all time. Their towels are beyond the beyond—soft, absorbent, and beautifully constructed with cotton that meets standards set by the International Federation of Organic Agriculture Move-ments. Coyuchi goes beyond the standards by commissioning cooperative family farm-ers in India to grow their organic cotton, pay-ing a premium for small-scale production because it not only protects the environ-ment, it also supports farmers and their com-munities in a locally sustainable economy. I'm not their only eco-cheerleader—the United Nations honored Coyuchi with an award for environmental excellence in the fashion industry. They deserve it. FYI, their organic sheets are also supreme.

*Available:* online at www.coyuchi.com

## GAIAM

Organic Cotton Towels: bath towel, bath sheet, hand towel, washcloth

Colors: natural, butter, shell pink, co-coa, persimmon, kiwi, aqua, French blue, lilac, mulberry

Organic Cotton Thick and Thirsty Towels: bath towel, bath sheet, hand towel, washcloth

Colors: white, azure, teak, chili, amber, moss, flax

Gaiam is a great go-to site for all kinds of green-living products, including towels made with 100 percent certified organic cotton and fin-ished without chlorine or formaldehyde. Both of the two lines available have a rich rainbow of colors achieved using certified low-ecological-impact dyes.

*Available:* online at www.gaiam.com

## INDIKA ORGANICS

Anastasia (a rich, raised paisley jacquard design): bath towel, bath sheet, hand towel, wash-cloth, bath mat

Colors: blanc, pale blue, mid-putty

Ode'on: (a textured Art Deco design): bath towel, hand towel, washcloth

    Colors: mulberry, bisque, limestone and bisque, jade and mid-putty

Linea' (a variegated wave-striped design): bath towel, bath sheet, hand towel, washcloth

    Colors: jade and mid-putty, bisque and paprika, bisque and mulberry

Bamboo (a bamboo stem motif, made from organic cotton, not bamboo): bath towel, hand towel, washcloth

    Colors: natural, limestone and Umbria, jade and bisque, pale blue and mid-putty

Indika Organics produces a few signature lines of exceptionally plush and handsome, dobby, hand-loomed Turkish towels. All are dyed with vegetable and plant dyes for a rich palette of color options. Indika's organic bedding and textiles are also worth looking into.

*Available:* online at www.indikaorganics.com

## NATIVE ORGANIC COTTON

Bath towel, bath sheet, hand towel, face towel, yoga towel, bath mat, terry kimono, terry robe, children's robe

Colors: white, café colorgrown (a varietal grown for its natural brown color and left undyed), café and white stripe, café and white jacquard, green, green and white stripe, green and white jacquard, blue, blue and white stripe, blue and white jacquard

Native Organic Cotton uses US-grown, certified organic, long staple Pima cotton to make all its top-shelf products. All of its cotton is grown on small family farms and the company manufactures all the products itself. It is all about having a direct relationship with the consumer, without the middleman. Also check out Native Organic Cotton bedding and kitchen furnishings for more green goods.

*Available:* online at www.nativeorganic.com

## WILDFLOWER ORGANICS

Luxury Organic Cotton Towels (luxurious, heavy, Turkish, and certified organic cotton, in white only): bath towel, bath sheet, hand towel

Legna Towels (made from a silky cellulose wood fiber harvested from managed forests and 100 percent biodegradable): bath towel, bath sheet, guest towel, hand towel, washcloth, bath mat

    Colors: cream, glacier, khaki, mink, parchment, white

Turkish Organic Towels (produced with no toxic dioxin bleaches, heavy metal or azo dyes, or formaldehyde finishing): bath towel, bath sheet, hand towel, washcloth

    Colors: blue, green, mustard, white

*Available:* online at www.wildflowerorganics.com

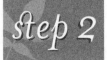

# step 2     Tub, Tile, and Basin Cleaners

Tubs, tiles, and basins are prone to building up scum from the oils in soap and personal care products, hard-water minerals, and the dirt and grime we slough off ourselves. Yuck. But much more gross are the chemical formulas that are pushed on us with the promise of giving us spanking clean bathrooms. The ads can easily lead you to believe that cleaning is a fun spectator sport because the products practically do the work themselves—no elbow grease required! They work so effortlessly because they are loaded with extremely harsh chemicals. Yikes. The question is, Is it worth using chemical products that yield good-looking results but risk your health? What about your kids' health? How about the fresh water we all need to drink? When there are oodles of green, eco-smart options available, the resounding answer is, Not in a million years ('cause that's about how long some of the chemicals will stick around).

Tub and tile cleaners are basically full of the same stuff as all-purpose cleaners. Conventional products favor solvents, ammonia, or bleach for corrosive cleaning action and usually contain synthetic fragrances to mask the smell of the chemicals (covering chemicals with chemicals—now that's a nifty idea!). You can get into real trouble if you use one product that contains ammonia and another that has chlorine bleach in it because the result will be chlorine gas, which, though odorless, can actually kill you. No kidding. Check out what's in some of this stuff. Then recognize that all of it is avoidable—there are plenty of nontoxic green solutions!

## Eco-Clean Tubs, Tiles, and Basins

The main sources of grime on tub, tile, and basin surfaces are buildup and residues from soap and personal care products and hard-water minerals. Bathroom cleaning products are specifically designed to tackle this stuff. The challenge is to scrub that stuff off without scratching the bathroom surfaces to smithereens. Porcelain tubs and sinks are fairly impervious to scratching, but tile, marble, hardware (faucets and the like), and some synthetic surfaces are more prone to scratching—hence the popularity of "nonscratch" abrasive cleaners and creamy cleaners that promise to polish.

You don't have to inflict harsh chemicals on your skin and lungs to get sparkly tubs, tiles, and basins. There are nontoxic products to use instead. They work great and won't hurt your body or the planet.

## COMMON INGREDIENT HAZARDS: TUB, TILE, AND BASIN CLEANERS

**Butyl cellusolve, aka 2-butoxyethanol.** This irritant of the eyes, skin, and lungs[29] can be absorbed through the skin.[30] Prolonged or chronic exposure can damage the liver, kidneys, lymphatic system, blood, and blood-forming organs.[31]

**Sodium hypochlorite (chlorine bleach).** This is an irritant of the eyes, skin, and lungs;[32] contact with the eyes may cause irreversible injury,[33] contact with the skin may cause severe irritation and burns,[34] and inhalation may cause severe immediate or delayed irritation of the respiratory tract and lung edema.[35]

**Ammonia.** This irritant of the eyes, skin, and lungs[36] is a severe corrosive due to its alkalinity, and it will burn any tissues it contacts.[37] Inhalation is extremely destructive to the mucous membranes and respiratory tract, and may be fatal.[38] It is extremely poisonous.[39] If absorbed through the skin, it may have systemic effects.[40] Prolonged or repeated exposure to it may damage the liver and kidneys.[41] It should not be mixed with other materials.[42]

**Diethylene glycol monobutyl ether.** This compound may be absorbed through intact skin,[43] and it is an irritant of the eyes, skin, and lungs.[44] Chronic exposure may injure the kidneys,[45] and repeated exposure may damage the central nervous system.[46] Repeated topical contact may discolor the skin.[47]

**D-glucopyranose, aka decyl octyl glycosides.** The toxicological properties of this irritant of the eyes, skin, and lungs have not been fully investigated.

**Trisodium nitrilotriacetate.** This is a severe irritant of the eyes, skin, and lungs. Contact with the skin may cause painful blisters,[48] and inhalation may cause immediate or delayed burning of the respiratory tract and shortness of breath.[49] It may also affect the kidneys[50] and be carcinogenic to humans.[51]

**Quaternary ammonium compounds, aka alkyl dimethylbenzyl ammonium chlorides.** These compounds irritate the eyes, skin, and lungs.[52] Prolonged inhalation may cause loss of motor skills and disorientation.[53]

**Sodium hydroxide.** Extremely caustic and corrosive,[54] sodium hydroxide is an irritant of the eyes, skin, and lungs.[55] Contact with the skin may cause burning and deep, penetrating ulceration of the skin and/or rashes,[56] and it may discolor skin.[57] Inhalation may cause chemical pneumonia, chemical burning, and/or severe irritation of the lungs and possibly coma,[58] in addition to possible systemic effects.[59]

While there are a flock of excellent nontoxic, biodegradable bathroom cleaners on the market (see the "Green Thumb Guide: Bathroom Cleaners," on page 158), there is a lot to be said for homemade formulas—they're cheap and they work really well. Here are three to try.

# Antibacterial Soft Scrub "Frosting"

*Soft scrubs work well on just about any nonglass surface in the bathroom—bathtubs, sinks, shower stalls, and counters—and on kitchen surfaces too! Baking soda is abrasive enough to get grit off, but it will not scratch tile or laminated plastics like Formica. Adding essential oils with natural antibacterial properties offers added action, and they smell wonderful too.*

½ cup baking soda

2 to 3 tablespoons liquid detergent or castile soap

12 to 20 drops antibacterial essential oil of lavender, lemon, orange, rosemary, thyme, and/or tea tree

In a bowl, mix together the baking soda and liquid detergent or castile soap with a fork until the consistency is like frosting. Detergents and soaps vary in their thickness, so add it a little at a time, mixing all the while until it looks good enough to eat (but don't eat it!).

Mix in the essential oils. Scoop some of the soft scrub onto a sponge and scrub. Rinse the surface well, then step back to enjoy the good job you've done.

# Porcelain Stain-Be-Gone Soft Scrub

*Minerals in hard water and rusting hardware can stain a tub. A good tub is a clean tub—though the stains won't hurt you, they don't look very nice. This formula dissolves stains with an item that lives in the pantry—cream of tartar! It's a pure by-product of winemaking that's used as a stabilizer in cooking and is a main ingredient in baking powder (which is different from baking soda).*

2 tablespoons cream of tartar

1 to 2 teaspoons 3 percent hydrogen peroxide

Mix the ingredients into a frothy paste.

Scoop some onto a sponge or scrubber sponge and scour the stain thoroughly.

Rinse. For stubborn stains, let the paste sit on the stain for 15 minutes, then scour.

Note: *Use this recipe within a few hours of preparing it or the hydrogen peroxide will become inactive.*

## SAVING THE PLANET
## ONE SPRITZ AND SCRUB AT A TIME

According to the Seventh Generation company, if every American household replaced just one 32-ounce bottle of chlorine-based bathroom cleaner with an eco-friendly, chlorine-free product, it would prevent *1 million pounds* of chlorine from entering our environment.[60]

# Baking Soda Scouring Powder

*Baking soda is the perfect material for scouring and scrubbing bathtubs and sinks. It rinses away completely without leaving grit, unlike commercial scouring powders. That's much nicer for the skin on your back if you are a fan of baths, like I am.*

> Baking soda (nothing else!)

Lightly sprinkle baking soda on the surface. Scour with a scrubby sponge, then rinse thoroughly.

*Note: Confectioners' sugar shakers (with medium-large holes), available at grocery and culinary stores, are handy for sprinkling baking soda.*

## Shower Cleaners: Preventing Scum

The sight of scum in the shower isn't very appetizing, and it doesn't seem very hygienic, either. But, its presence is inevitable. Scum mainly from soap and other products builds up in the shower and then mineral deposits from hard water cement it on the wall. To cut through all that crud, conventional products use the brute strength of harsh chemicals. They certainly do the job, but they certainly are also harmful to humans and the ecosystem.

The number-one way to avert buildup is to prevent it with regular wiping. I know, it's not that exciting, but it works. Wiping down the shower with an eco-friendly all-purpose or shower cleaner every few days will nip crusty buildup in the bud. But if and when the soap scum gets terribly caked on, you might want to break out the eco-friendly or homemade soft scrub. Go get it!

## Nontoxic Shower Curtains

Imagine cracking open a brand-new plastic shower curtain or liner: It's so fresh and clean and, boy, does it smell like intoxicating plastic—like a new car!

That smell is the plastic emitting its poisonous gases. Yup, it's really toxic, and it's a gift that keeps on giving—some plastic continues to emit gases for the whole of its existence. That means you breathe in and absorb it for as long as it lives in your home, even when you can't smell it anymore. It's definitely not something you want to inhale in a nice steamy shower.

Most plastic shower curtains are made from vinyl or polyvinyl chloride (PVC), both of which are highly toxic and hazardous to humans and the environment. These plastics are harmful throughout their life cycle, starting with their manufacture, continuing during their stay in our homes, and proceeding to their final resting places in landfill or incinerator. The PVC and vinyl used to make shower curtains are laden with chlorine, which creates dangerous dioxins during processing and degradation. The thing is, it's not just the PVC that's so terribly nasty, it's the plethora of additives that make it stable yet pliable, such as phthalates, that are just as bad, if not worse. Di(2-ethylhexyl) phthalate, a phthalate that is commonly used in shower curtains, is a probable carcinogen, and it may disrupt hormones and cause reproductive problems.[61] To add insult to injury, plastic curtains typically are treated with chemical fungicides for mildew resistance. Yikes! And on top of that, PVC isn't readily recyclable because of all of the toxic additives. It ends up in the dump, where it leaches into the ground, or it gets torched at an incineration plant, where it releases all kinds of horrible dioxins and mercury into the air. What to do? Avoid it completely. There are plenty of alternatives.

Fabric shower curtains are the green way to lean, but beware of curtains that have a water-repellent coating, which may contain the persistent contaminants used in nonstick coatings (for more on nonstick coatings, see page 107). Though convenient, water-repellent nonstick chemicals are relentlessly persistent in the environment and are detectable in most people's bloodstreams because of their pervasive use for everything from cookware to clothing.[62 63]

## Greener Solutions

If you like the convenience and low price of plastic shower curtains, go for 100 percent nylon or PVC-free plastic models.

Nylon shower curtains are available from many sources, such as Satara (www.satara-inc.com; their Pack Cloth Shower Liners are not cheap, but may last a lifetime).

PVC-free shower curtains are made of polyethylene vinyl acetate (vinyl made without the chlorine) or polyester. One source is IKEA (www.ikea.com).

Uncoated fabric curtains are a healthy green solution. Fabric curtains are more expensive than nylon or plastic, but they can be washed. With the right care, they will last a lot longer than plastic curtains.

Cotton and canvas shower curtains can be found at EcoPlanet's EcoChoices Web store (www.ecobathroom.com), Gaiam (www.gaiam.com), Green Home (www.greenhome.com), Satara (www.satara-inc.com), and Tomorrow's World (www.tomorrowsworld.com).

Hemp shower curtains are naturally mildew resistant and strong enough to be used for a boat's sail. You can find them at Earth Runnings (www.earthrunnings.com), Green Home (www.greenhome.com), Rawganique (www.rawganique.com), and Satara (www.satara-inc.com).

# Shower Filters: Get the Chlorine out!

Installing a shower filter is a simple way to improve the indoor air quality, treat your lungs kindly, and keep your skin and hair from drying out.

Unless you have your own well, it's highly probable that the water that comes out of your faucets is chlorinated. Chlorine is an effective disinfectant, but it's toxic to breathe and tough on skin and hair. Though the amount of chlorine in tap water is deemed "safe," reducing and eliminating even low-level exposure is a good idea. You don't have to be a fish to breathe water—humans inhale minute amounts of water via the humidity in the air. Under normal conditions chlorine is a gas, which is liquefied and then mixed with water to purify it. When chlorinated water is sprayed (like in a hot, steamy shower), run through a faucet, or allowed to sit in a tub, much of the chlorine vaporizes into a gas. We absorb more chlorine by showering in chlorinated water than we do by drinking it.[64] Yikes! That takes the fun and pleasure out of a nice, warm hosing down.

But it's not just chlorine that we absorb and inhale in showers. The water that makes its way through our showerheads also contains volatile organic compounds, chlorinated hydrocarbons that form when chlorinated water reacts with naturally occurring organic substances such as the humic remnants of decaying vegetation that are invariably present in tap water,[65] as well as a mess of other stuff.

A good shower filter will nip all this in this bud and likely improve the luster of your skin and hair in one shot. A shower filter is a good deal that doesn't cost much. Filters are easy to install, with most screwing onto any kind of showerhead without affecting the water flow.

Bunches of these filters are available on the market. Many hardware and home stores and even some natural markets stock them. To save water, install a low-flow showerhead, too!

A few noteworthy online sources for shower filters include Aquasana (www.aquasana.com), Custom Pure (www.custompure.com), Filter Water (www.filterwater.com), Gaiam (www.gaiam.com), New Wave Enviro Products (www.newwaveenviro.com), the Shower Filter Store (www.showerfilterstore.com), and Wellness Filter (www.wellnessfilter.com).

*For eco-friendly, spic-and-span results for bathroom surfaces, check out this spectrum of nontoxic products.*

## EARTH FRIENDLY PRODUCTS

### Creamy Cleanser
16-ounce squeeze-top bottle

Suitable for use on stainless steel, porcelain, hard counter surfaces, and Corian, this nonabrasive tub, tile, and basin soft scrub cleanser is for deep cleaning and polishing without scratching.

*Ingredients:* The biodegradable, nontoxic, plant-based ingredients include natural lemon oil fragrance.

### Shower Kleener
22-ounce trigger spray bottle

This shower cleaner helps eliminate and prevent hard-water stains and soap scum.

*Ingredients:* The biodegradable and nontoxic formula includes essential oil of lavender and tea tree fragrance.

*Available:* at natural markets and online

www.ecos.com

## ECOVER

### Limescale Remover
16-ounce trigger spray bottle

This all-purpose bathroom cleaner removes lime scale and soap scum from all bathroom surfaces.

*Ingredients:* It's biodegradable, nontoxic, and plant based, including the fresh fragrance.

### Cream Scrub
16-ounce squeeze-top bottle

This tub, tile, and basin soft scrub is a mild abrasive that cleans up mildew and soap scum. It's suitable for use on sinks, tubs, pots and pans, countertops, and stove tops.

*Ingredients:* It's biodegradable, nontoxic, and mineral and plant based.

*Available:* at natural markets and online

www.ecover.com

## METHOD

### Daily Shower Spray Cleaner
28-ounce trigger spray bottle

This cleaner is to be applied after each shower to prevent soap scum, mildew, and hard-water and lime stains.

*Ingredients:* It's biodegradable and nontoxic and includes a natural ylang-ylang fragrance.

*Available:* at most grocery stores and retail chains and online

www.methodhome.com

## MRS. MEYER'S CLEAN DAY

### Shower Cleaner
22-ounce trigger spray bottle

This product is designed for daily application to keep surfaces clean, but not for removing mold, mildew, or stains.

*Ingredients:* The biodegradable and nontoxic ingredients include a natural fragrance derived from essential oils.

*Available:* at natural markets and online

www.mrsmeyers.com

## NATURAL VALUE

### All-Purpose Cleaning Paste
12-ounce tub

This tub, tile, and basin soft scrub paste removes soap scum, hard-water mineral deposits, scuff marks, ink, heavy dirt, and food stains from virtually any surface, including acrylic, brass, chrome, porcelain, marble, stainless steel, vinyl, and plastic.

*Ingredients:* It's biodegradable and nontoxic.

*Available:* at natural markets and online

www.naturalvalue.com

## SEVENTH GENERATION

### Natural Tub and Tile Cleaner
32-ounce trigger spray bottle

This all-purpose bathroom cleaner is formulated to remove stains and soap scum.

*Ingredients:* It's biodegradable, nontoxic, and plant based.

**Natural Citrus Shower Cleaner**
32-ounce trigger spray bottle

This is a specially formulated cleaner for removing and preventing the formation of soap scum, stains, mold, and mildew.

*Ingredients:* It's biodegradable and nontoxic and contains natural citrus oil for aroma and grease removal as well as active hydrogen peroxide for stain removal.

*Available:* at most natural markets and some grocery stores and online
www.seventhgeneration.com

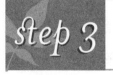

## step 3 — Clean, Green Toilets

There is no elegant way to discuss toilets. They are what they are, and they are much more pleasant when they're sparkling clean.

You don't need bleach, solvents, or harsh chemicals to deodorize your toilet and make it sparkle. And you can certainly do without the dyes that many conventional toilet cleaners also contain. Nontoxic, biodegradable toilet bowl cleaners are the best bet all around—for you, your family, and the environment.

Here are some homemade formulas for toilet cleaners.

# Basic Soda Fizz Toilet Scrub

*This great scrub has a little grit and fizz to remove funky gunk from the bowl without scratching it. It fizzes like something fun and effective. For extra disinfectant power and a lovely lingering smell, add a few drops of pure essential oils. Any of the antiseptic essential oils may be used (see page 64 for ideas).*

YIELD: LESS THAN 1 CUP

1 tablespoon castile or other liquid soap

⅓ cup baking soda

⅓ cup distilled white vinegar

8 drops essential oil of lavender, rosemary, or both

Squirt the soap into the bowl, douse it with baking soda, then pour in the vinegar and essential oils. Let it fizz and sizzle for 2 to 3 minutes, then scrub the bowl with a toilet brush and flush. Ta-da!

# Clean That Funky Toilet Brush!

A nice, clean toilet brush makes cleaning the toilet a more agreeable duty. A good toilet brush is not a huge investment, but they are generally made of plastic (unless you go for an engraved sterling silver model), which can't be recycled and ends up in a landfill. That's not very green-minded. So, to get the most out of a toilet brush, first, buy a good, sturdy one and, second, clean and disinfect it now and then. Here's how.

## FIZZY TOILET BRUSH DISINFECTOR
### YIELD: ABOUT 4½ CUPS, ENOUGH FOR 1 TOILET BRUSH

3½ cups water
½ cup white distilled vinegar
2 tablespoons castile soap
¼ cup powdered oxygen bleach
Small bucket or container to soak the brush in

Mix together the water, vinegar, and castile soap in a small bucket or container. The idea is to submerge the brush in the solution, so pick an appropriately shaped bucket or container that's not too wide.

Add the powdered oxygen bleach. It will fizz!

Submerge the toilet brush. Swish the brush around and rub it against the sides of the container to get more action.

Let it soak for 30 to 60 minutes.

Rinse the brush, then let it dry and stow it away.

Note: *I rinse the brush in the utility sink in my laundry area rather than in the kitchen sink or the bathtub.*

# Oxygen Bleach Toilet Scrub

*Oxygen bleach powder is a great disinfectant, deodorizer, and stain remover. For extra antibacterial action and a pleasant scent, add essential oils.*

1 tablespoon castile or other liquid soap
2 tablespoons oxygen bleach powder
2 tablespoons baking soda
8 drops essential oil of lavender, lemongrass, rosemary, and/or sweet orange

Squirt the soap into the bowl, sprinkle it with the oxygen bleach powder and baking soda, then add the essential oils and scrub the bowl with a toilet brush. For tough stains, let the solution sit in the bowl for 15 minutes and scrub it again. Flush and be merry.

*If you are a fan of clean, green toilets that sparkle, look for these plant-based toilet cleaners that don't contain bleach or harsh chemical solvents.*

## EARTH FRIENDLY PRODUCTS

### Toilet Kleener
24-ounce screw-top squeeze bottle

*Ingredients:* This biodegradable, nontoxic cleaner has plant-based surfactants and a natural cedar oil scent. It contains no chlorine, artificial fragrances or dyes, or caustic or chemical solvents.

*Available:* at most natural markets and online

www.ecos.com

## ECOVER

### Toilet Bowl Cleaner
25-ounce screw-top squeeze bottle

*Ingredients:* It's biodegradable and nontoxic and has plant-based surfactants and a natural pine fragrance. It contains no chlorine, no artificial perfumes or dyes, and no caustic or chemical solvents.

*Available:* at most natural markets and online

www.ecover.com

## RESTORE

### Toilet Bowl Cleaner
32-ounce screw-top squeeze bottle and 64-ounce refill bottle

*Ingredients:* This biodegradable, nontoxic cleaner contains plant-based surfactants and soy and citrus natural solvents. It has no chlorine, no artificial fragrances or dyes, and no caustic or chemical solvents.

*Available:* at select natural markets and online

www.restoreproducts.com

## SEVENTH GENERATION

### Emerald Cypress and Fir Natural Toilet Bowl Cleaner
32-ounce screw-top squeeze bottle

*Ingredients:* This biodegradable, nontoxic cleaner contains coconut-based surfactants and whole and natural plant essences. It has no chlorine, artificial perfumes or dyes, or caustic or chemical solvents.

*Available:* at most natural markets and online

www.seventhgeneration.com

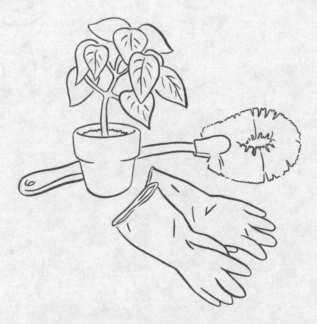

# Low-Flow Toilets: Save Water, Save Money!

Toilets guzzle water; it's their job. Almost one-third of the water used indoors is flushed down the toilet.[66] Standard toilets swill 3.5 to 7 gallons per flush—adding up to thousands of gallons in no time. That's a heavy footprint for perfunctory duties!

Low-flush toilets (also called *low-flow toilets*) use significantly less water—1.6 gallons per flush—reducing water waste by more than 50 percent. That's a big deal ecologically, and it will save you fistfuls of cash on water utility bills, too.

## TOILET REPLACEMENT SAVINGS

*Replacing an older toilet with an ultra-low-flush toilet (ULFT) adds up to big savings in water (and on your water bill!). Replacing just one standard 3.5-gallon toilet with a 1.6-gallon ULFT will save a family of four almost 25,000 gallons of water a year!*

| LARGE TOILET | MEDIUM TOILET | SMALL TOILET |
| --- | --- | --- |
| Replacing a pre-1980s toilet that uses 7 gallons per flush will save you 5.4 gallons per flush, or 77% of the water you would have used. | Replacing a pre-1980s toilet that uses 5 gallons per flush will save you 3.4 gallons per flush, or 66% of the water you would have used. | Replacing a pre-1980s toilet that uses 3.5 gallons per flush will save you 1.9 gallons per flush, or 54% of the water you would have used. |

## WHAT TO LOOK FOR IN A TOILET (not your reflection in the water, silly!)

*Ultra-low flush.* If your toilet is more than 10 years old, it probably is not a ULFT. In 1994, federal standards prohibiting wasteful plumbing fixtures from being manufactured went into effect. The 1.6-gallon toilet became the standard, so if your toilet is less than 10 years old, you have no worries, it probably is a ULFT.

*A fully glazed trapway (outflow).* Although it's not a prerequisite for a good toilet, a glazed trapway improves waste removal and reduces staining.

*A larger trapway.* The larger the trapway, the better the performance. One that is larger than 2 inches in diameter is best.

*A Uniform Plumbing Code symbol.* This should be printed on the toilet. Toilets with this symbol have been certified by the International Association of Plumbing and Mechanical Officials.

## RETROFIT AN OLDER TOILET TO BE LOW FLUSH!

The problem with replacing older toilets with low-flow toilets is disposing of them. Other than making an old toilet a great avant-garde planter for the garden, there is no way to recycle them. Solution? Make that old toilet a low-flush model yourself!

Displacing some of the water in a toilet's reservoir is a simple, easy trick that saves water every time you flush. There are a few good ways to go about adapting an older, water-guzzling toilet to be more water efficient.

*Toilet dam.* This inexpensive device is designed to prevent the reservoir from filling completely without affecting the toilet's performance. They usually come in a set of two, cost about 10 bucks, and will save more than a gallon of water per flush. A toilet dam is easy to install—simply place it in the toilet tank. Check on it every few months to be sure it has not slipped out of place. They are available at hardware and plumbing stores and online at www.amconservationgroup.com.

*Submerge a full plastic water bottle in the reservoir.* Yes! This is called *water displacement*. One full 1.5-liter water bottle submerged in the tank will conserve that amount with every flush. Most older toilets can handle two 1.5-liter water bottles. I put a little gravel in the bottle to ensure that it doesn't slip around too much, though I check on it every few months just to be sure.

Life without toilet paper and facial tissues would be messy. There is no way around the stuff being made from paper, and therefore trees. However, cutting down virgin trees for a quick wipe doesn't make much sense, nor does contaminating the planet with the horrendous dioxins generated by bleaching paper goods with chlorine.

The good news is that if you love trees *and* fluffy, snowy white toilet paper and tissues, you can have them both. The answer (drumroll, please): Naturally bleached, recycled tissue products!

The average American uses at least 100 rolls of toilet paper a year, so it makes sense to buy the good stuff. You might think that the very white papers on supermarket shelves are just paper, with no other ingredients. But you should know that this paper is bleached with chlorine or chlorine-containing chemicals that create dioxins and furans (pollutants that bioaccumulate, travel up the food chain, and cause severe health problems such as cancer, reproductive disorders, genetic damage, birth defects, and immune system dysfunction). See "Dioxins" on page 42 for details.

At the other end of the spectrum is brown, unbleached toilet paper that's not as pretty and feels a little rough, but is very eco-sensitive.

Toilet paper that is labeled as being chlorine free or whitened without chlorine is the ecologically savvy best of both worlds. It is bleached with oxygen, ozone, or hydrogen peroxide; no chlorine or chlorine compounds are used in the processing.

## GREEN TIP

To print an eco-smart wallet-size guide to tissue products you can keep with you for on-the-go consulting, go to http://nrdc.org/land/forests/tissueguide/walletcard.pdf.

## SAVING THE PLANET
## ONE ROLL OF TOILET PAPER AT A TIME

According to the Seventh Generation company, if every household in the United States replaced just one four-roll pack of 260-sheet virgin toilet paper with 100 percent recycled toilet paper, it would save:

- More than 1,000,000 trees
- 2.7 million cubic feet of landfill space, which is about 4,000 full garbage trucks' worth
- 356 million gallons of water—that's a year's supply for 11,200 people
- 60,600 pounds of pollution[67]

*If you are in the market for greener toilet paper and tissue, look for these products made from recycled content and processed chlorine free.*

# TOILET PAPER

## ATLANTIC PACKAGING

### April Soft toilet paper

This 100 percent recycled paper has 80 percent postconsumer content and is processed without chlorine.

### Fiesta toilet paper

This 100 percent recycled paper has 80 percent postconsumer content and is processed without chlorine.

*Available:* at grocery stores

## CASCADES TISSUE GROUP

### Cascades toilet paper

This paper has 100 percent recycled content, but less than 40 percent is postconsumer content. It's processed chlorine free.

### Pert toilet paper

This paper is also 100 percent recycled with less than 40 percent postconsumer content and processed chlorine free.

*Available:* at most grocery stores

## CVS

### Toilet paper

Seventy-five percent of this paper is recycled content, and 40 percent postconsumer content.

*Available:* at CVS stores

## EARTH FIRST (ROYAL PAPER CONVERTING)

### Toilet paper

Of this paper's 100 percent recycled content, 80 percent is postconsumer. It's processed without chlorine.

*Available:* at most natural markets and grocery stores

## EARTH FRIENDLY PRODUCTS

### Toilet paper

This paper is 100 percent recycled, with 10 to 25 percent postconsumer content.

*Available:* at most natural markets

## GREEN FOREST (PLANET)

### Toilet paper

This 100 percent recycled paper is 40 percent postconsumer content and processed without chlorine.

*Available:* at most natural markets

## MARCAL PAPER MILLS

### Marcal toilet paper

This paper is 100 percent recycled, 40 percent postconsumer content. It's processed chlorine free.

### Sofpac toilet paper

This paper's 100 percent total recycled content is 40 percent postconsumer content. It is processed chlorine free.

*Available:* at most grocery stores

## NATURAL VALUE

### Toilet paper

This toilet paper has 100 percent recycled content and 10 to 25 percent postconsumer content. It is processed without chlorine.

*Available:* at most natural markets

## SEVENTH GENERATION

### Toilet paper

This paper is 100 percent recycled and 80 percent postconsumer content, and it is processed chlorine free.

*Available:* at most natural markets and grocery stores

*(continued)*

## TRADER JOE'S

### Toilet paper

This paper is 100 percent recycled and 35 percent postconsumer content. It is processed chlorine free.

*Available:* at Trader Joe's stores

## WHOLE FOODS

### 365 Everyday Value toilet paper

This paper is 100 percent recycled, 80 to 95 percent of it postconsumer content, and processed chlorine free.

*Available:* at Whole Foods markets

# FACIAL TISSUES

## GREEN FOREST (PLANET)

### Tissues

These tissues are 100 percent recycled, 40 percent postconsumer content, and processed chlorine free.

*Available:* at most natural markets

## MARCAL PAPER MILLS

### Fluff Out

These tissues are 100 percent recycled content, with 40 percent of that postconsumer content. They are processed without chlorine.

### Hankies

These tissues are also 100 percent recycled content, with 40 percent of that postconsumer content, and processed without chlorine.

### Marcal

These tissues are also 100 percent recycled content, with 40 percent of that postconsumer content, and processed without chlorine.

*Available:* at most grocery stores

## SEVENTH GENERATION

These tissues are made with 100 percent recycled content, 80 percent of which is postconsumer content. They are processed chlorine free.

*Available:* at most natural markets and grocery stores

---

### SAVING THE PLANET ONE TISSUE AT A TIME

According to the Seventh Generation company, if every household in the United States replaced just one box of virgin fiber facial tissues (175 sheets) with 100 percent recycled ones, it would save:

- 163,000 trees
- 226,500 cubic feet of landfill space (about 330 full garbage trucks' worth)
- 31 million gallons of water, which is a year's supply for 960 people
- 5,300 pounds of pollution![68]

# CHAPTER 5

# Natural Beauty: The Simple 7

**Beauty** *noun*

1. the quality or aggregate of qualities in a person or thing that gives pleasure to the senses or pleasurably exalt the mind or spirit (*Merriam-Webster's Collegiate Dictionary*)

1. a combination of qualities that delights the aesthetic senses (*Oxford English Dictionary*)

Personal care products have been used for eons. Humans have been using prized formulas and special solutions in chase of good hygiene, beauty, lovely skin, clean teeth, and good smells, and the potions and lotions have changed with the times, for the better and the worse. While ladies and gents have given up dusting their faces with powders made of lead and painting their lips with the deep red of mercuric sulfide like the Victorians did (and the Romans and Egyptians before them), today's personal care products and cosmetics have become a veritable laboratory loaded with chemicals.

They say true beauty comes from within, but good products definitely help.

Most of us groom ourselves from dawn to dusk, using more than a handful of products without giving a moment's consideration to just what is in the formulas that we apply to our most intimate nooks and crannies. It's not only beautifying agents, but also maintenance materials like toothpaste, deodorant, shaving cream, and soap that should concern us. The genius of modern marketing can make shaving look sexy, and the smooth results may indeed be sexy, but it's a chore for most. Whether personal preening is a pleasure or just a daily chore, choosing products with au naturel ingredients is a clean, wise way to green your regime.

## Regulations, Anyone?

In the personal care product and cosmetics realm, there is alarmingly little regulation. The legal definition of personal care products and cosmetics reads "articles intended to be rubbed, poured, sprinkled, or sprayed on, introduced into, or otherwise applied to the human body or any part thereof for cleansing, beautifying, promoting attractiveness, or altering the appearance."[1] Soap does not qualify. Virtually any ingredient can be used in soap,[2] whether it is chemical, synthetic, or natural.

No federal laws require companies to test personal care products for safety before they hit the shelves. The Food and Drug Administration's Office of Cosmetics and Colors officially states that "neither cosmetic products nor cosmetic ingredients, other than color additives, need to be reviewed or approved by FDA before they are sold to the public. FDA cannot require companies to do safety testing of their cosmetics before marketing"[3]—so it's up to us and our purchasing reflexes to make clean, green choices. Taking care of our skin, hair, and teeth means knowing what we apply to them— what goes on our bodies gets into our bodies, and that's important. With just a little knowledge, we can pick personal care products and cosmetics that can do their jobs gracefully, without hazard or harm. Now we're talking.

## Skin Absorption

All the chemicals, additives, fragrances, and dyes in personal care products wouldn't be an issue if our skin wasn't so good at absorbing stuff. But it is. It's believed that our skin can absorb up to 60 percent of what's applied to it.[4][5][6]

## Skin Deep:
## What's in Your Products

Massive amounts of personal care products and cosmetics are on the market. Many are clean, green, and great, and many are worth avoiding like the plague.

If you want to find out what's what (as my grandma used to say), you can. The Environmental Working Group (EWG) is a Washington, DC–based public interest watchdog group that has compiled some of the most comprehensive research around. It is a team of scientists, engineers, policy experts, lawyers, and computer programmers who pore over federal data, legal documents, and scientific studies in their own labs to test and expose threats to human health and the environment. And, most important, they help find solutions. In short, they rock.

The EWG's database, Skin Deep, is the ultimate safety guide for personal care products and cosmetics. With research into 27,000 products (cross-referenced against 50 credible toxicity and regulatory databases), it is the largest and most definitive data resource anywhere. Products are rated on a 0-to-10 scale (with 0 being harmless and 10 being dastardly and hazardous) and their ingredients and possible health hazards are fully disclosed. It's brilliant as well as interactive and user-friendly, which is really nice of them. Thanks, EWG! To check out this dynamic piece of work, visit www.cosmeticsdatabase.com.

*BIG NOTE:* If you are keen to check products on this site, be sure to look at the ingredients that are responsible for a product's rating. For instance, certain natural ingredients like essential oils are flagged for their possible health effects. Also, the site does not differentiate between food-grade versus cosmetic-grade or organic versus regular ingredients. Some pure products made by trustworthy companies are flagged, so dig a little to find out the whole story. If you're in doubt about a product, contact the company directly—if it's a stand-up bunch, it will answer your concerns.

# Hazardous Ingredients: The Worst Offenders

In the wide world of personal care products and cosmetics, there are more synthetic and chemical ingredients than any one of us can shake a stick at, even in some product lines that look purely natural and nice. Avoiding lousy ingredients altogether is difficult, but there are a handful of really dodgy ingredients that are worth avoiding whenever possible.

Unfortunately, some of the most questionable ingredients are the most widely used. Preservatives, for instance, are necessary to keep products fresh. While synthetic preservatives like parabens (methylparaben, propylparaben, and the rest; see below) are cheap and work effectively in a broad range of products, their possible side effects on human health may be a big price to pay. The good news is that lots of products contain natural preservatives that cause no harm. Synthetic fragrances are also hugely popular because good smells are a pleasure, but the chemicals—like phthalates—lurking behind the vague term *fragrances* on product labels can be persistently harmful and linked to serious health hazards.

Choosing and using pure products with absolutely clean ingredients absolutely all the time is tough, but knowing which chemical bullies to avoid whenever possible will make a huge difference to your own and the planet's health.

## Parabens

**Use:** Parabens are synthetic preservatives. The cosmetics industry stands strongly behind the belief that parabens are safe, but a growing number of reputable studies say otherwise.

**Found in:** Hair shampoos, conditioners, and styling products; soaps and body washes; moisturizers; shaving creams and gels; cosmetics and makeup; toothpastes

**Linked with:** Studies link parabens with acute and chronic health hazards.

**Butylparaben:** This paraben may be linked with allergies and skin toxicity,[7] biochemical changes,[8] developmental and reproductive toxicity,[9] endocrine disruption and hormone mimicry,[10] tissue irritation,[11] and organ toxicity.[12]

**Ethylparaben:** It has been linked with cancer,[13] [14] developmental and reproductive toxicity,[15] endocrine disruption and hormone mimicry,[16] and organ toxicity.[17]

**Methylparaben:** This paraben is linked with allergies and skin toxicity,[18] biochemical changes,[19] cancer,[20] [21] endocrine disruption and hormone mimicry,[22] tissue irritation,[23] and organ toxicity.[24]

**Propylparaben:** Studies have linked it with allergies and skin toxicity,[25] developmental and reproductive toxicity,[26] endocrine disruption and hormone mimicry,[27] and organ toxicity.[28] It is also toxic to the environment.[29]

## Phthalates (Fragrance)

We met phthalates on page 70, when we talked about their use as plasticizers to make plastic softer, most notoriously in highly toxic polyvinyl chloride (PVC, #3) plastic. Independent studies by public health organizations reveal that about 70 percent of personal care products contain phthalates.[30] [31] Phthalates are included in a broad range of products. They're cheap and versatile—millions of tons are produced annually[32] for use in adhesives, building materials, cosmetics, films, personal care products, pesticides, plastics, and perfumes.

**Use:** On ingredient lists for personal care products and cosmetics, phthalates are regularly disguised as *fragrance*. They're used as solvents and to "fix" fragrance to make the aroma last longer, enhance skin penetration, lubricate other ingredients, and keep nail polish from chipping. Any product with synthetic fragrance may contain phthalates. Look for products with natural fragrances from plants and essential oils and those that disclose the sources of the fragrance.

**Found in:** Fingernail products; makeup, including lip products, eyeliners, eye shadows, blushes; deodorants; hair products, especially coloring products; feminine products; fragrances; perfumes

**Linked with:** Studies link phthalates with bioaccumulation in humans and wildlife;[33] cancer;[34 35] developmental and reproductive toxicity;[36 37] endocrine disruption;[38 39] neurotoxicity and neurodevelopmental disorders;[40] toxicity of the brain, kidneys, liver, and lungs;[41 42 43] and birth defects.[44] It is also toxic in the environment.[45]

Who's at risk? Like it or not, we are all exposed to phthalates. According to a study by the Centers for Disease Control and Prevention, *every* person tested—all of them!—had detectable levels of phthalates in his or her body,[46] though certain groups had higher levels and others were more susceptible to their ill effects. Women of childbearing age and kids, with their still-developing systems (especially the male reproductive system), are at the greatest risk.

# Sodium Lauryl Sulfate and Sodium Laureth Sulfate

**Use:** Sodium lauryl sulfate (SLS) and sodium laureth sulfate (SLES) are used because they're cheap and they work well as surfactants, making products lather up nicely. Like all surfactant detergents, they remove oils effectively, but they do so indiscriminately on the skin, which can cause dryness and contact dermatitis.

**Found in:** Anything that lathers: shampoos and conditioners, soaps and body washes/cleansers, toothpastes and whitening products, even moisturizers and mouthwashes

**Linked with:** Both are widely known to irritate skin,[47] but they also may be linked with deeper health concerns.

They enhance the skin's absorptive capacity.[48] SLS and SLES are used in part to increase the product's penetration through the skin and increase the skin's ability to absorb; in fact, they are effectively used for topical drug delivery to decrease skin resistance.[49] One concern with that is that other synthetic and chemical ingredients in the product will be delivered into our bodies more effectively too. *Tip:* Look at what other ingredients are in products that contain SLS or SLES to see what else will be absorbed thanks to that enhanced ability.

They lower the skin's immunological response.[50] The increased penetration by SLS and SLES messes with our skin's integrity and lowers its natural immune response.[51] Skin is an immunological organ, and when its innate immune response is compromised, skin inflammation and irritation can result.[52] This can also lead to a thickening of the skin.[53] Chronic, low-grade compromising of the immune system is not exactly helpful for overall health.

The jury is still out on whether SLS and SLES can act as endocrine disrupters and mess with hormones. While the studies are not conclusive, there is agreement in the scientific community that other chemicals known to contaminate SLS and SLES, like 1,4-dioxane and nitrosamines, do indeed wreak havoc with hormones[54] and may cause reproductive and developmental issues.[55] The best bet is to choose SLS- and SLES-free products for a long, healthy life.

## SLS and SLES and Cancer: Urban Legend or Real Concern?

There are controversial claims in the cosmetics industry that SLS and SLES are carcinogenic, meaning that they cause cancer.[56] The American Cancer Society states that the common belief is an urban legend, but the plot thickens. There are increasing numbers of studies revealing that SLS and SLES may be *indirectly* carcinogenic.[57] SLS and SLES are commonly contaminated with some pretty nasty substances that are accidental by-products of their processing.[58] While the FDA "encourages" manufacturers to remove the contaminants, the agency hasn't established a limit for allowable levels in cosmetics and there are no laws requiring them to be removed.[59] The two most common contaminants are:

- **1,4-dioxane.** The US Environmental Protection Agency (EPA) considers it a probable carcinogen[60] and the National Toxicology Program considers it a known animal carcinogen.[61] It's also linked with other serious problems like reproductive and developmental effects,[62] as well as being a persistent toxic pollutant in the environment.[63]
- **Nitrosamines.** These compounds are believed to cause cancer in humans[64] because they are known carcinogens in animals.[65]

*Tips:* To dodge these dastardly contaminants, avoid products that contain SLS, SLES, or ingredients whose names include *PEG*, *xynol*, *cetareth*, and *oleth*.

## Ethylenediamine Tetraacetic Acid

**Use:** Ethylenediamine tetraacetic acid (EDTA) is used as a stabilizer in cosmetics. It has this nifty chelating (binding) capability that acts like a sequestering preservative to keep all the atoms in order. It's used similarly to keep processed foods stable, and even in industrial cleaning to bind heavy metals for removal. That's actually a pretty neat and useful property, but it can run amok in the environment because it is fairly persistent at doing what it does. Given that EDTA is a stabilizer, it's quite stable itself and isn't very cooperative about breaking down or degrading in the ecosystem or even during conventional wastewater treatment. EDTA's chelating action is ecologically troublesome in waterways because it tends to remobilize dormant heavy metal sediments. In Europe, EDTA is considered one of the most abundant anthropogenic compounds found in surface water,[66] which means that it results from human activity and has heavy environmental effects. In the United States, it's among the top 10 measurable contaminants in the great Mississippi River.[67] To be fair, cosmetics production isn't the only place EDTA is used; it also has a bunch of industrial applications. But EDTA in cosmetics has its own set of concerns.

**Linked with**: On the skin, EDTA is yet another irritant[68] and may instigate allergies and contact dermatitis.[69] This begs the question of how useful it is to use chemical stabilizers in skin products if they cause skin problems, but EDTA is nonetheless found in plenty of formulas. Deeper concerns about EDTA are related to prolonged and repeated use. Potential chronic health effects include reproductive and fetal effects[70] and kidney damage.[71] Jeepers creepers, is that called for? Apparently, EDTA is a mutagen in animals,[72] but it's inconclusive whether it has that effect in humans.

## Formaldehyde

**Use**: Formaldehyde is not often seen on personal care product and cosmetic ingredient lists, but it's released by many commonly used preservatives. Formaldehyde is indeed a very effective preservative (remember those frogs we were supposed to dissect in high school biology class?), but it's also definitely carcinogenic.[73] A number of preservatives used in products are subject to either becoming accidentally contaminated with formaldehyde during processing[74] or to interacting with other substances to release formaldehyde during use.[75]

The most common formaldehyde-releasing preservatives are:

**Diazolidinyl urea.** This formaldehyde-releasing preservative is found in face and body moisturizers, cleansers and body washes, sunscreens, and hair conditioners and styling products. It's linked to mutagenic effects,[76] cancer,[77] allergic reaction,[78] skin toxicity,[79] and neurotoxicity in the forms of brain and nervous system effects.[80]

**Imidazolidinyl urea.** This compound contains and/or releases formaldehyde. It's found in face and body moisturizers, cleansers and body washes, sunscreens, feminine products, and cosmetics, including foundations, powders, eye shadows, and mascaras. It is linked to allergic reaction, contact dermatitis,[81] mutagenic effects,[82] cell toxicity,[83] and skin toxicity.[84]

**Dimethyl-dimethyl hydantoin.** A formaldehyde-releasing preservative, it's found in hair shampoos, conditioners, and styling products; face and body moisturizers, cleansers, and body washes; and sunscreens. It is linked to allergic reaction;[85] irritation of the eyes, skin, and lungs;[86] and organ toxicity.[87]

**Quaternium-15.** This compound contains and/or releases formaldehyde. It's found in face and body washes and cleansers, shampoos and conditioners, baby shampoos and soaps, sunscreens, and cosmetics. It is linked to allergic reaction,[88] skin sensitization,[89][90] reproductive effects,[91][92] and birth defects.[93][94]

**Bronopol (2-bromo-2-nitropropane-1,3-diol).** A formaldehyde-releasing preservative, it is found in face and body moisturizers, washes and cleansers; soaps; and hair conditioners and styling products. It's linked to allergic reaction, contact dermatitis,[95] skin sensitization,[96] birth defects,[97] severe skin toxicity,[98] and endocrine disruption.[99]

## Propylene Glycol

**Use:** Propylene glycol is a multitasking petrochemical wonder. In lotions, potions, and moisturizers, it works to retain moisture in the skin. Propylene glycol is also a wetting agent and solvent used to dissolve and combine ingredients in cosmetics and personal care goods like deodorants. But that's not all. It's a key ingredient in embalming fluids[100] and brake fluid.[101] It's also known as antifreeze (yes, for your car) and works brilliantly as a deicing solution for roads, planes, cars, and boats[102] and as a solvent in the paint and plastics industries.[103] The jury is out on how toxic it is in the environment, but generally, petrochemicals don't have a healthy reputation on that front.

**Linked with:** The FDA gives propylene glycol the GRAS (generally recognized as safe)[104] stamp of approval for pretty much any topical application. However, publicly registered Material Safety Data Sheets instruct users to "avoid contact with skin."[105] Hmm. In fact, propylene glycol seems none too friendly for skin in general. Beyond being a skin irritant[106] and common cause of allergies and contact dermatitis,[107] it's one of those chemicals that acts as a defatting agent,[108] especially with repeated or prolonged exposure. Yuck. If that's not enough to convict it, it's also measurably toxic to human cells[109] and may inhibit skin cell growth,[110] alter cell membranes,[111] and cause chronic surface damage.[112] Not exactly the qualities one looks for in a face cream or underarm deodorant.

## Toluene

**Use:** Toluene is a viciously toxic solvent that lurks in nail polishes, and its derivatives are found in some hair colorings and dyes. It's an ironically sweet-smelling VOC (volatile organic compound) that can cause a wide spectrum of adverse acute and chronic health effects.

**Found in:** Nail polishes and nail treatment products

**Linked with:** Severe irritation of the eyes, skin, and lungs;[113] central nervous system damage;[114] kidney and liver damage;[115] developmental effects;[116] and birth defects and brain damage[117]

## Talc

**Use:** Talc is a superfine powder that's used for its absorbency, anticaking and bulking properties, and ability to keep products like cosmetics from slipping.

**Found in**: Deodorants, antiperspirants, and body powders; cosmetics, including eye shadows, powdered concealers, foundations, blushes, and bronzers; sunscreens and SPF products

**Linked with**: One of the main concerns about talc is that it is commonly contaminated with asbestos,[118] a known carcinogen,[119] though talc is suspected to be a carcinogen in its own right.[120] Inhaling the superfine dust of talc is none too nifty for the lungs,[121] and there is also cause for concern about an increased risk for cancer with regular topical use.[122]

## Diethanolamine, Monoethanolamine, and Triethanolamine

Diethanolamine (DEA), monoethanolamine (MEA), and triethanolamine (TEA) are all types of ethanolamines (ammonia compounds), chemical constituents used for a broad range of applications, including as emulsifiers, pH balancers, and surfactants and foaming agents. They are made when one or more ethylene oxide molecules reacts with ammonia. MEA has one ethylene oxide molecule, DEA has two, and TEA has three. Since ethanolamines have the combined properties of amines and alcohol, they can react with tons of different substances like salts and acids for different uses.

The pervasive concern with amines is that they can include carcinogenic nitrosamines,[123][124] which are accidentally created by chemical reaction during manufacturing. Nitrosamines are known to cause cancer and can penetrate the skin.[125] The amine family is believed to be toxic, notably to the liver and kidneys, especially with repeated or chronic use. They all tend to be quite irritating and harmful to absorb through the skin,[126] which is ironic and disturbing since they are widely used in personal care products designed for the skin. One of the more confusing aspects of ethanolamine derivatives is that some are derived from natural sources, like cocomide DEA or cocamide MEA, which are derived from coconut. Though these compounds are synthesized from a "natural" source, these types of ingredients are still linked with the same health concerns.

**DEA**: DEA and its derivatives are used to boost foaming action and to improve viscosity. It's found in liquid soaps and hair shampoos. Though it yields a nice foam, it can be a severe skin irritant and harmful when absorbed though the skin.[127] Repeated use may also have adverse effects on the blood and cause liver and kidney damage.[128] None too friendly.

**MEA**: MEA (aka *ethanolamine*) and its derivatives are used to form foamy suds, increase viscosity, and adjust pH. It's not just irritating to the skin and eyes, it can actually cause burns.[129] MEA can be absorbed through the skin in potentially dangerous amounts,[130] and repeated and long-term exposure may cause liver and kidney damage.[131] It's been shown to be toxic to fetuses and retard growth in animals,[132][133] though human studies have yet to be documented.

TEA: TEA is widely used as an emulsifier and pH adjuster in personal care products. Along with the facts that it is a major skin irritant, can cause contact dermatitis,[134] and is harmful to absorb through the skin,[135] it also happens to be quite toxic,[136] and repeated exposure may cause liver and kidney damage[137] and necrosis or ulceration of the skin.[138]

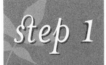

# step 1

# Clean Body Soap

Soap is a staple in even the simplest grooming routine. Whether you use a bar soap or a liquid on your skin, it's on one of two roads that diverge in the kingdom of soap—natural (plant based) or synthetic (petroleum based). However, the trickiest body soaps and the most important kind to look out for are those that have a natural oil base but are loaded with synthetic additives and fragrances.

Soap has been around since Babylonian times (from the 18th to the 6th century BC) and has always worked the same way—it acts as a surfactant to surround and suspend grime so water can get under it to slough it off—whether it's on your clothes, body, or dishes. All soap is made with some kind of fat or oil, and this is where the roads diverge. Natural soap is made with plant oils—like almond, coconut, olive, sesame, palm kernel—or animal oils. Synthetic soap is made with petroleum—yup, the stuff you fuel up with at the pump and that plastics are made of.

To make soap, a fat or oil is coerced into reacting with something very basic (meaning *alkaline*) in a process called *sapon-*

*ification*, which renders it into crude soap. It's useful and sudsy at this point, but typically subject to further refining, which may include stripping out the glycerin (which, though it moisturizes the skin naturally and beautifully, is more profitable for use in other products) or adding a slew of enhancing chemicals, fragrances, and/or dyes. The FDA simply doesn't regulate soap,[139] so anything goes.

Of course, not all soap is malicious. There are plenty of great soaps on the market that lather and cleanse beautifully without synthetic ingredients and chemicals. Many of them have fantastic smells that are gotten by way of plant-based fragrances and essential oils, because life is too short not to smell good.

Soap is such a basic product that it's easy not to give it too much thought. In an ideal world, we wouldn't have to. Soap is soap is soap, right? Well, soap is soap until other ingredients are added to it, some of which are cause for concern. Minor concerns include skin irritation, itchiness, or allergic reaction. Major concerns include ingredients that can cause the immune system to malfunction or developmental and reproductive toxicity, like endocrine disrupters. Would you believe that some of the major soap brands that Americans know and trust contain ingredients that may cause cancer? How about just a little bit of neurotoxin with your soap? Yes, soap. No fooling, they smell good.

So what's the difference between natural and synthetic soaps?

## Tricky Mix: When Natural and Synthetic Ingredients Mingle

It's rare to see a totally synthetic body soap—whether a bar, liquid, wash, or gel. It is, however, incredibly common to see natural and synthetic stuff mingling on the ingredient list of body soaps and washes. Synthetic constituents are most popular as lathering agents (the sulfate family, including SLS and SLES), preservatives (the paraben clan, including propylparaben and methylparaben), and fragrances (many of which contain phthalates and other nasties).

So what's the big deal with a little bit of synthetic chemicals in your suds? The industry claims it's no big deal. But some pretty reputable evidence links synthetic ingredients with a large spectrum of health effects ranging from minor inconveniences like irritation and allergy[140][141] to major problems like hormone disruption,[142][143] reproductive and developmental toxicity,[144][145] biochemical changes,[146][147] and even cancer.[148][149] See page 169 for the deplorable details.

See "Green Thumb Guide: Skin Care Products" on page 180 for a guide to pure products.

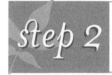

# step 2      Face and Body Care

Whether it's an effort undertaken out of vanity or a deep-seated biological drive for preservation, taking care of the skin on both our bodies and our faces is worthy of using pure products.

Skin is the largest and one of the most precious organs to cleanse, nourish, and protect. The tissues of our skin keep our innards in, serve as an immunological line of defense, and perform an essential role in respiration. It's also good fun when it feels great and looks good. The skin on our faces is perhaps the most precious and delicate of all. Taking care of that beloved mug with clean-ingredient products is a right good thing to do for immediate and long-term benefits. Choosing products made with pure ingredients is an eco-valiant pursuit. Everybody wins—you, the planet, and the good companies that produce the untainted formulas that keep everyone in the green.

# From the Inside Out

The skin reflects what's going on inside our bodies. Putting pure, clean stuff inside—by eating heaps of organic fruits and veggies and guzzling plenty of water—shows up on the outside like sunshine follows rain. Since the skin is an exit point for toxins in our bodies, the less junk there is to evacuate, the more our skin can glow with supple splendor. Even the most sophisticated and pure skin products can improve the appearance of only the outer layer of the skin. To reach deeper, to the living cells, we need to nourish them from within.

*Shifting perspective.* Focusing on what you love and does your body good is much more fun than getting hung up on denial. Including in your diet plenty of goodies that nourish your body to grow beautiful skin provides much more pleasure than hacking out all of the treats and snacks that you love but know do little good for you (other than a moment of recreational delight). Life is too short to live in renunciation. Go for the good stuff with unabashed jubilance.

*Beautifying indulgence.* It's great to live in a world where chocolate and wine are good for you. Yes, it's true—dark chocolate contains a wealth of age-defying antioxidants[150] and red wine is laden with resveratrol, a compound that is believed to lower the risk for heart disease.[151] My motto is: All things in moderation, including moderation—indulging in the finer things can have fabulous effects.

Here are some skin-beautifying foods to enjoy.

*Green tea.* It's abundant in antioxidants that combat free radicals (unstable molecules that bang around, wrecking cells and tissues that are trying to become stable). Free radicals from pollution, stress, and junk food take a toll on health and viciously age the skin.[152] Green tea can help you get a grip on them. It's also especially high in a catechin (a polyphenol), which is an antioxidant, that is believed to inhibit cancer and tumor growth.[153] Green tea can keep the metabolism burning at a healthy clip to aid weight loss,[154] and it may even improve cognitive function for clearer thinking.[155] It's a winner all around.

*Berries.* Blueberries, strawberries, raspberries, and other berries are abundant in antioxidants and phytochemicals that support and nurture beautiful skin and a great body. Berries are loaded with vitamin C, which is yet another antioxidant that may reduce or repair wrinkles[156] and regulates collagen,[157] which is essential for perky, supple skin.

*Pomegranate.* Both the juice and the whole fruit have long been hailed as a beautifying food. Pomegranates are filled with precious goods for great skin, like flavonoid antioxidants and tons of vitamin C. They're also rich in nifty compounds called anthocyanins (which are responsible for the fruit's ravishing crimson color) that effectively inhibit photoaging (sun damage).[158] The antitumor and anticancer properties don't hurt, either.[159] And pomegranates taste incredible.

*Good oils.* Extra-virgin olive oil, cold-pressed sesame oil, flax oil, and others, as well as raw nuts and seeds, olives, and avocados contain high-quality oils that are vital for health down to the cellular level and prerequisites for lustrous skin. Uncooked oils have the most to offer because the unique nutrients are damaged or destroyed by heat—the fresher the better, and the least refined is best of all.

*Tip:* Store oils away from light and heat, which damage them and diminish their good properties for beautiful skin. Darker glass bottles protect the oil better than clear glass.

*Green veggies.* Cruciferous vegetables (collards, broccoli, brussels sprouts, and kale) and leafy greens (lettuces, spinach, and swiss chard) give you more nutrients in fewer calories than any other food. Green is good. The crucifer family is loaded with skin-beautifying compounds like sulfur-containing phytonutrients, which boost the body's natural detoxification enzymes[160] to combat potentially carcinogenic invaders.[161]

*Red wine.* This is a feel-good medium for obtaining beautiful skin and a healthy heart. Loaded with beneficial antioxidant and antiinflammatory flavonoids, red wine is a fabulous source of resveratrol, which is concentrated in the skin of grapes and widely valued for its anticancer properties.[162] Red wine also shows great promise in protecting skin from sun damage.[163] Cheers to that!

*Dark chocolate.* Oh, yes! Prized for millennia as the "food of the gods," chocolate has now been blessed by science for its unique and evocative properties. Chocolate is wealthy in antioxidants. It contains catechins like those found in green tea, and it's the greatest food source of procyanidins.[164] These compounds counter skin damage and encourage cancer-free, heart-happy health.[165] New research is ablaze about chocolate's ability to improve circulation,[166] so it's a delicious way to keep your skin looking young and aglow. Dark chocolate offers optimal benefits all around (fair trade and organic are plusses), and it's best shared with someone you love.

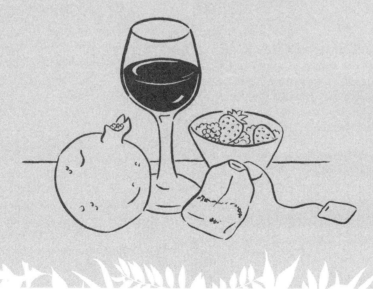

*Browsing the aisles for pure products can be dizzying. There are a few routes to aid the process of choosing the right stuff. Stopping everything to get a master's degree in biochemistry is one route—effective, but none too convenient. Another is to tote around an encyclopedia of cosmetic ingredients to reference—also effective, but you might throw out your back. The last, and most realistic, path is to learn about a reasonable smattering of ingredients to avoid (like petrochemicals and synthetic preservatives and fragrances) and which trustworthy companies abstain from using them (at least for the most part). Like everything in life, it involves a learning curve, and scouting out good products made with clean ingredients gets easier with practice.*

*The companies and products listed below are good places to start on the road to better skin care.*

## ALBA

**Facial cleansers, scrubs, moisturizers, day creams with sunscreens, lip balms, soap, body lotions, hair care, and intensive skin conditioners**

Formed under the banner of Avalon Organics, many products made by Alba contain a wide spectrum of natural and organic plant-based ingredients, botanicals, and essential oils—but not all are free of synthetics. Some contain paraben preservatives, SLS, and vaguely identified fragrances. Overall, it's a good company to look to for products—and it's committed to ecology at the corporate level—but be sure to read the ingredient list before buying.

*Available:* at most natural markets and online

www.albabotanica.com

## ANNEMARIE BORLIND

**Facial moisturizer/cream, facial cleanser, facial toner, facial serum, facial mask, scrub/exfoliant, eye treatment, lip treatment, body moisturizer/lotion, body wash (liquid and gel), men's line, SPF products**

Annemarie Borlind of Germany produces an epic spread of the finest natural beauty and skin care products and natural cosmetics. Committed to producing only the highest-quality natural skin care products, the company scouts the world for the most unpolluted, organic sources of plants and has established long-term commitments with farmers to ensure the high-quality ingredients meet strict standards. Using beneficial herbs and botanicals based on herbal folklore traditions, the company integrates state-of-the-art processing and techniques with natural ingredients. Made with high-quality ingredients—including only the first pressing of plant extracts and natural springwater from a protected region in Germany—all products contain only natural emulsifiers and preservatives and are free of artificial fragrances and colorings. Annemarie Borlind is at the top of the game for quality and masterfully formulated natural products. Look for her new line—Anne Lind—of natural shower gels and body lotions.

*Available:* at select spas, salons, and natural markets and online

www.borlind.com

## ASTARA BIOGENIC SKINCARE

**Facial moisturizer/cream, facial cleanser, facial toner/hydrator, facial serum, facial mask, scrub/exfoliant, eye treatment, body moisturizer/lotion**

Astara formulas are derived from the finest raw botanical ingredients—potent antioxidant extracts, raw organic plants, flower essences, and sea plant extracts—that feed the skin, supply nutrients to cells to prevent signs of aging, repair tissues, and hydrate deeply. All of the products are manufactured using low-temperature processing to preserve the efficacy of the ingredients. Astara avoids synthetic ingredients—only essential oils are used for fragrance. The company uses natural preservatives mostly; a few products do contain a wee bit of paraben, but at levels it believes to be safe for applying to the skin.

*Available:* at select spas and salons and online

www.astaraskincare.com

## AUBREY ORGANICS

**Facial moisturizer/cream, facial cleanser, facial toner/hydrator, facial serum, facial mask, scrub/exfoliant, eye treatment, face and body oil, body moisturizer/lotion, body wash (liquid and gel), bar soap, shaving cream, men's products, babies' products, SPF products**

All Aubrey Organics products are completely natural, being formulated with herbs, essential oils, and natural vitamins—the emphasis is on organic ingredients. No synthetic ingredients or petrochemicals of any kind are used. Only natural preservatives are used (which is huge)! All formulas are handcrafted in small batches, which is good for both the body and the earth. Products are not tested on animals.

*Available:* at most natural markets and online

www.aubrey-organics.com

## AVALON ORGANICS

**Facial moisturizer/cream, facial cleanser, facial toner/hydrator, facial serum, scrub/exfoliant, eye treatment, lip treatment, body moisturizer/lotion, bar soap, babies' products, SPF products**

Avalon Organics has a great range of natural products made "with deep respect to the process of body care" that are formulated with natural plant botanicals and many organic ingredients. No parabens, harsh preservatives, synthetic fragrances, or artificial colors are included, and no animal testing is done.

*Available:* at most natural markets and online

www.avalonorganics.com

## BURT'S BEES

**Facial moisturizer/cream, facial cleanser, facial toner/hydrator, facial serum, facial mask, scrub/exfoliant, eye treatment, lip treatment, body moisturizer/lotion, body wash (liquid and gel), bar soap, body powder, babies' products, SPF products**

Burt's Bees products contain natural ingredients "harvested from nature." No synthetic or chemical ingredients are used in the company's formulas—no petroleum, SLS, propylene glycol, phthalate fragrances, or artificial colors. Some products contain animal ingredients like beeswax, royal jelly, and milk, but none are tested on animals. Burt's Bees has led the way in using postconsumer recycled content in packaging (even plastic bottles!).

*Available:* at all kinds of markets and drugstores and online

www.burtsbees.com

## DR. HAUSCHKA SKIN CARE

**Facial moisturizer/cream, facial cleanser, facial toner/hydrator, facial mask, eye treatment, lip treatment, face and body oil, body moisturizer/lotion, body wash (liquid and gel), body powder, SPF products**

The vast majority of ingredients in Dr. Hauschka's Skin Care line are organically and biodynamically (beyond organic) grown and harvested, so the company's pure, effective natural products deliver the nurturing qualities that result from these holistic aesthetics. With a history and philosophy that are in line with a holistic approach, the formulas are based on the way skin works and use only natural, botanical preservatives. There are no chemical additives of any kind, and no animal testing is done.

*Available:* at most natural markets and online

www.drhauschka.com

*(continued)*

## DRUIDE

**Facial moisturizer/cream, facial cleanser, facial toner/hydrator, face and body oil, body moisturizer/lotion, body wash (liquid and gel), bar soap, babies' products**

Inspired by both the ancient work of herbalists and brand-new techniques, Druide uses a wide spectrum of organic and wild-crafted ingredients in its purely natural body care products. Pure processed ingredients and rigorous ecologic ethics make Druide products a beautifying collaboration between nature and humanity. They contain no synthetic ingredients or preservatives, GMOs (genetically modified organisms), or artificial coloring agents or perfumes.

*Available:* at select markets and online

www.druide.ca

## ECCO BELLA

**Facial moisturizer/cream, facial cleanser, facial mask, eye treatment, lip treatment, body moisturizer/lotion, body wash (liquid and gel), bar soap**

Ecco Bella's face, body, and cosmetic products are made with gentle, mostly natural ingredients that are tested on people, not animals. The company uses some organic ingredients, natural fragrances, and, mostly, natural preservatives, though some products contain synthetic paraben preservatives and vaguely identified fragrances, so be sure to read the ingredient list. The company's cosmetics contain delicate flower wax for longer-lasting wear, and none contain talc.

*Available:* at most natural markets and online

www.eccobella.com

## ÉMINENCE ORGANICS

**Facial moisturizer/cream, facial cleanser, facial toner/hydrator, facial serum, facial mask, scrub/exfoliant, eye treatment, lip treatment, body moisturizer/lotion, body wash (liquid and gel), SPF products**

One of the most remarkable companies, Éminence Organics uses the greatest possible amounts of hand-harvested, all-natural organically grown herbs, fruits, and vegetables in its complete line of premium products. All of the products are handmade in small batches without heating or hydrogenation. They contain no artificial or synthetic colors, fragrances, or preservatives. These are professional, spa-grade products I can't live without.

*Available:* at select spas and salons and online

www.eminenceorganics.com

## EXHALE

**Facial cleanser, facial serum, facial mask, scrub/exfoliant**

The GRN (grow, restore, nurture) line is eco-conscious and mindfully designed skin care. Exhale's dedication to improving inner and outer well-being by harmoniously balancing mind, body, and environment is evident in the company's approach to skin care. Intended to combat physical, emotional, and environmental stresses on the skin, these products work to produce visible results with pure, potent, certified organic food-grade ingredients like blue chamomile, white tea, bearberry, avocado, and pomegranate and without synthetic preservatives, fragrances, or colorants. *Note:* I helped to design this line, including the eco-friendly packaging, and it rocks!

*Available:* at Exhale Spas and online

www.exhalespa.com

## JOHN MASTERS ORGANICS

**Facial moisturizer/cream, facial cleanser, facial toner/hydrator, facial serum, facial mask, eye treatment, lip treatment, body moisturizer/lotion, body wash (liquid and gel), bar soap, men's products**

John Masters has created a luxurious beauty line using the purest ingredients that treat the earth with respect. With its extensive use of organic ingredients of the highest quality—cold-pressed oils and steam-distilled essential oils—and a deep commitment to sustainability, the company has developed fair-trade partnerships with small farmers around the world. All products are free of SLS, GMOs, petrochemicals, and artificial fragrances and colors. John is the man and his products are the real deal.

*Available:* at select natural markets, spas, and salons, including John's own salon in New York City, and online

www.johnmasters.com

## JURLIQUE

**Facial moisturizer/cream, facial cleanser, facial toner/hydrator, facial serum, facial mask, scrub/exfoliant, eye treatment, lip treatment, face and body oil, body moisturizer/lotion, body wash (liquid and gel), SPF products**

This is truly one of the most exceptional, fabulously pure product lines on the market. Jurlique formulates a full line of skin care products as well as some hair care products, all of which are absolutely natural and made using the finest-quality ingredients and phenomenal processes. The company's production methods are said to capture the "life force" of the plants used as ingredients. The products are formulated with a potent fusion of organic and biodynamically grown plants and herbs and their extracts, many of which are grown and harvested by hand on the company's farms under strict quality control measures. No synthetic or chemical ingredients are used, and none of the products contain animal products or are tested on animals. The line includes products suitable for every skin type, and I would spend my last dime and go to the ends of the earth for them.

*Available:* at select spas and salons and Jurlique stores and online

www.jurlique.com

## KIMBERLY SAYER OF LONDON

**Facial moisturizer/cream, facial cleanser, facial toner, facial serum, scrub/exfoliant, eye treatment, SPF products**

Kimberly Sayer offers an exquisite collection of hand-blended skin care and body care products made with the purest organic ingredients. All products are carefully formulated following the traditions of ancient apothecaries and contain the highest-grade organic ingredients, extracts, and essential oils. With their simple, clean approach to proper cleaning, cellular renewal, pH balancing, and hydration, Kimberly Sayer products are naturally brilliant.

*Available:* at select natural markets, spas, and salons and online

www.kimberlysayer.com

## KISS MY FACE

**Facial moisturizer/cream, facial cleanser, facial serum, facial mask, scrub/exfoliant, eye treatment, lip treatment, body moisturizer/lotion, body wash (liquid and gel), bar soap, shaving cream, SPF products**

Kiss My Face makes effective all-natural body care products that are formulated with ingredients from nature—vitamins, minerals, and botanicals—many of which are organically grown. They contain no artificial colors, chemical additives, or animal ingredients, and no animal testing is done. Many of the products use only natural preservatives. Many also use only pure essential oils for fragrance, though others contain vaguely identified fragrances that the company swears are derived from natural sources. Some formulations include synthetic paraben preservatives, so read each product's ingredient list to get the best of what the company has to offer, which is a lot.

*Available:* at most natural markets and online

www.kissmyface.com

*(continued)*

## KORRES NATURAL PRODUCTS

**Facial moisturizer/cream, facial cleanser, facial toner, facial serum, facial mask, scrub/exfoliant, eye treatment, body moisturizer/lotion, face and body oil, body wash, men's line, SPF products**

Korres's natural products hail from Greece and have their roots in an ancient homeopathic school of beauty. Offering a complete range of skin care products, Korres chooses naturally derived active ingredients and plant extracts and broadly avoids using synthetic components. The company uses high-quality vegetable oils that are compatible with healthy skin and nixes the mineral oils and petrochemical derivatives. The products are free of propylene glycol (a chemical solvent prevalent in conventional products, though it has been linked to allergies). I would say that two-thirds of the company's products are formulated with completely pure, clean ingredients, though the remainder contain questionable chemicals like parabens, vaguely identified fragrances, and other ingredients that it's best to steer clear of. Read the ingredient lists thoroughly!

**Available:** at natural markets and spas and online

www.korres.com

## MYCHELLE DERMACEUTICALS

**Facial moisturizer/cream, facial cleanser, facial toner/hydrator, facial serum, facial mask, scrub/exfoliant, eye treatment, lip treatment, SPF products**

MyChelle products are pure, plant based, and nontoxic. They are made using high-grade active ingredients like botanicals, fruit pulps, essential oils, and antioxidants. No harmful chemicals or preservatives, such as parabens, artificial colors, or synthetic fragrances, are used. The products are tested only on willing human beings, never on animals, and they serve all skin types. The company even donates a portion of all sales to charity.

**Available:** at most natural markets and online

www.mychelleusa.com

## NATURE GIRL

**Facial moisturizer/cream, facial cleanser, facial mask, body moisturizer, body wash, face and body oil**

Nature Girl is hip and mindful. The company's widely ranging products contain ingredients that are organically grown on small, family-run farms and ethically wild-crafted. All of the nut, seed, and flower oils are cold pressed and refined the old-fashioned way using paper filters and natural clays, and all of the essential oils are organic or sustainably harvested in the wild and steam distilled. No synthetic preservatives, fragrances, or colors are used in anything.

**Available:** at select natural markets and spas and online

www.nature-girl.com

## OLE HENRIKSEN

**Facial moisturizer/cream, facial cleanser, facial toner, facial serum, scrub/exfoliant, eye treatment, lip treatment, body moisturizer, body wash, men's products, SPF products**

Ole Henriksen goes hand-in-hand with natural beauty and celebrity clientele—his day spa on the Sunset Strip in LA has served beauties of the silver screen for 30 years. Ole Henriksen products, once exclusive to spas, are now available on the retail market at department stores and specialty boutiques around the world. With a broad, inviting range of products for all skin types, the formulas are rich with botanical extracts, antioxidant-heavy plants, high-quality oils, vitamins, and nutrients.

**Available:** at select spas, department stores, and specialty boutiques and online

www.olehenriksen.com

## PANGEA ORGANICS

**Facial moisturizer/cream, facial cleanser, facial toner/hydrator, facial serum, facial mask, face and body oil, body moisturizer/lotion, body wash (liquid and gel), bar soap**

Pangea Organics products are handcrafted, state-of-the-art formulations that use high-quality plant-based organic ingredients, herbal extracts, and botanicals. They contain no synthetic preservatives, SLS, petrochemicals, parabens, or artificial fragrances or dyes. Pure essential oil blends are used to benefit different skin types. These are pure, organic, great-smelling products for full-body skin care.

*Available:* at most natural markets and online

www.pangeaorganics.com

## RED FLOWER

**Facial toner/hydrator, scrub/exfoliant, face and body oil, body moisturizer/lotion, body wash (liquid and gel)**

By using regional ingredients, cultural influences, and sustainable sourcing in its two treatment collections, Red Flower celebrates purity with natural ingredients. Products for the face and body contain carefully selected, unique ingredients and the highest grade of essential oils. The company also formulates other lovely goodies like flower candles, teas, and organic essential oil room diffusers encased in recycled glass (see the "Green Thumb Guide: Candles" on page 338 for more information).

*Available:* at select spas and salons and online

www.redflower.com

## SENSUOUS BEAUTY

**Facial moisturizer/cream, facial cleanser, facial toner/hydrator, facial mask, scrub/exfoliant, lip treatment, face and body oil, body moisturizer/lotion, men's products**

All Sensuous Beauty products are made entirely with fresh food- and plant-based ingredients. The company uses the finest wild-crafted or certified organic herbs, botanicals, and grains and the highest-quality carrier oils and steam-distilled or organic pure essential oils. All of the products are formulated by hand "from scratch" in small batches to maintain their integrity. Absolutely no chemical or synthetic ingredients, fragrances, or preservatives are used.

*Available:* at select markets and online

www.sensuousbeauty.com

## SPA TECHNOLOGIES

**Facial moisturizer/cream, facial cleanser, facial toner, facial serum, facial mask, scrub/exfoliant, eye treatment, face and body oil, body moisturizer, body wash (liquid and gel), bath salts**

Spa Techologies has a remarkable range of highly effective, completely natural skin care products that integrate pure essential oils, botanicals, sea salt, and seaweed to protect, detoxify, nourish, and regenerate skin. The company's products are designed to fight environmental stress caused by scavenging surface radicals, maintain skin tone, replenish lost minerals, and heal damage. The core elements in these outstanding products are seaweed harvested from the pure waters of Brittany and Iceland, marine proteins, aloe vera, and essential minerals. Seaweed is an abundant storehouse of vital minerals, vitamins, enzymes, and plant elements that are essential for cell function and regeneration. All of the moisturizers and serums are formulated by blending natural active ingredients with a 70 percent seaweed base. The results are evident in the skin. Spa Technologies uses only pure, natural ingredients—no artificial fragrances or synthetic preservatives are used.

*Available:* at select spas and online

www.spatechnologies.com

*(continued)*

## SUKÍ

**Facial moisturizer/cream, facial cleanser, facial toner/hydrator, facial serum, facial mask, eye treatment, lip treatment, face and body oil, body moisturizer/lotion**

Sukí products are pure, holistic, 100 percent natural formulas made with organic, food-grade, botanical ingredients and extracts and pure, premium, steam-distilled essential oils. All products are ethically and thoughtfully made by hand in small batches for fresh, lively results. No synthetic ingredients of any kind are used in any of the company's products.

*Available:* at select markets, department stores, and spas and online

www.sukipure.com

## WELEDA

**Facial moisturizer/cream, facial cleanser, facial toner/hydrator, facial serum, face and body oil, body moisturizer/lotion, body wash (liquid and gel), bar soap, shaving cream, men's products, babies' products**

All of Weleda's products are made with the purest, finest ingredients, including organic and biodynamically (beyond organic) cultivated and naturally wild-crafted plants. (It was the first company to do the biodynamic thing, beginning in 1921.) The company grows some ingredients itself and has close fair-trade partnerships with farmers around the world. All of the products are formulated with strict quality control. Using pure fragrances obtained exclusively from essential oils, all products are free of petroleum ingredients and synthetic additives, colorants, and fragrances, and they are never tested on animals.

*Available:* at most natural markets and online

www.usa.weleda.com

# At-Home Spa Formulas

Formulating pampering products doesn't require a high-tech lab or an extensive bio-dynamic garden, just a few simple ingredients and a pause in activity to stop and smell the flowers (or at least use their essential oils on your skin). Some of the most sophisticated natural products on the market, indeed, evolved from homemade formulas. These simple formulas are some of my favorites for at-home spa treatments for face and body bliss. I keep a bottle of the Fresh Face Spray both on my desk and in my purse at all times for a hydrating pick-me-up. There's a certain feeling of pride and independence in making your own beauty formulas that is well worth its weight in gold. These also make admirably thoughtful gifts—particularly the Fresh Face Spray, Homemade Rose Water, Sea Salt–Peppermint Foot Scrub, Rejuvenating Face Serum, and the Sugared Vanilla-Coconut-Salt Body Scrub—because they all have a long shelf-life. Blending and devising your own formulary recipes is a savvy way to curb all the packaging and shipping of commercial products, and can save you fistfuls of dough.

# Homemade Rose Water

*Roses have long been hailed for their beauty, aroma, and beautifying properties—they hydrate, cleanse, and are anti-inflammatory. And they smell lovely, too. Pure essential oil of rose is among the priciest of oils, so making your own rose water is a way to indulge in its benefits without hitting up your wallet. It's excellent as the base of a facial spray or a toner to splash on or apply with a cotton ball (organic, of course!).*

*BIG NOTE! For goodness sake, use the petals of only roses that have been organically grown or that you know have not been treated with pesticides. Roses purchased from florists typically are loaded with nasty chemicals.*

Petals of 3 or 4 fresh, organic roses or 1 cup dried rose petals

2 cups filtered water

**For fresh rose petals:** Place the petals in a glass jar big enough to hold the 2 cups water. Bring the water to a boil and pour it over the petals. Seal the jar tightly with a lid, shake the jar gently, and let the mixture stand overnight. Strain the rose water and squeeze the petals to extract as much liquid from them as possible.

**For dried petals:** Place the dried petals and water in a saucepan and bring the mixture to a boil. Reduce the heat and simmer for 3 to 5 minutes. Remove the pan from the heat and let the water cool to room temperature. Strain the rose water and squeeze the petals to extract as much liquid from them as possible.

Store the rose water in a tightly capped jar or bottle in the fridge.

# Honey Face Treatment

*Honey is a venerable ingredient that has been valued for ages for its nourishing and beautifying effects on all skin types. It cleanses and tightens pores and hydrates skin. The active enzymes in raw honey slough off dead skin, which may make this treatment feel a bit tingly. After applying the honey, try fanning your face—it will feel deliciously warm.*

1½ tablespoons raw honey (ideally from a local or regional source)

Cleanse your face. Heat water in a pot until it is steaming slightly, then hold your face over the steaming pot for 2 to 5 minutes to open your pores. Alternatively, you can drench a washcloth with steaming hot water, wring it out, let it cool until it is comfortable to the touch, and then cover your clean face with it for 2 minutes.

Spread the honey evenly over your face. Make sure not to get it in your eyes, but do get some on your lips so you can sample the sweetness. Leave it on for 15 minutes. Wash it off with warm water, followed by a cool water rinse. Apply toner or face spray and moisturizer.

# Fresh Face Spray

*A misty spritzing of face spray is a terrific way to keep your skin hydrated and to wake up wandering senses. I recommend using distilled water or bottled mineral water for optimal shelf life and rewarding results.*

*Note about essential oils: Follow your sense of appeal when using oils for scent. Start slowly with mixing and matching—some of the best blends are simple, so try just one or two at first. High-quality essential oils cost a pretty penny, but just a wee bit is needed and they have an indefinite shelf life. Happy blending!*

1 cup distilled or mineral water (Fiji and Volvic are great brands to pick), or homemade Rose Water (see the recipe on page 187)

10 drops pure essential oils of lavender, rose, chamomile, and/or sweet orange (examples: 4 drops rose, 3 drops lavender, 2 drops chamomile, 1 drop sweet orange; 5 drops each lavender and chamomile or lavender and rose)

Place all of the ingredients in a glass jar. Cap the bottle tightly and shake well. Pour the mixture into a 1- or 2-ounce spray bottle (available at natural markets and online). Store the remainder in the fridge and refill the spray bottle as needed; it will keep indefinitely. Lightly spray your face whenever your skin or outlook needs refreshing.

**VARIATIONS**

For dry skin: Add ½ teaspoon vegetable glycerin (a humectant that draws water from the air to condition the skin and is available at natural markets) or 1 teaspoon avocado or almond oil.

For sensitive skin: Choose the soothing essential oils of rose and chamomile over those of lavender and sweet orange.

For oily skin: Add 1 teaspoon witch hazel and try the essential oils of lavender and grapefruit.

> *Fresh, organic fruits and veggies + plenty of water + ample exercise + sound rest = health, happiness, and beyond*

# Honey–Avocado Masque

**For normal or dry skin**

*Honey and avocado are a scrumptious blend for nourishing skin. Avocado is a gorgeous emollient that's rich in oils, vitamins, and minerals, and honey is packed with antioxidants and enzymes. Lemon juice is a natural source of alpha hydroxy acid (AHA), which renews skin. Together, they yield velvety skin.*

1 avocado
1½ tablespoons raw honey
1 tablespoon lemon juice

Mash the avocado meat and blend it with the honey and lemon juice until smooth in a small food processor or blender. Cleanse your face, then steam your pores open over a pot of hot water for 2 to 5 minutes or by drenching a washcloth with steaming hot water, wringing it out, letting it cool until it's comfortable to the touch, and draping it over your clean face for 2 minutes.

Apply the avocado and honey mixture evenly over your face. Let it stand for 15 minutes. Wash it off with warm water, then follow with a cool water rinse. Apply toner or face spray and moisturizer.

**VARIATIONS**

Exfoliation for dry skin: Mix 2 tablespoons rice flour thoroughly with the avocado and honey. Apply to the face as directed above. Wash off the mixture gently with warm water and a cloth, being mindful not to rub too hard, and follow with a cool water rinse.

Exfoliation for oily skin: Mix 2 tablespoons ground oatmeal thoroughly with the avocado and honey. Apply to the face as directed above. Wash off the mixture gently with warm water and a cloth, being mindful not to rub too hard, and follow with a cool water rinse.

# Organic Cotton Swabs, Balls, and Rounds

Choosing organic versions of little cotton helpers like swabs, balls, and cosmetic rounds to wipe and cleanse is a fine green way to treat bodily details and mind the planet at the same time. Cotton is a highly versatile natural fiber, though the difference between conventionally and organically grown cotton is drastic on the ecological front. Conventionally grown cotton is one of the most chemical-intensive crops on the planet—cotton is grown on less than 3 percent of viable farmland, but it accounts for about 25 percent of insecticide use worldwide.[167] Holy kamole, that's a lot. And the chemical pesticides applied to cotton are truly mephitic—7 of the 15 most commonly used pesticides are known human carcinogens.[168] Organically grown cotton, on the other hand, is a green alternative. Growers do not use chemical pesticides or defoliants, reyling instead on natural fertilizers, beneficial insects, and crop rotation to grow human- and eco-friendly fibers. That's good sense.

Conventional cotton accoutrements—like swabs, balls, and rounds—are as low as it gets on the totem pole of quality. They're made from *gin trash*, the low-grade by-products—the leaves, stems, and short fibers stripped from the cotton boll. In most agri-ventures, by-products like those in gin trash are valuable as good eats for cattle, but conventional cotton waste is so contaminated with pesticides that it's illegal to feed it to cows in some states like California.[169] Instead, it's used to make pillows, tampons, mattresses, and, you betcha, cotton swabs, balls, and the like.

When reaching for little cotton helpers, opt for organically grown goods. They're better for you and for the planet.

The one company that does it all is Organic Essentials, which offers 100 percent certified organic cotton products (balls, swabs, and rounds). The company goes the extra mile by obtaining organic certification from both the USDA and the Texas Department of Agriculture. Its products are available at most natural markets and online at www.organicessentials.com.

# Sea Salt–Peppermint Foot Scrub

*This lively scrub might make you want to play footsie. Soaking your feet first in warm saltwater not only feels heavenly, it also softens tough skin for maximum benefits.*

1 cup salt
⅓ cup almond oil or olive oil
1 tablespoon castile soap
6 drops pure essential oil of peppermint

Mix all of the ingredients thoroughly in a bowl. Soak your feet first if desired: Use 3 quarts of hot water directly from the faucet or warmed on the stove top to a comfortable temperature. Pour the water into a basin and mix in ¼ cup table salt or Epsom salts. Soak those lovely feet for a good 15 minutes. Then, scrub your dear feet with the mixture because they work so hard. Rinse them off and rest.

# Rejuvenating Face Serum

*This recipe is borrowed from my dear friend Liz, who, in addition to being a rock star manager, is a wizard in the kitchen at making food and natural beauty brews. With a clean, fresh feel that's good for all skin types, this serum is ultra-hydrating without oils—the glycerin is an emollient humectant that actually pulls water from the air to moisturize the skin. Aloe is an all-around skin healer that hydrates deeply without having a greasy feeling. Liz used to use royal jelly in the serum, but it's really expensive and hard to find, and it must be refrigerated at all times (as the serum must be, too). She finds that this blend stands spectacularly on its own. I agree.*

⅔ cup pure aloe vera (Liz and I use Lily of the Desert brand; just make sure you use a pure one that doesn't have other ingredients or preservatives)

2 tablespoons pure vegetable glycerin

3 drops pure essential oil of rose or lavender

Combine the ingredients in a glass jar. Cap the jar tightly and shake it well.

Put the mixture in a small, clean glass pump dispenser (one a store-bought product came in or one purchased online). The serum may also be stored in a small jar. It keeps indefinitely, but be sure to keep it in the fridge!

Spread the serum lightly over cleansed skin. An excellent time to apply it is before going to bed—it's light enough to let your skin breathe while you snooze.

# Sugared Vanilla–Coconut–Salt Body Scrub

*Salt has purifying properties that make the skin glow and sugar is an age-old beauty ingredient. The grains of both are natural exfoliants that slough off dead skin, allowing supple, young skin to emerge. Coconut oil is an emollient that hydrates and nourishes deeply. Jojoba oil comes closer than anything else to the natural oils our skin produces, so it feels really good and absorbs deeply. The salt and oil balance each other, rinsing off cleanly and leaving the skin radiant and soft all over. Vanilla is optional, but it smells darned good; nonalcoholic vanilla is extracted in glycerin, which is a plus for contributing moisture. Or, add or substitute other essential oils.*

½ cup sea salt

½ cup organic sugar

½ cup coconut oil

1 tablespoon jojoba oil

2 teaspoons pure vanilla extract, or 6 drops essential oil of your choice (optional)

Mix all of the ingredients in a glass jar. Using your hands or a cloth, rub the scrub over the skin in a circular motion. Store the remainder in a sealed container, and stir before using. It keeps indefinitely, with no refrigeration needed.

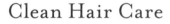

# Clean Hair Care

**step 3**

Hair is part of what makes us human (or mammals, at least). Anthropologists have long speculated about the functional significance of humans growing long hair on the head—perhaps it's a by-product of runaway natural selection marking a healthy stock of genes. Regardless, the grooming and styling of hair is not a newfangled trend, it's been going on worldwide for ages. Whether hair is of significant or marginal importance in cultural or evolutionary terms, maintaining it is pretty much mandatory.

## Picking Battles and Rotating Products

Every head of hair is different. It's worth it to navigate through the zillions of products on the market to find those that are safe and green and really work for your particular type of hair. From completely unscientifically based observations, I've noticed that different products work well for different people, and that certain products work brilliantly for a while and then lose their luster. It seems that with hair, rotating products can be helpful.

Finding products that perform well on your tresses without harming you or the planet is an eco-savvy goal that also benefits your health. To find the right fit, read the ingredient lists on labels, ask green-

leaning, beautiful-haired people for suggestions, and try out different products.

Here's the hair product conundrum: In the bigger of the two camps, the shampoos, conditioners, and styling aids are awash with a slew of synthetic and chemical ingredients that no one really wants to absorb through their skin. All that stuff is best avoided, but unfortunately—and I hate to admit it—some of it performs really well. In the smaller camp is a group of super-natural hair products that are made with such clean ingredients that you could practically snack on them. That's fantastic, but they don't always work well. It's hard to live having a perpetual "bad hair day" with flat, lifeless locks, even if we're taking one for the team. Somewhere in the middle, there is a camp of pretty natural products that hair responds to with bounce and appeal. They are formulated for the most part with clean, natural ingredients, but also contain some questionable ingredients, which, though they are not ideal, seem to perform with zest and zeal. This is where a little compromise, along with experimenting and rotating products, can be a good strategy.

### It's a Sliding Scale

It's easy to find certain types of products that are made with pure and natural ingredients and perform with poise. For

# A Word about Dandruff Shampoos

A flaky scalp is not much fun. Dandruff can be caused by yeasts and fungi in the body, so cleaning up your diet by steering clear of sugary and refined foods is a fundamental place to start to bust flakes. Cold, dry climates aggravate the condition, but ironically, two of the most common ingredients found in conventional shampoos are major contributors to dryness—sodium lauryl sulfate (SLS) and sodium laureth sulfate (SLES). Yet another reason to sidestep hair products with SLS or SLES is that those compounds are notorious skin and scalp irritants. Before reaching for a dandruff-busting shampoo, make sure the regular shampoo you're using doesn't contain SLS or SLES. If it does, try one that has neither and see if your scalp is happier.

Dandruff shampoos are riddled with super-toxic ingredients like coal tar. Yes, it's actually coal tar, and yes, it's highly carcinogenic. Other synthetic active ingredients that are weaseled into name-brand dandruff shampoos are pyrithione zinc, which may sound benign but is highly toxic to aquatic wildlife,[170] irritates the skin and eyes,[171] and may have teratogenic and reproductive effects;[172][173] benzyl alcohol, which is at the top of the toxic Richter scale (see "Beauty Not Worth Dyeing For: Common Ingredient Hazards" on page 200 for more); and selenium sulfide, which has been shown to cause cancer in animals[174] and to have serious and long-term environmental effects.[175]

*Natural dandruff solutions.* An SLS- and SLES-free shampoo made with tea tree oil or rosemary can help curtail the flaky itch. Or, try adding a few drops of antifungal essential oils, like oregano, rosemary, or tea tree, to a palmful of natural shampoo. An old-school scalp rinse calls for applying a solution of 1 part apple cider vinegar to 2 parts warm water before shampooing. Massaging in pure aloe vera is another soothing tonic for a cool, clean head

instance, a number of naturally luscious shampoos achieve terrific results without including a ton of synthetic additives. Conditioners, too. But when it comes to some styling products, the slope is slipperier. For example, I'm not usually one for stiff, hair-sprayed dos, but sometimes when I make appearances, I use the stuff to tether down a coiffure that won't behave. I don't know of a hair spray with ingredients clean enough to eat that performs with any staying power, but some that have better ingredients (abstaining from the worst offenders, at least) do the trick. I choose those, and I hope you do too. Check out the "Green Thumb Guide: Hair Care Products" on page 194 for leads on companies whose products lean in this direction.

The same is true for hair colorings and dyes. Most of them are thoroughly synthetic and notoriously toxic, especially deep-coloring browns and black. To get color to stick, unfortunately, chemicals work. Conventional hair dyes are laden with a mess of chemicals that are no picnic for humans or the planet. But there are degrees of purity, and coloring products

*(continued on page 198)*

*For naturally lustrous locks and eco–smart, spiffy styling, look for these products.*

## ALBA

**Shampoo, conditioner, leave-in conditioner, styling gel, finish/shine/texturizer, hair spray**

Alba's hair products contain lots of natural and organic ingredients and extracts. They don't have SLS or SLES, but some do include some questionable, though less harmful, ingredients such as sodium lauroyl sarcosinate. The ingredients vary by product—some contain no paraben preservatives whereas others do, as well as vaguely identified fragrances, so read labels carefully. Overall, choosing one of this company's products is a fairly pure pick.

*Available:* at most natural markets and online

www.albabotanica.com

## AUBREY ORGANICS

**Shampoo, conditioner, leave-in conditioner, repair treatment, styling gel**

All of the company's hair care products are ultra-pure, plant based, and made with an emphasis on certified organic ingredients. They contain only natural preservatives, and no synthetic or chemical ingredients, such as SLS, SLES, parabens, or artificial fragrances or colors. This is one of the cleanest product lines on the market.

*Available:* at most natural markets and online

www.aubrey-organics.com

## AVALON ORGANICS

**Shampoo, conditioner**

Avalon Organics shampoos and conditioners are formulated with a good spread of natural botanicals, organic ingredients, vitamins, and nutrients. Only natural fragrances derived from essential oils and flower

extracts are used, and they steer away from SLS and harsh synthetic preservatives.

*Available:* at most natural markets and online

www.avalonorganics.com

## AVEDA

**Shampoo, conditioner, detangler, leave-in conditioner, repair treatment, scalp treatment, straightener/frizz control, curl enhancer, mousse (nonaerosol), styling gel, pomade, finish/shine/texturizer, hair spray**

Aveda has one of the widest, most versatile selections of natural-leaning hair products. They're made with botanicals, plant extracts, vitamins, nutrients, and some organic ingredients. When Estée Lauder purchased the company, questionable ingredients were added to many of its products, though lately some of the formulas are returning to their natural roots. Aveda's hair care and styling products are skillfully formulated and work fantastically well. The company believes it makes the best ingredient choices for optimal performance, though they may not be absolutely pure. As always, read the ingredients to know what you're getting. Products are packaged in postconsumer materials like recycled plastic, and the company is ecologically minded at the corporate level. At 93 to 99 percent plant based, Aveda Concept Salons offer some of the most natural hair coloring processes around.

*Available:* at select salons and Aveda salons, Aveda retail stores, and online

www.aveda.com

## BELEGENZA

**Shampoo, conditioner, leave-in conditioner, scalp treatment, straightener/frizz control, curl enhancer, styling gel, finish/shine/ texturizer**

Belegenza (the *g* is soft; in Italian, the word means *genesis of beauty*) offers extraordinary hair care products made with a patent-pending fusion of food-grade organic ingredients that contain nutrients like vitamins, antioxidants, botanicals, and sea plant extracts. Belegenza is as good as it gets. I first tried these products in little sample bottles without ingredient lists that a savvy friend gave to me. When my hair dried with a lustrous bounce, I thought, "There is no way this is natural, it works way too well." After investigating and meeting the company's owner, Keith, I learned that indeed, all of Belegenza's products are super-natural—free of petroleum, silicone, and synthetic preservatives. Since then, my life and locks have changed and I am one happy-tressed camper. Note that some of Belegenza's newly formulated products are packaged with ingredient lists from older formulas; they now don't contain paraben preservatives and the like. This is a revolutionary line of products that I can't live without (and no, I don't own stock in the company!).

*Available:* at select salons and online www.belegenza.com

## BURT'S BEES

### Shampoo, conditioner, repair treatment

Burt's Bees formulates au naturel hair shampoos and conditioners using plant-derived ingredients. The company isn't keen on using synthetic or chemical ingredients—none contain SLS, SLES, paraben preservatives, or artificial colors. For the most part, it uses essential oils for fragrance (though a few vaguely identified fragrances find their way into products here and there, so read the labels).

*Available:* at all kinds of markets and drugstores and online www.burtsbees.com

## COLLECTIVE WELLBEING

### Shampoo, conditioner, straightener/frizz control, finish/shine/texturizer

Collective Wellbeing uses lots of natural, organic, and botanical ingredients and extracts in its hair products, and the company has a charitable core. None of the products contain synthetic paraben preservatives, and the natural fragrances all come from essential oils, though some synthetic and questionable ingredients are included. The company's philanthropic program enables customers to choose which nonprofit organizations it donates to from the profits on sales. The products are a pretty pure pick with a great heart.

*Available:* at natural markets and online www.collectivewellbeing.com

## DR. HAUSCHKA

### Shampoo, conditioner, repair treatment, scalp treatment

Shampoos and conditioners made by Dr. Hauschka contain ample amounts of organic or biodynamic (beyond organic) ingredients and high-grade botanicals and extracts. They are 100 percent natural—only pure essential oils are used for fragrance, and no synthetic preservatives are included.

*Available:* at most natural markets and online www.drhauschka.com

## DRUIDE

### Shampoo, conditioner, detangler, leave-in conditioner, styling gel, hair spray

Druide hair products are formulated with pure, ecological ingredients. Plant based, biodegradable, organic, and wild crafted are the name of the game at Druide. Only natural fragrances, preservatives, and colors are used. There are no synthetic ingredients or GMOs. Made in accordance with a rigorous ecological ethic from the first stages of production to the finished product, Druide is a treat for your hair.

*Available:* at select markets and online www.druide.ca

*(continued)*

## GIOVANNI ORGANIC HAIR CARE

**Shampoo, conditioner, detangler, leave-in conditioner, repair treatment, scalp treatment, straightener/frizz control, curl enhancer, mousse (nonaerosol), styling gel, pomade, finish/shine/texturizer, hair spray**

Giovanni makes a great portfolio of natural hair care and styling products. The company's plant-based formulas include lots of organic ingredients, botanicals, and extracts. Only natural preservatives and fragrances from essential oils are used. They contain no synthetic or petrochemical ingredients such as paraben preservatives, SLS, SLES, or artificial colors or fragrances.

*Available:* at most natural markets and online

www.giovannihaircare.co.nz

## HAMADI

**Shampoo, conditioner, leave-in conditioner, repair treatment, pomade, hair spray**

Hamadi makes a lovely range of pure hair care products with 100 percent organic essential oils and plant extracts. All are completely biodegradable and absolutely luxurious. Hamadi products embody a modern and intelligent sensibility without compromising their quality with synthetic stuff. I must say, the company's owner and founder, Jamal, is a brilliant cookie and hair guru to many of the beautiful cats and kitties on the red carpet. There are no artificial ingredients, perfumes, or colors in these products, ever. The line includes delicious formulas like Honey Soymilk Hair Wash, Shea Rice Milk Conditioner, and Shea Spray. All of them are natural, truly fabulous, and "Tested on Actresses; Never on Animals."

*Available:* at select spas, salons, and department stores and online

www.hamadibeauty.com

## JOHN MASTERS ORGANICS

**Shampoo, conditioner, detangler, leave-in conditioner, scalp treatment, straightener/frizz control, styling gel, pomade, finish/shine/texturizer**

John Masters is the man. His organic line of hair care products is brilliantly formulated using the purest, highest-grade ingredients and botanicals (emphasizing organic and wild-crafted plants), cold-pressed plant oils, and steam-distilled essential oils. The company has also engaged in fair-trade partnerships with small farmers around the world. Absolutely no synthetic or chemical ingredients are used—no SLS, SLES, paraben preservatives, petrochemicals, artificial fragrances or colors, or GMOs. John Masters Organics is New York City's only "clean air" salon, which means that all of the colorings used there are ammonia-free herbal- and clay-based products and the salon offers no chemical services, such as perms, relaxers, or bleaches—so there are none of the awful odors that come with them. I have been a loyal, long-time customer. These are among the purest and finest hair care products on the market.

*Available:* at select natural markets and John Masters's New York City salon and online

www.johnmasters.com

## JURLIQUE

**Shampoo, conditioner, repair treatment, scalp treatment**

Jurlique's shampoos and conditioners are formulated with herbal extracts, essential proteins, and vegetable oils to cleanse, hydrate, and moisturize hair purely and naturally. No synthetic ingredients, petrochemicals, or artificial colors or fragrances whatsoever are used. This is one of the best all-around companies going.

*Available:* at select salons and Jurlique stores and online

www.jurlique.com

## NATURE GIRL

### Shampoo, conditioner

Nature Girl's all-natural hair products contain nutrient-packed ingredients such as natural, organic, and wild-crafted botanicals, extracts, and pure plant oils. The company's products are free of SLS, SLES, and artificial fragrances and dyes.

*Available:* at select spas, beauty supply stores, and hair salons and online

www.nature-girl.com

## OLE HENRICKSEN

### Shampoo, conditioner

Ole Hendicksen's natural hair care line is formulated with vitamins, minerals, and amino acids to restore natural moisture balance and ensure smooth, healthy manageability. All of the company's products are free of SLS, SLES, synthetic paraben preservatives, and artificial dyes.

*Available:* at beauty supply stores, Sephora stores, select salons, and department stores and online

www.olehenricksen.com

## RED FLOWER

### Shampoo, conditioner

Red Flower has formulated a handful of deliciously natural shampoos and conditioners from the world's botanicals. Seductive blends and scents like Italian blood orange and Icelandic moonflower are derived from pure essential oils. The company's products are free of synthetic ingredients like paraben preservatives and artificial fragrances and colors. All are luxuriously natural.

*Available:* at select spas and salons and online

www.redflower.com

## SUKÍ

### Shampoo, conditioner, repair treatment, scalp treatment

Sukí has scouted the world to find the safest, most effective ingredients for its shampoo and conditioner formulas. They contain high-quality organic oils and extracts, herbal botanicals, and steam-distilled essential oils, and absolutely no synthetic or chemical ingredients—no SLS, SLES, parabens, or artificial fragrances or colors. All of the products are made by hand in small batches.

*Available:* at select markets and online

www.sukipure.com

## WELEDA

### Shampoo, conditioner, scalp treatment

Weleda pioneered the use of organic and biodynamic ingredients in personal care products, including the company's handful of hair care formulas. Using essential nutrients and extracts from plants, all Weleda products are absolutely natural and contain no synthetic ingredients or chemicals.

*Available:* at natural markets and online

www.usa.weleda.com

range from heavily chemical to less chemical to less chemical to pure and natural, and you have options that will let you avoid swaddling your lovely head in a toxic stew. There are products that contain less of the harmful stuff and salons that use them—like Aveda Concept Salons, where they use the company's semipermanent and permanent dyes, which are 93 to 99 percent plant based. Big fan here. Natural- and organic-product salons with sense and style are sprouting up, such as John Masters Organics Salon in New York City's SoHo neighborhood (www.johnmastersorganics.com), of whom I've long been a client; and Mode in Seattle (www.modehairart.com). See the "Green Thumb Guide: Natural and Ecological Salons" on page 203 for more information. If you don't have access to any of these fine shops and you are among the one in three women or one in 10 men who colors her or his hair on a regular basis, ask the colorist at your salon what they use, what's in it, and if there are lower-impact alternatives. Life is too short not to have great, natural hair.

You may be thinking, "But we just use this stuff on our hair, we're not eating it, for goodness sake!" True, but guess what's under your hair? Your beautiful scalp, and your brain beneath that. And what's more, where do these products go when they're rinsed out in the shower? They run down your body, where all those luscious pores are open and absorbing everything, then down the drain and into the ecosystem. Remember, what goes on the body gets in the body, and what goes down the drain doesn't really go away.

So think beyond the drain. Chemicals in hair colors and dyes are not only hazardous for humans, they're toxic in the environment—especially to the fishies and aquatic critters. Some of the chemicals are persistent, meaning that they stubbornly stick around. Where do they end up? You guessed it: Traveling right up the food chain.

## Hair Color: Dyes to Live For

Who doesn't love great-looking hair? Dye, color, streak, highlight, lowlight, cover at all costs.

Most hair dyes and colorings are scandalously toxic. I mean, *really* toxic. Unfortunately, they work and look great. Even though the outrageous dangers of dyes are unquestionable, the "right results" often trump safety, even when the stakes are high. I have more than a few health-conscious, eco-minded lady friends and a growing number of male buddies who admit to using hair dyes and colorings that they know are toxic. The general consensus on these noxious-but-effective colorings and dyes is to grin and bear it. People rationalize their use by thinking that, first, no other really good options exist (not true—it does take scouting to find better products, but you are worth it!), and second, because

# "Caution" Statements: Beware of Disclaimers

Because there is little or no federal regulation of hair colorings and dyes, products can contain non-FDA-approved coal tar if a simple cautionary statement appears on the package. Products that carry this disclaimer are exempt from FDA control over coal tar, but clearly they can cause serious adverse reactions and are known to cause cancer.[176]

The cautionary statement reads:

*Caution: This product contains ingredients which may cause skin irritation on certain individuals and a preliminary test according to accompanying directions should first be made. This product must not be used for dyeing the eyelashes or eyebrows; to do so may cause blindness.[177]*

coloring is only done a few times a year, the exposure to toxins is low (but there is no safe level of exposure with some of the monstrous chemicals that are found in hair dyes and colorings; even once can be too much).

The good news is that we are living in a great time. A growing number of less toxic and nontoxic products are on the market. Whether you do it yourself or go to a salon, there are more and better earth- and body-friendly options than ever. And boy, are they worth finding.

Conventional hair dyes are liberally laden with some truly malevolent stuff. They're among the most virulent products in the personal care product and cosmetic realm. How on earth some of this stuff is legal and remains largely unregulated is unclear, but what is clear is that you need to look out for your own health. Let's take a tour of what's lurking behind the labels of hair colorings and dyes.

## Hair Bleaching

Lightening hair is generally a less harmful process than dyeing it. Chemical lighteners typically include hydrogen peroxide, which isn't too bad—it's eco-friendly, biodegradable, and can be used to clean counters and clothes. It's commonly mixed with ammonia, which is a severe skin and lung irritant and is highly toxic to aquatic life, so look at ingredient labels and ask for ammonia-free brands. Good old lemon juice and sunshine will lighten locks au naturel.

## Smarter Picks for Hair Colorings and Dyes

There are two categories of choice for hair colorings and dyes that are better for you and the planet. One is a less toxic breed; the other, a nontoxic variety.

*I investigated a spread of conventional hair dyes and found that an alarming host of toxic chemicals are consistently used in many formulas. Here are the hazardous ingredients that I found to be common.*

**Ammonia.** This compound is toxic and corrosive. It prepares the hair by opening the shaft to receive the color. It's been linked with severe skin and lung irritation[178] and is toxic in the environment, especially to aquatic life.[179]

**Benzene** is toxic, as are its derivatives, such as benzyl alcohol, m-aminophenol, and resorcinol. It's used as a solvent, to help the color stick to the hair and stay there. It's absorbed through the skin and by inhalation.[180] It is toxic to bone cells[181] and bone marrow[182] and causes changes in the blood.[183] It damages the central nervous system and the immune system[184] and has been linked to reproductive and developmental issues.[185] Benzene is a class A carcinogen, and its derivatives may also be.[186] All contaminate water and the environment in general.[187]

**Coal tar.** Found in aniline dyes, it's a thick liquid by-product of processing bituminous coal. It's used in dark-colored dyes especially, and in dandruff shampoos. It's a known carcinogen[188] that is toxic in the environment.[189]

**Lead acetate.** It's highly toxic, and there's no safe level of exposure according to the Agency for Toxic Substances and Disease Registry.[190] It's approved for use as an active ingredient in hair dyes, and if it's used within FDA guidelines, no labeling requirements are necessary to indicate that it is hazardous. This probable human carcinogen[191] has been linked with tumors.[192] It also damages the central nervous system,[193] is neurotoxic and disrupts brain function,[194] and has been linked to brain damage[195] and developmental and learning disorders.[196] It's also toxic in the environment.[197]

**p-Phenylenediamine.** Also known as p-diaminobenzene, oxidation dye, amino dye, and para dye, this compound is highly toxic and a severe irritant. It's used to make the color stick to the hair, and is more prevalent in dark hair dyes like brown and black. It is absorbed through the skin and via inhalation.[198] It's a carcinogenic substance that has been strongly linked with cancer and/or may increase the risk of cancer,[199] [200] especially of the breast and bladder.[201] It can also cause skin sensitization.[202] It's highly toxic in the environment, especially to aquatic life.[203]

**Toluene** is toxic and an irritant, as are its derivatives, like toluene-2,5-diamine and 2,4-toluenediamine. It's used as a solvent to improve the adhesion of the color and gloss to the hair. Repeated exposure to toluene affects the central nervous system,[204] liver, and kidneys.[205] It's been shown to be mutagenic,[206] causing genetic changes and increasing the incidence of mutations, some of which cause cancer. It has been shown to cause cancer in animals,[207] and it contaminates water and the environment.[208]

**Less toxic hair colorings and dyes.** The stock of better, safer coloring and dye products for home and professional use has improved in performance and availability in response to concerns about conventional colorings and dyes. This less toxic bunch contains much lower amounts of the insidious chemicals, and many call on the rainbow of hues available in the plant kingdom. This alternative breed is not necessarily chemical free, but its products do yield long-living color results that are better for you and the planet.

**Nontoxic hair colorings and dyes.** One of the oldest, most traditional, and most widely used plant-based dyes that's been used worldwide for ages is henna. You can't lighten hair with it, but it's great for coloring the full range of brunette, black, auburn, and graying heads of hair. Henna is a semipermanent dye made from the leaves of a shrub that is native throughout Sri Lanka, India, and Northern Africa. It actually stains the hair, coating and sealing the strand, which brilliantly protects hair from the elements as a result. Cleopatra was a big fan, and henna is still used around the globe as a color enhancer for hair and as ink for body art on skin and nails.

A new generation of sophisticated nontoxic hair colorings and dyes are worth looking into. By using plant botanicals, these products are free of synthetic and chemical ingredients, but they achieve a wide spectrum of results. Wow! European companies are leading the charge, but some brands are made in the United States, and European products are widely available for purchase here.

## GREEN TIPS for Safer Hair Coloring

1. *Dye less frequently.* Stretching out the time between color processing reduces your exposure to chemicals, which is a good thing even with less toxic products and especially with conventional products.

2. *Choose safer coloring products.* Try plant-based demipermanent and semipermanent colorings and dyes with low levels of or no p-phenylenediamine, or henna-based products.

3. *Shorter processing.* To reduce your exposure, don't leave coloring products on for longer than necessary (and wear gloves if you do it yourself). If you go to a salon for professional treatment, mention to your stylist that you'd like to limit the processing time.

4. *Rinse thoroughly.* There's no need to let product residue sit on your head until the next time you shampoo. If you go to a salon, ask for an extra-thorough wash and rinse after processing.

5. *Less-intensive processing.* Streaking and foiling processes expose your precious scalp to a lot less of the product and typically need less maintenance and upkeep.

6. *Seek out a natural salon.* If there isn't a natural salon in your area, ask your regular salon to carry safer dyes and colors or if you can bring your own for them to apply.

*Whether you color your hair at home or have it done at a salon, choosing less toxic or nontoxic hair dyes is a smart practice for your own health and for the planet.*

## LESS TOXIC PRODUCTS

These colors aren't completely natural, but they use a lot of natural, safe ingredients and very little of the nasty stuff that's in conventional hair dyes.

### ECOCOLORS

This permanent colorings line has a nutrient-rich soy and flax base that makes it close to p-phenylenediamine (PPD) free; there are trace amounts of PPD in the base, but the company believes that the nutritive soy–flax blend prevents it from being absorbed. The products contain flower essences, vitamins, and natural preservatives, but no ammonia.

Twenty-six colors are available for professional use at salons (check the Web site for locations) and 13 are sold for use at home.

*Available:* at select salons and online

www.ecocolors.net

### HERBAVITA

This company has two lines of semipermanent and demipermanent (lasting longer than semipermanent) colorings.

Herbatint, a less toxic product, is a semipermanent coloring that lasts for 4 to 5 weeks. It comes in 30 shades. The colorings in this line contain much less PPD than conventional products and no ammonia, though they do have a bunch of other weird chemicals. Still, it's a much safer pick for long-lasting results.

Vegetal is a nontoxic line of demipermanent colorings that begin to fade after six to eight shampoos. It comes in 13 shades and is plant based and chemical free.

*Available:* at natural markets and online

www.herb.it (in Italian) or www.herbavita.co.nz (in English)

### NATURCOLOR

These semipermanent colorings last for 4 to 5 weeks. They're plant based, have a low PPD level, and are ammonia free. Thirty-one shades are available. Some reviews say the color fades quickly, but these products are a better pick than conventional colorings and dyes for safer results.

*Available:* at natural markets and online

www.naturcolor.com

## NONTOXIC PRODUCTS

### IGORA BOTANIC

Made by Schwarzkopf Professional, these semipermanent colorings last 4 to 5 weeks. They're plant based and organic, and the pigments are made with natural raw dyes like chamomile, indigo, and walnut. The results can be natural or intensive. Choose from colors like Havana, Rosewood, and Bamboo.

*Available:* by phone at 800-234-4672

### LIGHT MOUNTAIN

These semipermanent colorings last for 4 to 5 weeks. They're completely natural and plant based, using only botanicals and henna. They contain no chemicals, PPD, ammonia, or peroxide. Twelve shades of reds, browns, and black are available, as well as the Color the Gray line, which comes in eight shades.

*Available:* at natural markets and online

www.light-mountain-hair-color.com

### LOGONA

These semipermanent colorings contain 100 percent natural pigments and conditioners—there are no synthetic components, chemicals, or preservatives. Colorants used: buckthorn, cassia, coffee, indigo, rhubarb, and walnut.

Herbal color powders are available in 10 shades. Herbal color creams come in five shades.

*Available:* at select natural markets and online

www.logona.com

Look for the growing sector of professional natural- and organic-product salons like these that offer a full range of less-toxic and nontoxic services.

## AVEDA CONCEPT SALONS AND LIFESTYLE SALONS

Locations: Nationwide

Aveda Concept Salons offer a full range of hair, skin, and makeup services. Aveda Lifestyle Salons, the company's flagship salons, also offer Aveda's signature spa services.

Aveda's wide spectrum of hair colorings and dyes are naturally derived from plants and nonpetroleum mineral bases.

To find salons nationwide, visit www.aveda.com.

## BELEGENZA—THE SECRET SALON

Locations: Houston and San Diego

Family owned and operated, The Secret Salon offers a full range of natural hair services including state of the art safe hair coloring in an eco-conscious atmosphere using nontoxic products. Specializing in corrective haircoloring, long-term color maintenanc,e and Belegenza products, this salon also offers make up services and lash tinting.

For more information visit www.thesecretsalon. net or www.belegenza.com or call 713-266-0099 (Houston) or 760-518-8823 (San Diego).

## ECOCOLORS— A NATURAL HAIR SALON

Location: Atlanta

This salon provides expert hair services, including coloring with nontoxic EcoColors permanent hair colorings.

EcoColors coloring and dye products are used in an impressive number of salons nationwide. To find one in your area, call 404-875-2620 or check online at www.ecocolors.net.

## JOHN MASTERS ORGANICS

Locations: SoHo, New York City

One of the first salons of its caliber and kind, John Masters Organics offers a wide spectrum of fine hair services and is New York City's only "clean air" salon. All colorings used in the salon are ammonia-free herbal- and clay-based products. The salon does not offer any chemical services—no perms, relaxers, or bleaches.

To find out more, go to www.johnmasters. com or call 212-343-9590.

## MODE—AN ORGANIC SALON

Locations: Two salons in Seattle

These boutique-style salons offer a full range of hair services with an emphasis on organic coloring. One location also offers organic facials and body care pampering, along with hair removal. Cosmetics and wedding services are available at both.

For more information, check online at www.modehairart.com or call 206-623-0195 or 206-527-7010.

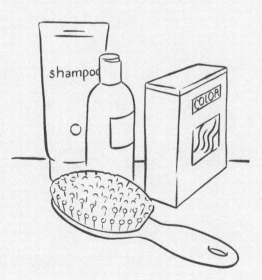

# Good Oral Care

Gorgeous pearly whites are a sign of good health and make smiling with confidence a pleasure. Good-smelling breath is a definite attribute when kissing and conversing intimately. Brushing and rinsing are motions many of us go through on autopilot, without giving them much thought. Gargling and flossing are also parts of the routine if dentists have their way. Regardless, taking care of our chompers is mandatory because we only get one set of them.

Blinded by our pursuit of gleaming white teeth, and by the products that achieve these sparkling results, it's easy not to think too much about what the heck is in all of this stuff. What exactly are we using to brush and swish with and then rinsing right down the drain?

## Mouthwashes

Gargling is a sure way to freshen breath and, though it's not a substitute for flossing, swishing mouthwash between your teeth is sort of a lazy man's way to floss, as far as I'm concerned. The question is, What's in mouthwash? In the conventional products camp, there's a lot of artificial junk, like synthetic dyes, low-grade solvents, and chemical sweeteners. The concept of swishing this stuff around in your mouth leaves a lot to be desired, and a lot of it is eco-toxic.

After looking into the ingredients of a number of big-brand mouthwashes, I have never felt more confident that choosing natural mouthwash is the clean, green, safe way to go. I found that they contain a

## What the Heck Is a Tongue Scraper?!

A tongue scraper is a nifty, low-tech device used to gently rake plaque and junk from the tongue. They've been used since ancient times in places like India and China as a cure for indelible and potent halitosis—yes, bad breath. This simple apparatus is made from either thin metal or hard plastic that is shaped like a long *U* or a bell-shaped triangle at the end of stick. The scraper is used to slough off crummy buildup on the tongue. Ancient use aside, in peer-reviewed studies, heavy-hitting dentists from New York University's College of Dentistry found that using a tongue scraper had significantly positive effects on reducing the numbers of nasty bacteria that thrive in the mouth.[209] Empirical evidence aside, I've been scraping my tongue every time I brush for years with results that my dentist finds impressive and my husband finds kissable.

Tongue scrapers are widely available at drugstores and natural markets, and online (two sources are www.amazon.com and www.tonguesweeper.com).

# The Dental Herb Company

The Dental Herb Company has a few professional oral hygiene products that are over the moon and unequaled. Only the purest high-grade materials are used, including certified organic or ecologically wild-crafted herbs, botanicals, and essential oils. No artificial chemicals, flavorings, preservatives, sweeteners, SLS, fluoride, or poloxamers are used. Formulated by a dentist, these products are absolutely brilliant. Unfortunately, the line is sold only through dental professionals. If you can't find one in your area who carries it, the company will sell it to you directly with a note from your dentist. It's worth the effort—this stuff is powerfully good. Go to www.dentalherbcompany.com for the details.

*Tooth and Gums Paste.* This creamy formula is chock-full of powerful botanical extracts; plant saponins; herbs like green tea, echinacea, and gotu kola; and lots of pure essential oils.

*Tooth and Gums Tonic.* This very potent mouthwash makes me want to sing to the hills. Full of pure extracts and essential oils in a vegetable glycerin base, a little bit goes a long way for tingling, fresh power. I put some in a 1-ounce glass spray bottle to use as an on-the-go mouth-freshening spritz. I never leave home without it.

*Under the Gums Irrigant.* Add a small capful of this almighty botanical blend to a home oral irrigator like a Waterpik for seriously healthy gums.

*Tooth and Gums Spritz.* This is a supreme mouth spray for freshening your breath when you're on the move.

slew of chemicals that I would never want to put in my mouth, and I doubt that you would want to, either.

But on the natural side of the fence are some effective mouthwashes that use botanicals and extracts for clean-as-a-whistle results without all the chemicals.

## Natural Mouthwashes to Look For

If you like to swish, these brands and products are human- and eco-friendly options worth looking into.

- **Jason Natural Mouthwash.** The botanicals, extracts, and essential oils in this four-variety line let you swish without synthetic or chemical ingredients.

- **Tom's of Maine Natural Cleansing Mouthwash.** Look for fluoride-free versions of peppermint, cinnamint, and spearmint. I'm not quite sure about the poloxamer 335 that's in all of them. It's a surfactant made from polyoxyethylene and/or polypropylene, which the label states is "processed from natural gas and oil." It's your call.

- **Weleda Ratanhia Mouthwash Concentrate.** Made from botanicals and extracts such as ratanhia (a root prized for its oral health properties) and myrrh, this swish will cleanse and purify. Alcohol is the first ingredient, and, though it disinfects, it may be intense and possibly irritating.

# COMMON INGREDIENT HAZARDS:
## TOOTHPASTES AND MOUTHWASHES

*The idea of using irritating petrochemicals, synthetic dyes, and saccharin to brush with is pretty bizarre, but they're in most toothpastes and mouthwashes, even some of the friendly looking brands at the health food store. Here are some ingredients to look out for.*

### FLUORIDE (SODIUM FLUORIDE, SODIUM MONOFLUOROPHOSPHATE)

We have long been told that fluoride is good for teeth and bones, but is it really? There is some question about how good certain types of fluoride—like the sodium fluoride found in toothpaste—really are. Sodium fluoride is poisonous[210]—meaning that it can kill you. Before being sold under the FDA-approved banner for healthy teeth, it was used as a rat poison.[211] The same stuff, albeit in lesser amounts, is used in toothpastes today, some 80 years later. It was also popular as an insecticide[212] for a while, but it was found to injure and kill plants.

Though approved as an ingredient in toothpaste, sodium fluoride has never been approved by the FDA for ingestion.[213] That's why those clear "do not swallow" warnings are found on dental products. This is a big deal for kids, who inevitably do swallow some of the stuff because it's sweet and they're just getting a handle on the coordination needed to spit on command. Kids' lower body weights put them at greater risk when they ingest poisonous materials—that's why they're advised to use only a pea-size lump of toothpaste.

Along with being poisonous, fluoride is linked to developmental issues like lower IQ levels.[214] Even though 98 percent of Europe has banned fluoride in drinking water,[215] about two-thirds of American drinking water is fluoridated.[216] The reason I bring up fluoridated water is because double-dosing fluoride with water and toothpaste may cause chronic overexposure and some terrible effects—like crippling skeletal problems,[217] bone cancer,[218] rashes, mouth sores, and discolored teeth.[219] Discolored teeth?! Yes. The most commonly accepted adverse effect of constant low-dose fluoride exposure is fluorosis, which can cause yellowed and mottled teeth. That doesn't sound helpful. Nor does the fact that it bioaccumulates in plants and animals.[220] Overall, fluoride is worth avoiding entirely in toothpaste. Keep your eyes peeled, though—it's included in some natural-looking brands. The best advice for parents concerned about preventing their kids from getting cavities is to make sure they eat a healthy diet, including lots of veggies and avoiding too many refined and sugary foods, brush after meals (or at least morning and night), floss, and make regular visits to the dentist for teeth cleaning.

### SLS

Sodium lauryl sulfate is hard to escape. This miraculous detergent and foaming agent seems to be in everything—toothpaste included. So what's the deal with this suds enhancer? First of all, it's a big irritant,[221] which isn't great for gums. Then there's the fact that it enhances the penetration of other substances into the body,[222] which is not a problem if all the other ingredients in the toothpaste are peachy keen. But if the toothpaste also contains potentially carcinogenic saccharin[223] or a synthetic dye, be prepared to have them more efficiently delivered into your bloodstream, as well. Then there's the whole indirect-cause-of-cancer concern,[224] which is that SLS can be contaminated with really nasty stuff during processing,[225] like 1,4-dioxane and nitrosamines, both of which are probable human carcinogens[226][227] because they are good at causing cancer in animals.[228][229]

Toothpaste doesn't have to foam up a storm to do its job. How can you get at your teeth through all that foam, anyway? I've been using Jason SeaFresh toothpaste for years; it's SLS free, and it foams just fine. In fact, my teeth feel so clean, I want to yodel.

## SACCHARIN

The safety of saccharin has been controversial for more than a century. One of the main concerns is that it's a potential carcinogen for humans because it causes cancer in animals.[230][231] After a number of influential studies were done on saccharine during the craze for diet soda in the 1970s, even the FDA proposed a ban on it in 1977.[232] But like most big-business chemicals, saccharin has staying power. And like many of the most notorious chemical inventions, it was discovered by accident. Not too long before the turn of the 20th century a scientist working with a toxic coal tar derivative, toluene (see page 174), noticed its sweet taste and started investigating the possibilities for using coal tar derivatives as sweeteners. Yup, saccharin is made from coal tar.[233] Well, nowadays, saccharin is also made using a host of other chemicals, including sulfur dioxide, chlorine, and ammonia.[234] The bottom line is that there is no need to brush your teeth with a product that contains it.

## SYNTHETIC DYES

According to the FDA, which regulates them, FD&C (food, drug, and cosmetic) colors are "manmade."[235] What do you think that means they're made of? You got it, chemicals and coal tar. Yum! By nature, coal-based substances are toxic and persistent polluters. Just which colors are lurking behind the major brands? Check it out.

*FD&C Blue 1.* Derived from coal, this dye was banned in 11 countries in Europe for a while. Apparently, a few of them lifted the ban because now it's considered safe. The FDA says not to worry even if hospital patients given feeding solutions tainted with the dye might experience toxicity or death,[236] it's harmless in toothpaste. Hmm.

*FD&C Red 3.* Use of this coal-based dye is restricted by the FDA because it has been linked with thyroid tumors.[237] Apparently, a little bit in toothpaste is acceptable. Why? It makes it pretty. Europe doesn't recommended Red 3 (E129 on European labels) for kids because it's linked to behavioral problems like temper tantrums, poor concentration, and hyperactivity.[238][239] America seems to like it in toothpaste.

*FD&C Red 33.* This coloring's use is restricted for cosmetics and not approved by the FDA for anything that's applied around the eyes,[240] but apparently it's A-OK for the mouth. It's a popular colorant for toothpaste, especially brands geared toward kids.

*FD&C Red 40.* This one is approved by the FDA for inclusion in cosmetics applied around the eyes even though it has been banned entirely in eight countries in Europe.[241]

*Yellow 10 Lake.* This bright yellow dye can be mixed with FD&C Blue 1 to make a pretty green. It's potentially genotoxic[242]—a fancy term for something that causes genetic mutations and the development of tumors. In Europe, it's not recommended as an ingredient in products for kids because it is believed to make them hyper, distracted, and prone to throwing tantrums.[243]

*Here's the good stuff—pure toothpaste you can use without fear. Treating your mouth to eco-friendly, chemical-free products will yield a brilliant, confident smile. They'll give you an untainted kisser and make the planet happier, too.*

## DESERT ESSENCE

Big on tea tree oil formulas for all kinds of personal care and hygiene, Desert Essence toothpastes blend tea tree oil with fresh, all-natural flavors like ginger, fennel, mint, neem, and wintergreen and whitening ingredients like baking soda for antiseptic brushing power. These products don't contain artificial colors, flavors, sweeteners, fluoride, or harsh abrasives. Unfortunately, SLS is included in all but one formula, Sparkling Sea Mint, which is sweetened with sorbitol, a natural sugar substitute. If you're okay with a little SLS detergent, all of these formulas are much cleaner picks than conventional brands for getting a smart, sharp smile. Desert Essence also makes good oral accoutrements like floss and naturally flavored tea tree oil and cinnamon toothpicks. For extra eco-consumer, feel-good power, all of these products are manufactured using renewable energy!

*Available:* at most natural markets and online www.desertessence.com

## JASON NATURAL

Jason Natural toothpastes and gels blend the art and science of natural oral health with the highest-quality ingredients. I give the company a big thumbs-up all around for these brilliant, pure formulas that contain no SLS, fluoride, synthetic ingredients, or artificial preservatives, colors, or sweeteners. Their 12 clean, innovative options include nifty and effective ingredients like bamboo powder, perilla seed, sea algae extracts, vitamins and nutrients, grapefruit seed extract (a natural preservative and antiseptic), and natural herbal sweeteners like organic stevia. They even use vegetable glycerin, which isn't derived from animal fats or, as synthetic glycerin is, from petroleum. I am passionate about having a naturally clean kisser, and Jason SeaFresh toothpaste is the only one I use.

*Available:* at most natural markets and online www.jason-natural.com

## NATURE'S GATE

Nature's Gate natural toothpastes come in a variety of formulas and flavors—minty, fruity, and anise crèmes and gels. The bummer is, they all contain SLS (and it's close to the top of all the ingredient lists, which means that a fair amount of it is included). The company argues that SLS isn't a big concern when you just brush with it, but you should decide for yourself. There are fluoride-free versions of both the crèmes and gels. All the "crème toothpastes" contain synthetic methylparaben preservatives, but the "natural gels" don't. If you don't mind partially synthetic tooth suds, Nature's Gate is a fairly clean option in comparison with conventional products.

*Available:* at most natural markets and online www.natures-gate.com

## PEELU

Peelu toothpastes are 100 percent natural and contain the soft fibers of the peelu tree—also known as *neem*—for gently effective dental care. No SLS, fluoride, harsh abrasives, or artificial sweeteners or preservatives are used in Peelu's products. Natural mints and cinnamon flavors round out these clean oral options that have the natural whitening power of peelu. They also make gum and toothpowder for extra action. The toothpowder can be used instead of or in addition to toothpaste. Overall, products in this line are pure, clean picks.

*Available:* at most natural markets and online

www.peelu.com

## TOM'S OF MAINE

Tom's of Maine is the largest natural tooth-paste company with products on the market. Its dental products are wholesome-looking and pretty natural, though the company stands by its inclusion of SLS in every single product, saying that it's not a big concern. Some ingredient lists specify that the SLS is derived from coconut oil, which, though better than its petrochemical sibling, has the same health concerns. The company is also big on fluoride, though it offers fluoride-free versions of a lot of its flavors. If you are okay with all of that then you are in luck, because Tom's has more than 50 kinds of toothpaste in pastes and gels to choose from. There's a full spread of natural flavors, including all kinds of mints, and some formulas contain great botanicals like fennel and myrrh and neat ingredients like propolis, a nutritive tree resin gathered by bees. Instead of artificial sweeteners, they use nifty naturals like xylitol, a sugar made from birch trees. If SLS doesn't concern you, the fluoride-free products are a good choice for cleaning your chompers.

*Available:* at many markets of all kinds and online

www.tomsofmaine.com

## WELEDA

For super-pure toothpastes, Weleda is a good company to look to. Its products are SLS free across the board, and fluoride free, too. The company uses herbs and botanicals like calendula, fennel, myrrh, and essential oils, and some even contain biodynamically grown ingredients like lemon. Weleda's products are absolutely pure picks for cleaning and protecting healthy teeth and gums.

*Available:* at most natural markets and online

www.usa.weleda.com

# Clean Deodorants and Antiperspirants

Sweating is a natural part of life. On its own, perspiration is pretty odorless, but when the bacteria that naturally grow on our skin go to work on it, mostly in the intimate depths of our armpits, odor gets the upper hand. The quest to smell good is often met by attempting to mask or arrest odors with chemicals, but there are naturally effective ways to stay as sweet as a fresh-picked peach.

The way the ads paint it, men are supposed to be strong and sweaty, but smell clean and sexy; women are supposed to be capable of doing everything backward in heels, like Ginger Rogers, and still smell shower-fresh. A chemical deodorant bath may help achieve this kind of ease, but its possible side effects may include much more than you bargained for.

## The Deal with Deodorants and Antiperspirants

Deodorants and antiperspirants are both used to battle body odor, but they work in different ways. Lots of us think of them as the same thing, but there are distinctive differences. Deodorants mask odor with perfume and usually contain ingredients to kill the bacteria that cause it. Antiperspirants use chemicals to stop sweating from happening. Most conventional deodorants contain antiperspirant chemicals, so they're referred to by either name and considered to be one category of products.

### Deodorants

Conventional deodorants work by killing the bacteria that eat sweat and cause the pungent aromas, or they simply overpower the odor with perfume. Most also contain antiperspirant ingredients to oppress the bacteria. Natural deodorants take advantage of the clean smells of plant extracts and essential oils and of the ability of some minerals to quell the growth of odor-causing bacteria.

### Antiperspirants

Deodorants that contain antiperspirant ingredients are actually classified by the FDA as over-the-counter drugs because they chemically affect the functioning of the body. The active ingredients in conventional antiperspirant deodorants tamp down the flow of perspiration with metal chelators,[244] particularly aluminum, and kill off the bacteria that cause the stink with antibacterial chemicals like triclosan[245] and ethanol.[246] In addition to this chemical cocktail are synthetic fragrances that likely contain phthalates and a crew of preservatives that usually contain formaldehyde. The result: one of the most volatile chemical soirées of all time, happening right in your armpits!

# Crystal Deodorants

Once upon a time, crystal deodorants were available only as small hunks of clear rock that you moistened and then rubbed in your armpits. Strange, but effective. Now, they are available as convenient roll-ons, pump sprays, and sticks.

## HOW DO THEY WORK?

A crystal deodorant (in any form) is composed of a variety of mineral salts that are collectively called *alum*. The salts are naturally nontoxic and highly effective at curbing BO. The molecules are too large to be absorbed into the skin, which is good because that way they stay on the outside of your body to do their job and don't get absorbed into your bloodstream. The mineral salts in crystal deodorants form a layer on the skin, creating an environment where it's impossible for odor-causing bacteria to thrive. No bacteria, no odor—it's as simple as that. Crystal deodorants don't stop sweat, they simply stop the accompanying smell.

## HOW ARE THEY USED?

Deodorant crystal stones and sticks need to be moistened with water for application; roll-ons and sprays are applied like any other deodorant. They are best applied to clean pits immediately after bathing. That will ensure that you have an optimally performing protective barrier built up before any odor-causing bacteria can form on the skin.

## HOW WELL DO THEY WORK?

In my opinion, crystal deodorants work brilliantly when they're applied immediately after bathing. Because of the way they work, they need to be applied to clean pits—they don't work well if you are already sweating. I've been using a roll-on crystal deodorant for years and am consistently pleased as punch.

Naturally effective deodorants capitalize on the ability of ingredients like naturally derived mineral salts and organic alcohols to affront malodorous bacteria. These products use pure fragrances from plant extracts and essential oils, which may do double duty as antiseptics and preservatives. Reading ingredient lists is the single most powerful tool in the consumer's toolbox for seeing what exactly is in deodorant products. Even some of the really natural-looking products on health food store shelves everywhere contain questionable ingredients like propylene glycol and the vague *fragrance*, which could be any number of chemicals.

Scouting out effective products made with safe, clean ingredients will become particularly inviting after we take a brief tour of the very real side effects of noxious conventional sweat-busting chemicals.

### ALUMINUM SALTS

The most widely used forms of aluminum are aluminum zirconium complexes that literally plug up sweat glands to stop the flow of sweat. The commonly used forms of aluminum salts in conventional deodorants react with the natural salts in sweat to form a little gel plug that simply prevents perspiration from being excreted. Less sweat may mean less smell, but it has potentially serious side effects.

While aluminum is the third most common element on Earth,[247] pasting armpits and plugging glands with it may be linked to consequences like breast cancer[248] and Alzheimer's disease.[249]

**Breast health.** While the debate rages on over whether there is a *direct* link between aluminum in deodorants and breast cancer,[250] there is evidence that there is, indeed, a relationship,[251] because aluminum-based compounds can mimic estrogen hormones.[252] [253] One thing's for sure: Aluminum is known to be not only just plain toxic,[254] but also to be genotoxic,[255] meaning that it may cause genetic mutations and tumors. The widespread, long-term effects of aluminum salts in deodorants remain unclear, but clinical studies showing high incidences of breast cancer consistent with what aluminum has been shown to do are raising a lot of scientists' eyebrows.[256] Add to that the concern that aluminum is quite capable of binding to and blocking hormone receptors[257] and you get a real nightmare.

**Brain health.** Aluminum is well documented to be a neurotoxin[258] [259] [260] that is adept at crossing the blood–brain barrier.[261] [262] That means that deodorants containing aluminum may get into the bloodstream and then into the brain. Investigation of the link between aluminum and Alzheimer's disease began more than 20 years ago, and includes suspicions about deodorants. While some details warrant further research, here's the deal: Alzheimer's patients generally have abnormally large concentrations of aluminum in their brains.[263] [264] [265] It's still controversial in scientific circles, but until the empirical evidence is clear, it's probably not a bad idea to avoid products that contain aluminum.

### TRICLOSAN

Triclosan is a synthetic broad-spectrum biocide (a chemical capable of killing a broad range of living organisms) that has become all the rage as an ingredient in a vast array of antibacterial products: soaps, socks, tissues, hand wipes—you name it. Conventional deodorant makers are big on triclosan because it kills off the bacteria that cause BO. That's all well and good, but because it's a phenol, triclosan is also pretty noxious for humans and acutely toxic to aquatic life.[266] Phenols are persistent organic pollutants (POPs) in the environment,[267] meaning that they're stubborn as hell and pretty much never break down. Rather, phenols accumulate in the fatty tissues of humans and animals and travel up the food chain, eventually even into breast milk.[268] Plus, they generally wreak havoc in the ecosystem because of their nasty habit of being reactive with certain compounds, like chlorine.[269]

When triclosan gets together with chlorine, which is found in treated water and wastewater, it forms a whole slew of carcinogenic compounds, including highly chlorinated dioxins[270] and chloroform[271]— both of which are known to cause cancer.[272] [273] For kicks, that horrible conversion into dioxins happens naturally when triclosan is exposed to sunlight.[274] This is unlikely to happen in your armpits, which might rarely see the light of day. But there's a different kind of reaction that happens when triclosan is manufactured—as a chlorinated substance, it's generally "suspected to be"[275] contaminated with dioxins during manufacture.[276] The EPA is not wild about that, and in fact it registers triclosan as a pesticide, but maybe because these products are big business, the number of triclosan-laden products on the shelves continues to grow. So, it's up to us to avoid it as much as possible.

## ETHANOL (SD ALCOHOL 40)

Ethanol, also known as *ethyl alcohol*, is a type of alcohol that is more like fuel than something you want to put on your skin. In fact, a car can run on it, and the government is now touting it as the biofuel of the future. Ethanol is by far a cleaner-burning fuel than petroleum, but applying it to your skin might not be advisable. It's not very friendly to human skin,[277] and Material Safety Data Sheet instructions for handling and storing ethanol clearly state to "wash thoroughly after handling"[278] and "wear appropriate protective gloves to prevent skin exposure."[279] So what's it doing in deodorants? Well, it works well as a volatile carrier, like a solvent, delivering other ingredients to your armpits and then evaporating.

If your armpits have stung after you applied a conventional deodorant, especially after shaving, it could have been the ethanol. It's an effective disinfectant, but it's also an irritant[280] that may also dry out skin and reduce its elasticity[281]—saggy armpits, anyone? It's a common allergen[282] and may cause contact dermatitis[283] before evaporating, sort of like a hit-and-run. But the trouble with ethanol goes far beyond irritation, unfortunately. It's not recognized as a carcinogen, but it seems to be a mutagen,[284] meaning that it messes around with genetic information and increases the odds that mutations will occur, some of which may lead to cancer.

Ecologically, ethanol is no picnic either. When it's released into the environment, it degrades pretty quickly,[285] though its hazardous decomposition products include irritating and toxic fumes and gases such as carbon monoxide.[286]

Overall, ethanol is definitely best avoided on your skin. In your car, however, it's a clean-burning, renewable fuel with significantly lower emissions that we all hope to see more of in the near future.

## TALC

Talc sounds pretty benign, like something found in baby powder, and it is. Talc is a super-fine powder that, though it's used for its absorbent, deodorizing qualities, is suspected of being a carcinogen.[287] It is sometimes contaminated with asbestos,[288] which is a definite carcinogen.[289] Given that it's a major lung irritant,[290] aerosol spray deodorants containing talc are the most hazardous variety. In stick and roll-on antisweat goods, breathing it in is not as much of an issue because it is in a solid form, but it is a skin irritant.[291] There are also concerns that applying talc to the skin can cause problems inside the body.[292] For instance, feminine sprays and powders are often loaded with talc, and regular users may significantly increase their risk for ovarian cancer.[293] Talc is also found in many powdery makeups like blushes, bronzers, face powders, and eye shadows.

## PROPYLENE GLYCOL

Propylene glycol is common in stick deodorants because of its multifaceted properties. It acts as a moistening agent as well as a solvent that marries and carries other ingredients. That would all be fine and well if that is all it did, but lo and behold, it's known to cause a bunch of skin- and cell-damaging side effects. Propylene glycol is the name of the game in antifreeze,[294] deicers,[295] and embalming solutions.[296] It's found in a wide spectrum of personal care products and cosmetics like face and body lotions and cleansers, shampoos, conditioners, and hair styling products. Its prowess as a solvent makes it popular in not just cosmetics, but in paints and plastics, too. Though commonly found in a wide range of personal care products like deodorants, propylene glycol is really irritating to the skin and perceptibly toxic and damaging to cells.[297] It may be a common cause of allergies and contact dermatitis.[298] While propylene glycol is not nearly as dangerous in deodorants as aluminum is, you can avoid it without forfeiting odor-busting efficacy. Look for natural products that instead use natural ingredients like glycerin for happy, healthy, deodorized pits. See the "Green Thumb Guide: Deodorants" that follows for recommendations.

*For fresh, healthy, good-smelling pits, check out these products with clean, green ingredients.*

## ALBA

### Clear Enzyme deodorant stick

Made with signature ingredients like antibacterial alpine lichen, absorbent baking soda, and pure essential oils, Alba's Clear Enzyme deodorants are skin-healthy picks for long-lasting protection. They're available in lavender, tea tree, and fragrance-free varieties. The line's new formulation contains no synthetic paraben preservatives.

*Available:* at most natural markets and online

www.albabotanica.com

## AUBREY ORGANICS

### Spray and roll-on deodorants

Aubrey Organics is as clean and natural as it gets for personal care products. The company's spray and roll-on deodorants harness the power of botanical extracts, antioxidants, and essential oils for clean, naturally good-smelling pits. Aubrey deodorants contain only natural ingredients, though they may not provide protection that's as long-lasting as you might need when wearing big sweaters.

*Available:* at most natural markets and online

www.aubrey-organics.com

## AVALON ORGANICS

### Roll-on deodorant

Made with organic plant extracts like green tea, calendula, and chamomile, Avalon Organics roll-on deodorants are completely natural. The glycerin-based formulas are enriched with aloe vera and great-smelling pure essential oils such as lavender, lemon, and peppermint. They contain no artificial, synthetic, or chemical ingredients such as propylene glycol, fragrances, or paraben preservatives.

*Available:* at most natural markets and online

www.avalonorganics.com

## BURT'S BEES

### Herbal Deodorant spray

Burt's Bees Herbal Deodorant spray is a simple denatured alcohol-based formula with essential plant oils like sage, lavender, and lemon that works to minimize and neutralize odors naturally. It contains no chemical ingredients or artificial fragrances or preservatives, period.

*Available:* at most natural markets, grocery stores, and drugstores and online

www.burtsbees.com

## CRYSTAL

### Body Deodorant

Crystal Body Deodorant is 100 percent natural mineral salts and nothing else. Mineral salts keep odor-causing bacteria from growing on the skin, preventing body odor before it starts. It's great for men and women, and it's fragrance free, paraben free, and nonstaining. I've been using this brand for years and won't change a thing.

*Available:* at most natural markets and online

www.thecrystal.com

## DESERT ESSENCE

### Stick and roll-on deodorants

Desert Essence is synonymous with tea tree oil. It's used in the company's deodorant products for its natural antibacterial properties, as are other pure essential oils and plant extracts. Desert Essence deodorants contain odor-busting sodium bicarbonate (baking soda) and soothing aloe vera gel. Unfortunately, all the stick deodorants contain paraben preservatives and all the roll-ons contain propylene glycol. If either or both pass in your book, then this is an effective pick.

*Available:* at most natural markets and some grocery and drugstores and online

www.desertessence.com

## DR. HAUSCHKA

### Roll-on deodorants

All Dr. Hauschka products are purely natural, including the deodorants. Zinc ricinoleate reduces odor without changing the way the skin functions, and plant extracts like neem and sage and light natural scents from pure essential oils deodorize.

*Available:* at most natural markets and online

www.drhauschka.com

## JASON NATURAL

### Stick and roll-on deodorants

Jason has a good spread of stick and roll-on deodorants, some of which contain 70 percent certified organic ingredients. All are made with deodorizing ingredients like baking soda and clay and enriched with soothing aloe vera. The company also uses great botanicals, plant extracts, and essential oils such as lavender and apricot, many of which are certified organic. Unfortunately, either propylene glycol or paraben preservatives are in almost all of them. If you're okay with one or the other, these products promise lasting efficacy. Read the labels, though, because there may also be a few other chemicals like ceteareth-20, which is one of those ingredients that can be contaminated with really bad stuff during processing.

*Available:* at most natural markets and online

www.jason-natural.com

## KISS MY FACE

### Stick and roll-on deodorants

Kiss My Face has a wide portfolio of natural plant- and mineral-based stick and roll-on deodorants. The company's new formulations of old favorites are now paraben preservative free. Hooray! Active Enzyme sticks utilize odor-neutralizing enzyme proteins from vegetables, baking soda, and purified clay; unfortunately, they also contain propylene glycol. Liquid Rock roll-ons use the power of natural mineral salts to prevent odor-causing bacteria from growing. Some of the deodorants contain vaguely identified fragrances, but the company promises that they are derived from natural sources. I've used their fragrance-free Liquid Rock for years and feel as clean as a fresh cucumber.

*Available:* at most natural markets and online

www.kissmyface.com

## NATURALLY FRESH DEODORANT CRYSTAL

### Crystal deodorants

Naturally Fresh Deodorant Crystal products are natural mineral salts, which curb odor extremely effectively. Mineral salts inhibit the growth of odor-causing bacteria instead of artificially stopping sweat or masking it with fragrances. Apply it immediately after bathing for best results.

*Available:* at most natural markets and online

www.tccd.com

## NATURE'S GATE

### Stick and roll-on deodorants

Nature's Gate offers an extensive spread of stick and roll-on deodorants. The company's original formulas are in white packaging—they are pretty clean, though some contain paraben preservatives or propylene glycol, and a few have vaguely identified fragrance oils, so read the labels thoroughly. The newer certified organic sticks are packaged in green and silver, and orange is the color for the newest ones of all. All of these are super clean, and none contain paraben preservatives or propylene glycol. A boon! My husband loves both the Lemongrass and Clary Sage and Tea Tree and Blue Cypress varieties and I love their effects—he smells great.

*Available:* at natural markets and online

www.natures-gate.com

*(continued)*

## NUTRIBIOTIC

### Stick Deodorants

This company pioneered the use of grapefruit seed extract 20 years ago—it's made from the seeds and pulp of certified organic grapefruit. The extract is highly effective in many applications, including when used as a totally natural preservative and for long-lasting protection against odor. The deodorants contain grapefruit seed extract along with certified organic aloe vera and witch hazel. The all-natural fragrances in the Lavender and Mango Melon varieties are from plant oils. All deodorants made by NutriBiotic contain propylene glycol. If you are okay with that, they are a good pick.

*Available:* at most natural markets and online

www.nutribiotic.com

## TERRESSENTIALS

### Roll-on deodorants

Terressentials deodorants are completely natural and made with a strong portfolio of certified organic ingredients. They contain odor busters like natural clay minerals, baking soda, and ecologically wild-crafted botanical tinctures, as well as soothing, cooling organic aloe vera gel. All three fragrances are from certified organic essential oils, and there's a fragrance-free variety too. None contain synthetic or chemical ingredients, preservatives, perfumes, or dyes.

*Available:* at natural markets and online

www.terressentials.com

## TOM'S OF MAINE

### Stick and roll-on deodorants

Tom's of Maine is a natural kind of company. In making its deodorants, it calls on the powers of plant extracts like hops to inhibit the growth of odor-causing bacteria and of natural botanicals to neutralize any odors that do arise. The deodorants contain only natural fragrances derived from a variety of essential oils and plant extracts. The company's new, long-lasting stick and roll-on formulas also use the odor-binding properties of zinc ricinoleate and encapsulate natural fragrance ingredients in silica to make them last longer. If you ask me, silica is questionable for applying to the skin (it's kind of like glass), and the propylene glycol also found in their products is something some of us want to avoid. Overall, these deodorants are pretty pure picks that carry the promise of long-lasting efficacy.

*Available:* at most natural markets, grocery stores, and drugstores and online

www.tomsofmaine.com

## WELEDA

### Spray deodorants

Weleda is dedicated to using natural, organic, and biodynamic ingredients in all of its personal care products, spray deodorants included. With their natural alcohol base and a broad spectrum of pure essential oils (many of them biodynamically grown), these sprays naturally rejuvenate and deodorize skin and neutralize odor-causing bacteria. The scents are lovely and light, though they may not be effective if you need hard-core protection.

*Available:* at most natural markets and online

www.usaweleda.com

# Natural Feminine Products

For women, not much is as intimate as feminine products. Sorry, guys. Disposable goods are par for the course at that time of the month. Whether you greet your flow with celebration, dread, or indifference, there are a few things to know about being green and healthy with feminine products.

## All about Tampons

Tampons have been around since the 1930s, and most of us give little thought to what they're made of or how safe they are. However, many women don't know what's lurking in a simple tampon. Many women are surprised to learn that synthetic rayon, pesticide-laden cotton, dioxins, formaldehyde-releasing preservatives, and artificial fragrances can all be found in conventional tampons. None of that sounds like anything worth inviting inside your body. They are *really* not good. On the other hand, tampons made with natu-

rally bleached, 100 percent organic cotton are as simple as that. It's clean, natural, no-fuss care that ladies of all ages should treat themselves to.

### Tampons and Toxic Shock Syndrome: Is It the Materials?

Back in the 1970s and 1980s, health issues associated with tampons emerged with a vengeance, including toxic shock syndrome (TSS). TSS is a potentially fatal disease reportedly caused by toxic bacteria that are said to grow when a tampon has been left in for way too long. While neglecting to change a tampon can create a breeding ground for bacteria that can cause TSS, a significant part of the problem might actually be the synthetic materials in some tampons. After all, tampons had been around for a good 40 or 50 years before TSS reared its head. Could the move from all-cotton to synthetic blends have had something to do with it?

To meet the demand for more absorbent products, tampon manufacturers turned to synthetic materials like rayon starting in the 1970s. Rayon is more absorbent than cotton, but that comes at a cost. Some serious concerns were documented as early as 1975, when an internal memo at Procter and Gamble disclosed that one of its tampon products contained cancer-causing agents and altered the organisms that naturally populate a woman's vagina.[299] That product

> *Look for TCF (totally chlorine free) feminine products—pads and tampons— for the greenest cycle possible.*

was pulled from the shelves, but even now, few safety regulations for feminine products are in place or enforced.

After that semipublic pickle passed, three of the four synthetic materials used in tampons were pulled—carboxymethylcellulose, polyester, and polacrylate rayon. Synthetic viscose rayon stayed in the loop—though less absorbent than the other three, it was the least problematic. But viscose rayon still causes problems and may amplify the amount of TSS toxin produced.[300] The trouble with synthetics like rayon is that they are viscous, or sticky, and deposit stuff that no woman wants in her precious insides. Try this: Take a conventional brand of tampons and stick one in a glass of water. Wait a few minutes for it to expand and then remove it from the glass. Check out what is left in the water. It's likely that you would not want to deposit that in yourself.

Today, leading brands of tampons are made with conventional cotton and undisclosed chemical fragrances along with rayon. The FDA insists that the tampons are safe, regardless of the fact that more than a billion *tons* of pesticides and herbicides are sprayed on conventional cotton every year. Many of them are carcinogenic, damage the nervous system, and disrupt hormones. Sadly, the statistics on TSS show that it is as rampant today as it was 20 years ago.

## Conventionally Grown Cotton Tampons: The Bottom of the Barrel

Conventional cotton ranks as one of the most destructive, chemical-intensive crops of all time. It's wickedly laden with some of the most notoriously toxic Class I and II pesticides, many of which are known carcinogens.[301] See page 269 for more information. The kind of cotton used to make tampons is the bottom of the barrel—the leaves, stems, and short fibers called *gin trash*. It's no secret that conventional gin trash cotton is loaded with concentrated levels of pesticides. In fact, it's so laden with toxic residues that it's illegal to feed it to cattle in states like California.[302] Instead, conventional cotton gin trash is used to make products like tampons! Disturbing, but true. If this kind of cotton is dangerous to a cow weighing half a ton, what might it do to a woman who wears it inside her precious tissues for days on end? What happens after thousands of conventional tampons are worn over a lifetime?

By choosing to wear tampons made entirely of organically grown cotton, you'll never have to find out. Organic cotton is grown without chemical pesticides, insecticides, weed killers, or defoliants. It's clean and safe—better for you, better for the planet—and you are worth it!

## Bleached Tampons

Chlorine is a chemical prized for bleaching all things white. Unfortunately, it's very toxic stuff. Chlorine bleaching releases oodles of toxins into the environment—namely, dioxins—and leaves detectable residues in finished products.[303] Dioxins are a serious cause of eco-injury as well as a cause for concern when putting tampons you know where.

# Dioxins in Tampons and Endometriosis:
## Is There a Link?

Endometriosis is a chronic hormonal and immune disease that affects millions of women. It's a case of misplaced tissue—the endometrial tissue that normally grows inside the uterus grows elsewhere, usually in the pelvic and abdominal regions. The trouble is that, unlike the uterus, which sheds the endometrial tissue with menstruation, the misplaced tissue has no way to escape, and the growths get larger over time. It's said to be terribly painful, and many women who have it also have heightened chemical sensitivity, allergies, and frequent yeast infections. There is an unfortunate, but still unclear, link between endometriosis and infertility. Infertility affects about 40 percent of women with endometriosis,[304] and those who are fertile may have more difficulty conceiving.[305] The mechanism is not completely understood, but the effects are evident.

The cause of the disease itself is not understood either, though a connection to chemical toxins, namely dioxins,[306] is becoming tangible. Studies on monkeys (poor monkeys!) in the last decade painted a very clear picture that dioxin exposure can cause endometriosis.[307] The studies showed that the severity of the disease varied in direct relationship to the amount of dioxin exposure,[308] though some of the poor creatures fed as little as 5 parts of dioxin per trillion developed endometriosis.[309] Imagine a trillion ping-pong balls, and 5 of them are dioxins; that's a minute amount! According to the FDA, "dioxin levels in the rayon raw materials for tampons are reported to be at or below the detectable limit of the state-of-the-art dioxin assay, i.e., approximately 0.1 to 1 parts per trillion."[310] The tampons being referred to here are the reputedly "dioxin-free" products bleached with elemental chlorine-free processing.[311] The difference between 1 and 5 parts per trillion is incomprehensibly minute. Something is wrong with this picture.

The only safe level of dioxins is *zero*. Certified organic, nonchlorine-bleached tampons are the only products that have verifiable stakes on that claim. It's a choice well worth making.

Cotton and rayon (made from synthetic cellulose fibers derived from wood) are bleached white to look nice. The EPA has been working to encourage wood-pulp manufacturers to use dioxin-free processes like elemental chlorine-free (ECF) bleaching, which uses chlorine dioxide instead of elemental chlorine gas,[312] for raw materials like rayon. It's a step in the right direction, but ECF can still generate dioxins, just less of them.[313] Dioxins are known to cause cancer in animals and are strongly believed to cause cancer in humans[314] because they act as a complete carcinogen that doesn't require another chemical to fully act.[315] The FDA says that ECF-bleached raw rayon in US-made tampons is considered dioxin free, even though trace amounts of dioxins may be detected.[316] Huh? Plus, dioxin monitoring seems to be in the manufacturers' court—the FDA only asks for test results.[317] If dioxins are reported to be "at or below the detectable limit,"[318] everything is A-OK. That might be cause for a collective sigh of relief, except the EPA says that, as for lead, there is "no safe level" for dioxins.[319] Dioxins are among those pesky, fat-loving, persistent chemicals that accumulate in body tissue.[320] They are wickedly toxic for humans and the environment. The amount of dioxins in tampons may very well be small, but since dioxins don't leave the body, even small amounts can add up to dangerous levels over a lifetime.

## Natural Tampons: Organic Cotton, Chlorine-Free Bleached

Natural tampons are the clean, green choice for women of all ages. Free of the hazards of synthetic materials and chemical additives, natural tampons that work just as well as conventional brands are available with and without cardboard applicators in a variety of absorbencies.

Considering that the average woman uses more than 11,500 tampons in her lifetime,[321] even trace amounts of dioxins and chemical fragrances and preservatives add up big-time. Organic, nonchlorine-bleached products are the only smart, green, healthy choice to make. And the good news is, organic tampons are super easy to find. See the "Green Thumb Guide: Feminine Products" on page 222 for the best of what's around.

## Oh-So-Feminine Pads

Choosing sanitary pads made from natural versus synthetic materials is an easy green move—better for you, better for the planet.

Commercial pads are basically wads of chlorine-bleached pulp, superabsorbent petrochemicals, and plastic seasoned with a few preservatives and fragrances for good measure. A synthetic pad is less cause for concern than a synthetic tampon in terms of chemical exposure, but they create a helluva mountain of waste—we're talking more than 10 billion pads a year. Choosing pads made of natural materials puts ladies lower on the food chain of petrochemical production, exposure, and disposal. It's good green sense all around.

Natural pads made with chlorine-free pulps and plant cellulose are a clean, green alternative to chemical- and plastic-laden conventional models.

### Fragrances and Preservatives

Scented feminine products seem about as useful as scented toilet paper. While many ladies (like myself) fail to see the point of how chemicals can make things freshly appealing, artificial fragrances are commonplace in pads and tampons. Synthetic fragrances can be made from just about anything—they're generally brewed up from petrochemicals and may contain viscous "fixers" like phthalates, which no one ought to expose herself to (see "Phthalates" on page 170 for information on how they bioaccumulate, disrupt hormones, and do other dastardly things).

Of the preservatives, formaldehyde-releasing imidazolidinyl urea is a popular industry pick. Not only does it rank as one of the most common causes of allergic reactions of all time,[322] it is also toxic on a cellular level[323] and believed to be a mutagen.[324] Not exactly something worth exposing your private parts to.

Since fragrances and preservatives aren't listed on feminine product packaging, look to trustworthy natural product brands that guarantee that none of this junk will appear in your pants.

## Tips for Emergency Drugstore Feminine Product Shopping

Stocking a good reserve of nonchlorine-bleached organic tampons is a smart, green preventive measure to avoid runs to the nearest drugstore for emergency supplies. But, in a pinch, here are some tips for greener purchases.

- Choose tampons with cardboard applicators instead of plastic.
- Choose tampons with no applicator, like O.B.
- Consider a sanitary pad instead of a tampon. Though they're more wasteful of materials, your exposure to the chemicals in commercial pads is way less than it is with commercial tampons—at least until you can get your hands on a chlorine-free organic brand.
- When choosing sanitary pads, pick the right size—bigger isn't always better.

## Feminine Sprays, Wipes, and Powders

Considering what kinds of sprays, wipes, and powders we use to feel and smell spring-fresh in the nether regions is worth a moment. For the most part, conventional feminine products in this arena are loaded with chemicals, fragrances, talc, petrochemicals, and preservatives. None of that seems very fresh or feminine at all.

**Conventional aerosol sprays** are riddled with the usual suspects—hydrocarbon propellants that are rough on skin and brutal on the environment, and toxic chemical fragrances. Various disinfectant alcohols are used in a lot of feminine deodorant products, but they can irritate the skin and be hostile to breathe. Petroleum mineral oils also prevail as carriers, but they don't let skin breathe, which seems to work against the purpose of freshening products. Even with thorough scouting, I haven't seen much available in the way of natural feminine sprays. If it's natural freshness you are after, I recommend any nonaerosol natural deodorant for doing the trick (check out the "Green Thumb Guide: Deodorants" on page 214 for some healthy leads).

**Feminine wipes.** Disposable wipes are the new marketing sensation in feminine sanitation. For the most part, they are simply wipes moistened with petroleum-based wetting agents and chemical carriers like propylene glycol, formaldehyde-releasing preservatives like imidazolidinyl urea, and synthetic paraben preservatives. Take a pass on those jobbies. For naturally clean mopping, go for the good stuff like Natracare's organic cotton feminine wipes, which are made with healing herbs like calendula and pure essential oils. Another

*Next time you are browsing the market shelves for safe, clean, green feminine needs, look for these products for trustworthy support.*

## PADS AND TAMPONS

### NATRACARE

Natracare products contain only organic and natural ingredients from ecologically sound sources. Whitened totally without chlorine, no chemicals or additives are used whatsoever. Natracare gets high green marks on all of its products. The company makes tampons, with and without applicators, in several absorbencies; pads and liners in several sizes and absorbencies; feminine wipes; maternity and nursing pads; and incontinence pads.

*Available:* at most natural markets and online

www.natracare.com

### ORGANIC ESSENTIALS

This company's tampons are made using 100 percent certified organic cotton, no chlorine bleach, no rayon, and no binders or fillers. They come without applicators in regular and super absorbencies.

*Available:* at natural markets and online

www.organicessentials.com

### SEVENTH GENERATION

Seventh Generation is synonymous with eco-friendly products. The company has a full line of totally chlorine-free feminine care products, and the tampon boxes are even made with 100 percent recycled material. Kudos to all! Tampons (without applicators) are available in three absorbencies and made with 100 percent organic cotton; no rayon, dyes, or fragrances are used. Pads and pantiliners, offered in three absorbencies, are made with an absorbent gel derived from wheat; they do contain some plastic.

*Available:* at most natural markets and some grocery stores and online

www.seventhgeneration.com

## BODY POWDERS

### BURT'S BEES

**Baby Bee Dusting Powder**

This talc-free powder gets its drying power from cornstarch, baking soda, clays, and slippery elm. Its all-natural fragrance comes from powdered rosebuds and myrrh.

*Available:* at most natural markets, grocery stores, and drugstores and online

www.burtsbees.com

### DR. HAUSCHKA

**Body Silk powder**

This powder is talc free, instead using silk powder and rice starch to dry. It has pure fragrances derived from essential oils and plant extracts like English oak.

*Available:* at most natural markets

www.drhauschka.com

### JASON NATURAL

**Aloe Vera and Tea Tree body powders**

Corn flour is what gives these talc-free powders their drying efficacy. They also use natural fragrances from plant extracts and essential oils in scents like aloe vera and tea tree. Some contain paraben preservatives, so read the ingredient listings.

*Available:* at most natural markets

www.jason-natural.com

## PERSONAL LUBRICANTS

For intimate moments that need a little lube-love, reach for natural products for eco-friendly pleasure that's safe and healthy for your precious tissues.

Conventional lubricants are loaded with petroleum, synthetic fragrances and colorants, and very questionable preservatives.

I personally find pure organic plant oils to be perfect for the private quarters, though you can't use them with latex condoms, which can only handle water-based lubricants. Any unscented massage oil works wonders—pure coconut oil, avocado oil, and apricot kernel oil are luscious picks. (Blends that contain essential oils may be too strong for sensitive skin.) Try adding a bit of jojoba oil for more viscosity.

For some good, latex-safe, organic lovin', try any of these natural anointments.

## EMERITA

**Natural Lubricant with Vitamin E**

This all-natural, water-based formula is paraben free, has no mineral oils or petroleum distillates, and is latex safe.

*Available:* at natural markets and select drugstores and online

www.emerita.com

## FIREFLY ORGANICS

**Intimate Botanical Moisturizing Creme**

This lubricant is 100 percent natural, petroleum and paraben free, and nonsticky (no glycerin).

It's made with smooth, soothing aloe vera. And it's safe for use with silicone, rubber, and latex.

*Available:* at natural markets and online

www.fireflylubricant.com, www.organiclubricant.com

## O'MY PRODUCTS

**Natural Lubricant, O Pleasure Gel**

These water-based natural formulas are paraben free, have no artificial colors or flavorings, and are latex safe, so they can be used with condoms.

*Available:* at select natural markets and online

www.omyonline.com

## SYMPATHICAL

**Personal Lubricants**

The all-natural, water-based homeopathic formula is certified organic and made with plant-based ingredients; its peach and raspberry flavors are certified organic. Both are paraben free, glycerin free (nonsticky), and latex safe.

*Available:* online at www.luckyvitamin.com, www.lovemenaturally.com

www.sympathical.com

green option is to exercise your maternal instincts and go with natural baby wipes like those made by Seventh Generation and Tushie Wipes; they even come in nifty, convenient tote pouches.

**Feminine powders.** Powders are a nice idea if they don't contain talc. Talc may be contaminated with asbestos, which is obviously no good to breathe. With or without asbestos, talc is considered a car-cinogen[325]—conclusive studies also show that frequent use of talc-containing products below the waist increases women's risk for ovarian cancer.[326][327][328]

Enough said. Instead of making powder your poison, opt for au naturel products made with cornstarch or rice starch and plant-based fragrances, like the powders from Burt's Bees, Dr. Hauschka, and Jason Natural.

*For ladies who wish to really reduce their generation of feminine product waste, there are a few options—reusable menstrual cups and pads. They aren't for everyone and involve a bit of interacting with fluid flow, but for advanced believers, here are some options to consider.*

## REUSABLE MENSTRUAL CUPS

These mini cups, made of either natural latex rubber or silicone, are designed to catch and collect the menstrual flow—kind of like a structured, inverted diaphragm. They've been around in one form or another since the 1930s, though when a dear, savvy friend first told me about them with foot-stamping glee, I was skeptical. I was concerned the cups would leak or get lodged in place and generally be a bummer, but I must say, they are fantastic. They perform well for heavy or light flow, are low maintenance, don't leak, are choice for active lifestyles, and are really comfy (most gals say they don't feel the cup at all). Depending on the flow, they are designed to be inserted and emptied two to four times a day. A menstrual cup can hold a good fluid ounce, whereas the average woman's flow is about 3 to 4 ounces over her entire cycle. While involving a wee bit of slippery interaction, reusable cups may be the least wasteful things going on the feminine product front. The only maintenance required is washing the cup with warm, soapy water. They cost a little bit up front, but will pay for themselves in 3 to 4 months for most ladies. Technically, they last indefinitely and will prevent a mountain of landfill waste. Most even come with a lovely little cloth pouch for safekeeping. Ladies allergic to latex should choose a silicone cup. I have to say, these have changed my life. Here are some brands to look for.

## THE DIVACUP

Made of medical-grade silicone, it's available in two sizes.

**Available:** at some natural markets and online www.divacup.com

## THE KEEPER

This company makes two menstrual cups. The Keeper is made of natural gum rubber and is available in two sizes. The Keeper Mooncup is medical-grade silicone and one size.

**Available:** at some natural markets and online www.thekeeper.com

## REUSABLE CLOTH PADS

For ladies who want to take the next green step with pads, reusable cloth pads are an advanced eco-option. They aren't for everyone, but will prevent a palisade of rubbish in landfills. Reusable pads are typically made of soft cotton—organic, conventional, or recycled fabric from clothing industry end runs—and last 5 or so years (they should be soaked in cold water to prevent stains and then washed in warm water to keep clean). They're very ecological, a little messy, and may be more user-friendly to use at home or for overnight protection. Some have nifty wings with snaps to secure them in place and others have extra inserts for heavy-duty flow. FYI, darker-color pads stain less.

## GLADRAGS

These pads are winged with snaps to secure them to panties and made with 100 percent cotton (organic or nonorganic). They have a flannel cover and an absorbent, layered terry flannel insert. They're available as day pads, night pads, and panty liners, as well as kits with all three, and in colored nonorganic cotton and undyed and colored organic cotton.

**Available:** at some natural markets and online www.gladrags.com

## LUNAPADS

Lunapads are winged with snaps and come with an additional liner for extra protection. Certified organic cotton pads are available, as are nonorganic cotton fleece pads. They come in many styles, sizes, prints, and colors. Lunapanties, with built-in pads, are also available in three styles.

*Available:* at some natural markets and online

www.lunapads.com

## MANY MOONS

These are winged pads with snaps and liners without snaps. They're made with 100 percent cotton (organic and nonorganic) and have a flannel cover and an absorbent layered terry flannel liner. They come in many styles, sizes, and fabric patterns.

*Available:* at some natural markets and online

www.manymoonsalternatives.com

## PANDORA PADS

The pads are winged with snaps; the inserts have no snaps. Both are made of 100 percent cotton (organic or nonorganic). The flannel cover and absorbent, layered terry flannel insert are available in three sizes and in white, colors, or a floral pattern.

*Available:* at some natural markets and online

www.pandorapads.com

## RAWGANIQUE WASHABLE MENSTRUAL PADS

These winged pads with inserts are made of 100 percent certified organic, US-grown cotton. Many sizes for all flow levels; kits and combination packs are also available.

*Available:* online

www.rawganique.com

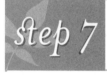

**step 7**      Cosmetics Worth Living For

Whether makeup is part of your daily ritual or saved for certain occasions, choosing clean, natural products will do your skin and the planet a world of good.

Cosmetic makeup has a long and scandalous history. At the zenith of the age of the pharaohs in ancient Egypt, aristocrats favored lead to paint their faces white, iron oxide as rouge, and dark kohl made from more neurotoxic lead for eyeliner. Lead remained the cosmetic foundation of choice for Greek women, though they opted for an ore of mercury for blushing their cheeks. Yikes. As the Common Era rolled around, Europeans caught the face-painting buzz by way of a substance called *ceruse*, a toxic mixture of lead and mercury that was haute couture for both men and women in France, though popular only with women in the rest of Europe. By the 17th century, it was determined to be toxic

*(continued on page 228)*

*True beauty may come from within, but pure products definitely help. Check out the fantastic spectrum of natural cosmetics available from these companies.*

## ANNEMARIE BORLIND

Annemarie Borlind of Germany offers an extensive line of natural makeup and cosmetics made with pure ingredients like jojoba oil, witch hazel, sage, and beeswax. Available in a wide range of classic and in-vogue colors and shades, all of the company's cosmetics contain natural preservatives and emulsifiers, are free of artificial colors and fragrances, and are not tested on animals.

*Available:* at select beauty stores and online

www.borlind.com

## AVEDA

Aveda is a leader in manufacturing high-performance plant-based products, namely hair products, but also a diverse range of cosmetic makeup. With its commitment to environmentally sound products and practices, Aveda has socially responsible fair-trade relationships with its ingredient sources and seeks out sustainable, renewable, or organic plant ingredients. Aveda has established a "Soil to Bottle" system to document sources and promote quality throughout the company's extensive supply chain. It uses only nonpetroleum minerals and GMO-free ingredients in all its products. Consistent with the "Cradle to Cradle" approach to design principles, Aveda uses postconsumer recycled content and is an EPA Green Power Partner, using 100 percent certified wind power in its manufacturing. The company is even pursuing the development of biodegradable and completely recyclable or reusable packaging for its emerging products. While some Aveda cosmetics have long lists of ingredients, some of which are questionable, Aveda is a good company to look to for a full range of makeup needs.

*Available:* at Aveda salons and retail stores and select salons and online

www.aveda.com

## BURT'S BEES

Burt's Bees is all about using ingredients from nature, and even the company's cosmetic formulations reflect that. It uses all natural ingredients like plant oils and waxes, beeswax, and mineral colors; no synthetic preservatives, fragrances, or colorants are used in any of these lovely products.

*Available:* at most natural markets and online

www.burtsbees.com

## DR. HAUSCHKA

At the core of Dr. Hauschka products is a profound respect for the planet and its inhabitants. Deeply commited to encouraging sustainable agriculture through organic, biodynamic, and ecologically sound practices and production methods, the company's cosmetics contain only plant- and mineral-based ingredients and botanical preservatives. No chemical additives, fragrances, or colorants are used. Dr. Hauschka products are "certified natural," meeting the highest European standards and selective criteria for purity. *Note:* Talc is used in a number of products.

*Available:* at most natural markets and online

www.drhauschka.com

## ECCO BELLA

Ecco Bella offers a lovely collection of cosmetics made with minerals and flower waxes. With a principle of formulating products using gentle, natural ingredients that are beneficial to the skin, Ecco Bella tests its goods on humans, never on animals. The cosmetics contain no talc and most are preservative free.

*Available:* at natural markets and online

www.eccobella.com

## ÉMINENCE ORGANICS

Éminence Organics makes one of the most innovative sun protection makeup powders with the purest ingredients. Suitable for all skin types, SPF 30 Sun Defense Minerals is housed in a nifty pump tube with a retractable brush. Loaded with bioflavonoids and vitamins A, C, and E, this water-resistant powder serves as a bronzer or finishing powder. It's available in six tones, and I can't live without it.

*Available:* at select spas and salons and online

www.eminenceorganics.com

## JANE IREDALE

Jane Iredale formulates state-of-the-art natural mineral cosmetics in an epic range of products that have a vast array of shades. With their highly sophisticated blend of micronized minerals and natural pigments, Jane Iredale cosmetics don't block pores and are said to be beneficial to the skin, allowing it to breathe and function normally while protecting it from environmental pollutants. All products pose virtually no allergy risk and are tested for skin sensitivity. With broad-spectrum UV-B and UV-A SPF protection, these products are naturally anti-inflammatory and wear extremely well, with long-lasting staying power and water resistance. The minerals used in Jane Iredale cosmetics are inert by nature, so they don't support bacterial growth and therefore require no synthetic preservatives. I must say, this line is revolutionary.

*Available:* at select beauty shops, spas, and salons and online

www.janeiredale.com

## KISS MY FACE

Kiss My Face makes a fantastic tinted moisturizer that gives you SPF protection from UV-A and UV-B rays. Available in six tones, the formulas are sheer, blend evenly and beautifully, and are oil free. The tints are made with minerals, not artificial dyes, and they don't contain artificial fragrances.

*Available:* at most natural markets and online

www.kissmyface.com

## KORRES

Korres provides an array of natural cosmetics that are friendly to and compatible with different types of skin. Made with natural emulsifiers and vegetable oils and fortified with botanicals, vitamins, and antioxidants, all Korres color products are free of petroleum derivatives, propylene glycol, and ethanolamines. Korres's wide selection of products and colors is suitable for a broad range of uses.

*Available:* at select natural markets, spas, and Korres stores and online

www.korres.com

## MIESSENCE

Miessence is part of the ONE Group (Organic and Natural Enterprise Group), which offers an innovative, comprensive range of products, including cosmetics, that are pure and effective and operates within an ethical and ecological business model. Claiming to be the world's first internationally certified organic line of cosmetics, Miessence uses independently certified food-grade ingredients. The company's cosmetics contain skin-beneficial organic ingredients made from plants, minerals, vitamins, and nutrients. Miessence does not use synthetic or chemical ingredients, emulsifiers, colorants, fragrances, or preservatives. The ONE Group is carbon neutral, offsetting the emissions generated by manufacturing and shipping through tree-planting programs.

*Available:* at natural markets, select stores, spas, and salons and online

www.miessenceproducts.com

*(continued)*

## MINERAL FUSION COSMETICS

Mineral Fusion offers a full range of mineral cosmetics that are free of artificial and chemical colorants and dyes and fortified with vitamins, minerals, and antioxidants to give you radiant skin. With their skin-friendly, moisture-balancing formulas, Mineral Fusion's cosmetics allow the skin to breathe and function normally. The company uses a quartet of unique antioxidant ingredients to protect skin against environmental conditions and stresses, and it features paraben-free formulations.

*Available:* at Whole Foods and select natural markets and online

www.mineralfusioncosmetics.com

## NVEY ECO

Nvey Eco organic makeup is where luxury and nature meet. The company's formulas are created using harmonious plant and mineral ingredients that are blended with botanical extracts, antioxidants, fortifying plant oils, vitamins, and nutrients to make pure, high-performance cosmetics in a broad range of colors and mediums. Nvey Eco makeup meets strict certified organic standards for ingredients, processing, and manufacturing. All of the company's products are paraben and preservative free and contain no SLS, propylene glycol, talc, or petroleum-based ingredients. It's naturally beautiful!

*Available:* at select stores and online

www.econveybeauty.com

## ZIA NATURAL SKINCARE

Zia Natural Skincare formulates sheer, natural-looking makeup that is made with mineral pigments—no artificial colorants are used. Zia's natural foundation is available in 10 shades and its pressed compact powder comes in six shades to match a wide variety of skin tones.

*Available:* at most natural markets and online

www.zianatural.com

and linked with a slew of serious problems including facial tremors, paralysis, and even death. Ceruse was snuffed out before European immigrants came to America, where whitewash rubbed from walls was favored for foundation, dust from red bricks emphasized cheekbones, and soot from burned matches or cork served as eye makeup.

While we have come a long way since using lead as a concealing foundation, lead kohl is still used today, and other ingredients are cause for equal levels of concern.

The crazy fact is that very few regulations exist for makeup formulas. It's crazy because facial skin is some of the most delicate and permeable skin on our bodies, and makeup is typically worn for hours on end. The chemicals, dyes, colorants, fragrances, and preservatives found in conventional cosmetics are seriously disturbing. Think about the vulnerable beauty of an eyeball, and about applying heavy-metal-laden products right at the edge of it, and you've got grounds for immediate evaluation.

Entirely too many synthetic and chemical ingredients are commonly found in cosmetics to address them all in one chapter of a book this size. We're talking thousands and thousands—a mind-boggling amount. In fact, if you read the ingredient list on a tube of most name-brand mascaras or concealers, you will likely need to bust out a magnifying glass because the print is so small and the list so extensive. It's not uncommon to find three- or four-dozen ingredients in one product alone.

You will also likely need to consult a chemical textbook to look up ingredients like triethanolamine, which works as an emollient and pH adjuster, but is likely to be contaminated with cancer-causing nitrosamines,[329] [330] is harmful to absorb through the skin,[331] may cause necrosis of the skin,[332] and may cause liver and kidney damage.[333] Here's another example: imidazolidinyl urea—a formaldehyde-releasing preservative[334] that may be toxic to the skin and cells,[335] cause allergies and contact dermatitis, sensitize the skin[336] and have mutagenic potential[337]—is used in facial powders, eye shadows, and mascaras. Goodness.

Four broad groupings of ingredients are found in conventional makeup and cosmetics products: the carrier (the bulk of the thing), colorants or dyes, fragrances (which are pervasive), and last, but certainly not least, preservatives.

As with all else, the river of ingredients diverges into either a synthetic (chemical) or natural (plant or mineral based) tributary. Now, not all natural and synthetic ingredients are respectively created equal—there's definitely a sliding scale. For instance, heavy metals like lead and mercury are natural—they are found in nature. But neither is advisable to apply near your eyes, or anywhere else.

As a kid, I was smitten with the theater. My dad was a member of a community theater group that captivated my every sense—the sets, the lights, the stage, the costumes, props, and makeup. I was a tomboy, but the theater stirred an excitement that I couldn't have ignored if I tried. I can still smell with somewhat nostalgic nausea the pancake makeup in the dressing rooms—that makeup wouldn't melt off even during fancy dance numbers performed in heavy costume under white-hot spotlights.

Makeup and cosmetics are very personal things.

To avoid lawsuits from the cosmetic companies, I will not name names. I will, however, strongly encourage—insist, really—you to simply take a look at the ingredient lists and consider if you want to apply that stuff to your beautiful face, eyelids, and lashes. Think about your reproductive organs, kidneys, liver, and the luscious blood pumping through your veins. Ask yourself how important all of it is. Is it necessary to use mascara that won't run even if you are caught in a monsoon? If it contains coal tar, liquid plastic, or mercury and it does run into your eyes, how do you feel about that? Or consider the lipstick or lip gloss that's likely made from petroleum and colored with synthetic dyes. How do you feel about eating it slowly day after day? What's the long-term effect of all of it?

Let it suffice to say that there's no need to walk around with a bare face—there's a bouquet of fabulous, natural cosmetics that perform fantastically and can meet every nuance and need in the makeup arena. While I don't think I am alone in thinking that less is more when it comes to makeup, choosing natural cosmetics is an absolute essential for long-term beauty.

# 6 Steps to Eco-Fresh Laundry

**Pure** *adjective*

**1b:** free from harshness or roughness and being in tune; **3a(1):** free from what vitiates, weaken, or pollutes (*Merriam-Webster's Collegiate Dictionary*)

**Free** *adjective*

**2a:** not determined by anything beyond its own nature or being; choosing or capable of choosing for itself (*Merriam-Webster's Collegiate Dictionary*)

Laundry is a constant chore. Just when the hamper is empty and all is clean, dry, and folded or hung, more clothes in need of laundering miraculously appear. But do it we must, and often, at that.

Every year, Americans wash about 35 billion pounds of laundry. That's a huge heap—about 50 pounds a week for every household—and it has a giant environmental impact. Just how big an effect depends on how wise and green we choose to be. The two main variables to consider if you're going to be green with eco-fresh laundry are laundry products and energy use.

Washers and dryers are ravenous consumers of energy. And most laundry rooms are stocked with a gaggle of products loaded with petrochemicals and toxic, synthetic compounds that are hazardous to humans and leave ecological disaster in their wake. So what can we do to keep our clothes and our planet clean? Plenty!

This chapter opens the laundry room door to five easy, effective steps you can take to get eco-fresh laundry. You'll save time and money, improve your health, and mind the health of the planet at large in the process.

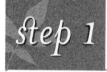 **step 1** Eco-Friendly Detergent

In stores across the country, dozens of laundry detergents beam at you with brightly colored bottles and boxes that make bold promises of spring-fresh smells and ultra-super action. While they may look like a domestic dream for achieving fluffy and spotless results, the reality is that most conventional laundry products are a stew of hazardous and toxic chemicals that create an ecological nightmare. This kind of detergent is not a good deal, even if it's on sale. But don't put your head in the washer on high spin. If you look in the right places, even the shelves of your local supermarket have nontoxic, eco-friendly laundry detergents. They're the first step to getting green, clean laundry.

Let's look at what a detergent is and does. Then, choosing a green product to get the job done will be a snap.

## The Difference Between Soap and Detergent

Soap and detergent are kindred products with distinctive differences. Both are surfactants (which is a nifty abbreviation for *surface-active agents*). My dad always says that soap and detergent make water wetter so it works better. It's true. Surfactants reduce the surface tension of water so it can spread out beneath dirt and grime to slough them off.

The difference between soap and detergent is how they are made. Before World War II and the petrochemical revolution, soap was soap and all of it was rendered from natural materials—natural oils, in fact. During the war, natural oils became expensive and scarce. In waltzed cheap, readily available petroleum and modern chemicals, and, with a little manipulation, synthetic soap and detergent were born. Newfangled detergent was embraced with great enthusiasm because it not only worked wonders to wash away grime, it didn't leave clothing with an unsightly residue that would make it stiff and eventually gray. Detergent was a boon! Detergent still works the same way today: Unlike soap, which reacts with the minerals in water (namely, minerals like calcium and magnesium found in "hard" water) and leaves an insoluble film, aka soap scum, most detergents don't react with those minerals. Since the vast majority of Americans have hard water, it's a problem that detergent seems to effortlessly solve.

Here's the thing, though: synthetic detergents are a nightmare for the environment. Petrochemical surfactants in synthetic detergents are a vengeful bunch; they cause imbalances in aquatic ecosystems, wreak havoc at large, and are reluctant to go away. Those aren't exactly the qualities you want in an invited houseguest, and the insult and injury don't stop there. Conventional detergents may also contain a nasty covey of vaguely disclosed toxic ingredients like bleaches, synthetic whiteners and brighteners, and artificial perfumes and fragrances. But behold! There are green options!

## What Is Eco-Friendly Detergent?

Green detergents are made from natural (that is, plant based) materials that readily biodegrade. The surfactants in natural laundry products are derived from materials like vegetable oils instead of from petroleum. This is big. Natural surfactants do their job effectively, and then quickly and quietly break down into harmless compounds without leaving persistent, low-grade ecological mayhem in their wake. Everybody wins.

## Powder or Liquid Detergent?

Which is better? Powder and liquid detergents work the same way. The only difference is the texture, and they work equally well.

**Powder Pros**

- Less detergent is required, because the active ingredients have not been dissolved into liquid form
- Lower cost per load
- Less packaging, because it usually comes in a cardboard box rather than in a thick plastic jug with a top or dispenser

### SAVING THE PLANET ONE LOAD AT A TIME

According to the Seventh Generation company, if every American replaced just *one* 1-gallon bottle of petroleum-based liquid laundry detergent with a vegetable-based product, it would save more than 250,000 barrels of oil—enough to heat and cool close to 15,000 homes for a year!

If every American replaced just *1 pound* of petroleum-based powdered laundry detergent with a vegetable-based detergent, it would save more than 150,000 barrels of oil, enough to heat and cool almost 9,000 homes for a year![1]

# COMMON INGREDIENT HAZARDS:
## LAUNDRY DETERGENTS

*Here is a typical list of ingredients you are likely to find in most conventional laundry detergents: cleaning agents or anionic and nonionic surfactants; buffering agent; stabilizer; brightening agent or optical brightener; and fragrance. If you are like me and persistently investigate, it becomes quite clear that many of the common ingredients are hazardous. Read on for more disclosure.*

**Linear alkyl sodium sulfonates.** These surfactants (sometimes listed as *anionic surfactants*) are contact irritants of the skin as well as lung and eye irritants, especially when in powdered detergents. Nonbiodegradable, they are very slow to break down. They're also toxic during manufacture because they release benzene (a carcinogen and reproductive toxin).

**Alkyl phenols, nonylphenols, nonylphenol ethoxylate.** These surfactants are hormone disrupters, bioaccumulative,[2] and potentially toxic.[3] They are persistent, not biodegradable, in nature; some slowly degrade into even more toxic compounds.

**Ethanolamines (triethanolamine, diethanolamine).** These are contact irritants of the skin, and may cause allergies; they're also lung and eye irritants (especially in powdered detergents). They are corrosive to tissues and carcinogenic. They absorb through the skin,[4] and may cause central nervous system depression[5] and liver and kidney damage.[6] They react with nitrates (which are sometimes used, but not disclosed, as preservatives) to form carcinogenic compounds.

**Sodium silicate.** This contact irritant of the skin may cause allergies and is a lung and eye irritant[7] (especially in powdered detergents). Corrosive to tissues,[8] it is not biodegradable.[9]

**Sodium sulfate.** This contact irritant of the skin may cause allergies. It is also a severe lung irritant and may cause asthma attacks.[10] It is corrosive to tissues.[11] Moderately persistent in the environment, it is slow to biodegrade.[12]

**Sodium hypochlorite.** This contact irritant of the skin is also a severe eye and lung irritant.[13] It is corrosive to tissues and can release toxic and corrosive chlorine gas.[14] It damages the liver, kidneys, blood, heart, and immune and respiratory systems and is especially hazardous to people with asthma or heart conditions.[15] It reacts with organic compounds in the environment to form toxic organochlorines like dioxins,[16] harms plant life, and is acutely toxic to aquatic life.[17] The Environmental Protection Agency (EPA) classifies it as Toxicity Category I, the highest degree of toxicity.[18]

**Sodium dodecylbenzene sulfonate.** Found in heavy-duty detergents, this compound is very hazardous to the eyes and skin[19] and may be toxic to the lungs, nervous system, and mucous membranes.[20] Its products of degradation are toxic in the environment.[21]

**Triethylene glycol.** Repeated exposure to this compound may cause central nervous system depression and liver damage.[22] It can leach into groundwater, where it will biodegrade but is toxic to aquatic life.[23]

**Trisodium nitrilotriacetate.** This known carcinogen[24] [25] [26] is an eye and skin irritant.[27] It also harms aquatic life.[28]

# What in the World Are Optical Brighteners?

Optical brighteners are a broad classification of newfangled chemicals found in a lot of conventional laundry detergents these days. They are also called *optical bleaches*, *whitening agents*, or *fluorescent whitening agents*, and they are all part of the same chemical bunch. They do just what they say they do and then some (which is not so good).

Optical brighteners are a group of colorless fluorescent chemicals that convert ultraviolet light into visible light, making freshly laundered clothes look "whiter" via an optical illusion. It's really just a cheap trick and doesn't improve the performance of the product or make clothes cleaner. What these brighteners do after being rinsed out is cause a mess in the ecosystem because they don't biodegrade for a long, long time. This posse of compounds is especially toxic to fish and wildlife and has a wicked propensity to cause bacterial mutations. They also have a tendency to cause contact allergic skin reactions, especially on skin that is later exposed to the sun.[29] Not nice. Unfortunately, a lot of optical brighteners in popular products are listed under trade names, so you won't know what they are without savvy Sherlock skills.

To be safe, avoid any conventional product whose label mentions a "brightening agent," "optical brightener," or other names and words that look suspicious (and are) and whose purpose in the product is not explained. Fortunately, most natural products that are biodegradable just don't include this kind of stuff. (Obviously, because they would no longer be biodegradable if they did.) If you long for whiter whites naturally, check out "Step 2: Nontoxic Stain Removal," on page 248, for information on oxygen bleach.

## Liquid Pros

- Already dissolved, so less risk of residue left on clothing
- Works well in cold water
- Good for dark clothes, because powdery residue shows better on dark fabrics

## Powder Detergent Tips

- **Dissolve first.** To avoid detergent residue (especially on dark fabrics), dissolve the detergent in the washing water first. Add powder detergent to the machine and let the water run for a few minutes—using warm water will help it dissolve more quickly, but it does eat up energy—then add clothing and continue filling. Carry on!
- **Use less detergent.** Don't overdo it. Using more detergent doesn't get clothes cleaner (pretreating stains does), it just requires more rinsing to remove it and prevent residue.

## GREEN TIPS for Washing and Drying Laundry

Here are some simple, smart ways to be greener when you do laundry.

## For Washing

- **CHOOSE YOUR WATER TEMPERATURE WISELY.** Hot water does not necessarily clean clothes better than warm water. That's good news, because 85 to 90 percent of the energy consumed in washing clothes is used to heat the water.[30] Hot water is also tough on clothes—it wears and tears them more quickly and makes colors fade faster. The biggest determinant of energy consumption and the overall environmental impact of doing laundry is the temperature of the washing and rinsing water.[31] Using warm instead of hot water for just two loads a week will prevent a huge amount of pollution—about 500 pounds a year for electric water heaters or 150 pounds for gas water heaters! Always rinse with cold—period.

- **SORT LAUNDRY SENSIBLY.** Separate lights, darks, and delicates. Sorting will simply help your clothes live longer, a long-term green choice. Closing zippers and buttons is also a smart move to extend the life of your threads.

- **PRETREAT STAINS.** It's a basic technique that works wonders (see "Step 2: Nontoxic Stain Removal" on page 248.

- **WASH FULL LOADS, BUT DON'T OVERLOAD.** It will save time, energy, and money. A washing machine uses the same amount of energy regardless of how full it is. A full load uses more water than a small load, but still less than two small loads. However, an overfilled machine won't perform well and usually requires longer wash and rinse cycles.

- **SELECT THE PROPER WATER LEVEL.** When washing a load that isn't full, set the water level for a small or medium load.

- **DISTRIBUTE ITEMS EVENLY AROUND THE WASH BASKET.** This gives you the most effective action in the shortest wash and rinse cycles.

- **USE LESS DETERGENT.** Using more detergent does not get clothes cleaner (I promise you!), it just requires more rinsing. Less detergent also means less residue left on clothing, which will grant it a longer life.

- **USE A SHORTER WASH CYCLE.** Detergents do all they are capable of in the first 10 minutes. After that, your clothes are just agitating in dirty water. It seems like just a small waste of energy, but over time it adds up.

## For Drying

Save energy, money, and time using your clothes dryer wisely with these smart green tips.

- **USE AN EXTRA SPIN CYCLE IN THE WASHING MACHINE FOR HEAVY MATERIALS.** Heavy stuff like towels will benefit when as much water as possible is centrifuged out. They'll need less time in the dryer.

# "Fresh" Synthetic Fragrances

The promise of springtime-fresh-smelling laundry may elicit nostalgic ideas of a pure and simple life, but if that smell were brewed up and put in a bottle, it could be downright dangerous for humans and the environment. Synthetic fragrances are petrochemicals, derived from petroleum. These kinds of chemicals have a nasty habit of contaminating water and are viciously toxic to fish and wildlife.[32][33] To add insult to injury, because they don't biodegrade, they don't go away for a very long time. They just keep on being toxic and accumulating and contaminating, on, and on, and on.

Synthetic fragrances can also be irritants for humans, especially of our skin and eyes. Constant contact (like you have with your clothes) may bring on allergic reactions and may also lead to a greater overall chemical sensitivity. That's no fun.

The safest bet is to avoid products with chemically derived scents. This doesn't mean you have to avoid smells altogether. Natural and nontoxic products can smell good too, and when you use them you don't have to get a rash and destroy the planet's coral reefs at the same time. A bunch of great biode-gradable detergents have delightful smells. Their scents are simply derived from natural (i.e., plant) sources. They're good stuff, so look for them.

- **CLEAN THE LINT SCREEN EVERY TIME.** This basic, effective trick maximizes airflow for optimal drying action.

- **HANG DRY AS MUCH AS POSSIBLE.** Lightweight fabrics, like T-shirts and underwear, dry quickly enough to hang. Colors and fabrics hold up longer when not subjected to tumbling heat.

- **DRY ITEMS OF SIMILAR WEIGHT TOGETHER,** so everything is dry at the same time. Heavier materials take longer, so don't waste the energy on lightweights that dry quickly.

- **THROW IN A BIG DRY ITEM,** like a towel, to absorb and distribute moisture for quicker drying time.

- **DON'T ADD WET STUFF TO A PARTIALLY DRY LOAD.** It will slow down drying and waste energy.

- **DRY TWO LOADS IN A ROW** to take advantage of the heat (energy) still in the dryer.

- **DRY FULL LOADS, BUT DON'T OVER-LOAD.** It takes the same amount of energy to run the dryer regardless of how much is in it. Air should be able to circulate easily around the clothes.

- **DON'T OVERDRY.** Excessive drying is a waste of energy and is tough on mate-rial. Set the timer for a shorter cycle. You can always run it longer if needed.

- **SET THE MOISTURE SENSOR.** Most machines have a moisture sensor that reads "less dry" or "more dry"; use it! Take clothes out when they are just slightly damp to hang them to dry and keep them from wrinkling (this is espe-cially good for cotton).

- **USE THE PERMANENT PRESS OR COOL-DOWN CYCLE.** Take advantage of the residual heat in the dryer by using a cool-air cycle at the end. It will also help prevent wrinkles—less ironing, more bettah.

- **CHECK THE OUTSIDE VENT REGULARLY.** Maximize the action and life of your dryer by keeping the outside vent clean and clear of lint and debris. (This is also a good safety measure to prevent fires.)

## Color-Saving Tips

Faded clothing is a bummer. Here are a few ways to keep colors perky as long as possible.

- **Separate light and dark colors.** This is basic and still true, especially the first time clothing is washed.

- **Brighten colors with salt.** Minerals in hard water (which most of us have) cause colored clothing to fade to dull and dingy. Add a couple of pinches of ordinary table salt along with the detergent, let the water run for a few minutes to dissolve it, then add clothing. Colors will come out brighter!

- **Set dark colors with salt and cold water at their first washing.** Salt helps dyes set, keeping them from bleeding. Add ½ cup salt along with the detergent to the first wash, let the water run for a few minutes to dissolve it, then add clothing.

- **Use cold water to preserve colors.** Warm and hot water cause colors to bleed and fade more quickly

- **Turn dark clothing inside out.** You'll get less wear and tear on the outside surface and color that way. It also keeps lint from other clothing from adhering to the outside. This technique is especially effective in the dryer.

- **Hang dry colored clothes.** The dryer's high temperature wears fabrics and fades colors quickly, so dry clothes on a clothesline or folding rack when you can.

## Switch from Hot to Warm or Cold

About 90 percent of the energy used to wash a load of laundry is for heating the water.

Using warm water instead of hot to wash just two loads of laundry a week over a year will save 500 pounds of carbon dioxide that an electric water heater would produce or 150 pounds of $CO_2$ that a gas heater would produce.[34]

*For clean, green laundry, look for these biodegradable detergents that are free from phosphates, and chemical and synthetic ingredients.*

## BIOKLEEN

### Laundry Liquid
32 ounces (32 loads), 64 ounces (64 loads), 5 gallons

This very concentrated (1 ounce for a full load) product has no irritating residue, so it's great for people with sensitive skin or allergies. It's good for hand-washables and delicates, and its low sudsing makes it suitable for front-loading machines.

### Laundry Powder
5 pounds (50 loads), 10 pounds (100 loads), 50 pounds (500 loads)

A concentrated (¼ cup for a full load) powder, it contains color-safe oxygen bleach and grapefruit seed extract. It works well in cold and hard water, leaving no residue or water deposits (minerals in the water that are deposited on clothing). It has only active ingredients—no fillers or additives. It's low sudsing, so it's suitable for front-loading machines.

### Premium Laundry Powder
5 pounds (54 loads), 50 pounds (540 loads)

This extra-strength cleaning powder contains color-safe oxygen bleach, natural enzymes, and grapefruit seed extract. It works well in cold and hard water, leaving no residue or water deposits. Low sudsing means it's suitable for front-loading machines.

All Biokleen products are nontoxic and biodegradable.

*Available:* at natural markets and online

www.biokleenhome.com

## CALDREA

### Laundry Detergent
64 fluid ounces (32 loads)

This liquid laundry detergent is mild, yet highly effective, containing powerful plant-derived surfactants and borax to get your whites white and colors bright. It's biodegradable and contains no phosphates. With a special formulation of essential oils designed to linger in your clothing longer, this detergent smells so delicious, it will make you want to wash your clothes as often as possible. In six enticing fragrances such as Sweet Pea, Citrus Mint Ylang Ylang, and Basil Blue Sage.

*Available:* in select home stores such as Sur la Table, Smith & Hawkin, and online

www.caldrea.com

## CITRA-SOLV

### Ultra Citra-Suds
### Concentrated Laundry Detergent
Liquid: 50 ounces (25 loads)
Powder: 7 pounds (42 loads)

The powder contains color-safe oxygen bleach and non–animal-derived enzymes. Biodegradable and with no artificial perfumes or dyes, these detergents use real citrus extract.

*Available:* at some natural markets and online

www.citra-solv.com

## COUNTRY SAVE

### Liquid Laundry Detergent
100 ounces (50 loads)

This concentrated (2 ounces for a full load) detergent has a natural fragrance and no enzymes or optical brighteners.

### Powdered Laundry Detergent
5 pounds (40 loads), 10 pounds (80 loads)

The formula was 25 years in the making, and it includes no fragrances. It won't leave residue on clothes, so it's good for use with cold and hard water and also for people with sensitive skin. Low sudsing makes it suitable for high-efficiency (HE) and front-loading machines. The box is made from recycled and postconsumer recycled cardboard.

All products are nontoxic and biodegradable and have no dyes or artificial fragrances.

*Available:* at natural markets and online

www.countrysave.com

## EARTH FRIENDLY PRODUCTS

### Baby Laundry Soap
53 ounces (26 loads), 128 ounces (64 loads), 5 gallons (320 loads)

This liquid is hypoallergenic and good for sensitive skin. It's suitable for hand washing silk, wool, and delicates, and its pure fragrance comes from the essential oils of chamomile and lavender.

### Ecos Free and Clear Liquid Laundry Detergent
53 ounces (26 loads), 128 ounces (64 loads), 5 gallons (320 loads)

A concentrated (2 ounces for a full load) liquid, it contains no fragrances, optical brighteners, or dyes. It's low sudsing, so it's suitable for front-loading machines.

### Ecos Liquid Laundry Detergent
53 ounces (26 loads), 128 ounces (64 loads), 5 gallons (320 loads)

This concentrated (2 ounces for a full load) detergent includes a soy-based fabric softening agent and a cellulose-based optical brightener. It comes in three natural, plant-based scents: Magnolia and Lilies, Lavender, and Lemongrass. It's low sudsing, so it's suitable for front-loading machines.

### Ecos Powder Laundry Detergent
54 ounces (25 loads)

This is a concentrated, fragrance-free detergent that's suitable for front-loading machines.

All products are nontoxic, plant based, and biodegradable.

***Available:*** at natural markets and online
www.ecos.com

## ECOVER LAUNDRY DETERGENT

### Ecological Laundry Powder
3 pounds (19 loads), 6 pounds (37 loads)

This powder is good for cold and hard water, leaving no residue. The carton is made of 95 percent recycled cardboard.

### Ultra Laundry Wash
51 ounces (20 loads), 100 ounces (40 loads)

This liquid has a plant-based fragrance.

All products are biodegradable, nontoxic, and plant based. Over 20 years, Ecover's scientists have replaced the harsh petrochemical ingredients used in conventional detergents without sacrificing performance.

***Available:*** at natural markets and online
www.ecover.com

## METHOD

### Laundry Detergent
32 ounces (32 loads)

This biodegradable, nontoxic, highly concentrated (1 ounce for a full load) liquid contains active enzymes. It's formulated for use in standard and HE washers and comes in Morning Bloom, Sweet Water, and Free and Clear scents, as well as a Lullaby Scent baby variety.

***Available:*** at many grocery stores and chain stores and online
www.methodhome.com

## MOUNTAIN GREEN

### 3X Concentrate Refill
20-ounce pouch of concentrate (20 loads)

It's available in Free and Clear (fragrance free), Original Citrus, Free and Clear Baby (for sensitive skin, fragrance free), and Ultra Baby (for sensitive skin, with fragrances from essential oils).

Biodegradable, nontoxic, and plant based, this liquid detergent has no dyes or artificial fragrances.

***Available:*** at natural markets and online
www.mountaingreen.biz

## MRS. MEYER'S CLEAN DAY

### Laundry Detergent
64 ounces (32 loads)

Biodegradable, nontoxic, plant based, and concentrated, this detergent contains natural enzymes, but no artificial fragrances or dyes. Instead, the fragrances in its four varieties are

*(continued)*

derived from the essential oils of, among others, geranium, lavender, and lemon verbena.

*Available:* at natural markets and online

www.mrsmeyers.com

## NATURALLY YOURS

### Liquid Laundry Detergent

32 ounces (32 loads), 1 gallon (128 loads)

Biodegradable, nontoxic, and plant based, this product is highly concentrated (1 ounce for a full load). The bottle's labels and literature are made from postconsumer recycled paper and printed with soy-based inks.

*Available:* at some natural markets and online

www.naturallyyoursclean.com

## SEVENTH GENERATION

### Natural Liquid Laundry 2X Concentrate

50 ounces (32 loads)

This low-sudsing formulation comes in Blue Eucalyptus and Lavender, White Flower and Bergamot Citrus, and Free and Clear varieties.

### Liquid Laundry Detergent

50 ounces (16 loads)

Unscented Delicate Care and Baby varieties are available.

### Laundry Powder

48 ounces (18 loads), 112 ounces (42 loads)

Free and Clear or Natural Citrus Scent is available. These powders contain color-safe oxygen bleach and non–animal-derived enzymes. Good for cold and hard water, they'll leave no residue.

All of these detergents are biodegradable, nontoxic, and contain no chlorine, phosphates, optical brighteners, artificial fragrances, or dyes. Seventh Generation discloses all ingredients.

*Available:* at many grocery stores and natural markets and online

www.seventhgeneration.com

# What's the Deal with Phosphates?

Phosphates are becoming more widely known as an ingredient on the eco no-no list. There is a huge effort (by state governments, even) to restrict or ban them altogether. In the right context, phosphates are fine—and even good. Phosphates are derived from phosphorus, a naturally occurring mineral that is essential for the maintenance of all plant life. Plants *love* phosphorus. So what's all the fuss? Too much of a good thing is still too much.

Phosphates have been hugely popular in detergents as water-softening agents (to keep the detergent from leaving scum all over everything). Phosphates are cheap, and they make detergents work better. Phosphates even have nifty deflocculating action, which means that they keep dirt and grime from settling back on the clothing during washing. Sounds good, right? Phosphates are even relatively nontoxic to humans and the environment. So what's the deal? Well, here's the thing. Plants, including algae, are just crazy for phosphates. They can't get enough of them. Feed algae phosphates and they will thrive and explosively bloom all over the place, in lakes, rivers, and oceans, throwing the whole system out of whack. Given a chance, algae will eat up all of the oxygen in the water, leaving nothing for other aquatic creatures, which will then suffocate and die. The process is called *eutrophication* and it is a *major* problem in waterways worldwide. No coral reefs, no fish, no food

# Boost Laundry Detergent with Baking Soda

Baking soda creates a better pH level in the wash, getting clothes cleaner, fresher, brighter, and better deodorized. Add ½ cup baking soda along with your laundry detergent to each load of laundry.

means collapse of the aquatic ecology and, eventually, worldwide disaster.

The good news is that phosphates are being phased out. Even major laundry detergent manufacturers are finding alternatives. That's how big a problem phosphates have become. However, something else must take the place of the crummy phosphates. After all, a detergent requires some sort of surfactant to actually *be* a detergent. The industry has come up with synthetic phosphate substitutes, for better or for worse. The question is, what's the tradeoff?

The new wave of synthetic phosphate substitutes raises a lot of questions because they are so new that it's hard to say what kind of long-term impact they will have. The industry claims they are relatively nontoxic and don't cause explosive growth of aquatic plants. That's good. But guess what they are made of? Petroleum. That means they take a long time to biodegrade. That's not good. Inevitably, this stuff causes problems because it sticks around for so long and causes a mess. To be safe, it is best to avoid synthetic detergents, period. Here are four phosphate substitutes to look out for.

**Polycarboxylates.** Among the newer phosphate alternatives, these compounds are, chemically, a lot like plastic and acrylic compounds. Initial tests show that they are nontoxic, but they haven't been around long enough to register their effects on human and environmental health. Made from petroleum, they not biodegradable.

**Ethylenediamine tetraacetic acid (EDTA).** Used to reduce minerals in hard water and as a foaming stabilizer, this synthetic phosphate alternative does not readily biodegrade, but it does do something uniquely troublesome. Like all detergents, EDTA ends up in the aquatic ecosystem, where it has a special ability to free up toxic heavy metals (like mercury) and reintroduce them into the environment (namely, the food chain).

**Alkyl phenoxy polyethoxy ethanol.** This phenol takes a long time to biodegrade, and breaks down into even more toxic compounds in the ecosystem (see "Common Ingredient Hazards: Laundry Detergents" on page 233 for the dastardly details).

**Nonylphenol ethoxylate.** This is another phenol that bioaccumulates and doesn't biodegrade in a hurry (see "Common Ingredient Hazards: Laundry Detergents" on page 233).

If you like your white clothes to be pure, snowy bright but don't want to expose yourself and your family to the dangers of household chlorine bleach, there is one simple choice: oxygen bleach.

Household bleach is a type of chlorine (sodium hypochlorite, to be exact) and it's hugely popular in the laundry room for whitening clothes and removing stains, as well as elsewhere in the house as a cleaner and disinfectant. But it's actually dangerous stuff. Another place where it's perennially popular is at poison control centers, where they field many calls about it.

## What Is Chlorine Bleach, Anyway?

Chlorine is a popular chemical agent that sits at #17 on the periodic table of elements. It's a yellow-green gas that is highly reactive and notoriously toxic. The chemical industry forces chlorine into liquid or powdered form, rendering it into bleach as we know it, because it is none too convenient to go about whitening your undershirts with a gaseous substance. However, chlorine is much happier and more stable as a gas, which is a big part of the problem that we will get to in a minute.

Chlorine is very strong stuff. With a pH of 11, household bleach (sodium hypochlorite) is extremely basic, or alkaline (as opposed to acidic). It's a benchmark in chemistry because it is the strongest base that can exist in a water solution without wreaking serious chemical havoc.

It is also extremely reactive, which is why it does what it does. Chlorine bleach works on stains by oxidizing them (via chlorine radicals) and breaking them down so they will separate from the fabric. Presto, clean clothes! But the reactions don't stop there.

## Chlorine at Large

Chlorine bleach also reacts with all kinds of materials for a multitude of horrific results—especially when it comes to organic matter in the environment and the dirt in our clothes. One of the truly unforgiving results when chorine mixes with naturally occurring materials is the formation of a particularly nasty class of compounds called chlorinated hydrocarbons.

This class includes carcinogens like dioxins, which, at 300,000 times more carcinogenic than DDT, are the *most* toxic substances known to man, as well as chlorinated furans and trihalomethanes like the poisonous gas chloroform. Let me be clear—when I say *carcinogen*, I mean a substance that is *known* to cause cancer. And, these substances don't go away. In fact, the reality is quite the opposite: they *accumulate* in the environment and in our bodies.

# Chlorine Bleach Profile

*Synonyms:* Bleach, household bleach, Clorox

*Active chemical:* Sodium hypochlorite (NaOCl)

*Human hazards:* Dangerous to inhale; severe irritant of the eyes, skin, and lungs; severe corrosive, topical contact will chemically burn skin

*Household hazards:* Indoor air pollutant; highly reactive, and dangerous when it mixes with other chemicals and cleaners. For example, ammonia or urine + bleach = deadly chloramine fumes, and acidic compounds like vinegar + bleach = toxic chlorine gas

*Environmental hazards:* Not biodegradable, persistent in the environment; reacts with organic matter to form organochlorines and carcinogenic chlorinated hydrocarbons, including dioxins, furans, and trihalomethanes (see "Dioxins" on page 42 for more information).

*Fabric safety:* Not for use with colored fabrics; weakens fibers and fabrics

*Green solution:* Oxygen bleach!

Though it might seem like using a little bit of bleach can't be all *that* harmful to the environment, think again.

## Hazards to Humans and the Environment

Just how hazardous is chlorine bleach? The dangers affect us both directly and indirectly.

Acute (direct) hazards from chlorine bleach include the following.

- **It is extremely corrosive.** Remember that chlorine works because it reactively oxidizes stuff. Technically, fast oxidation is called *burning*, and that is just what chlorine does—including burning your skin and eyes. Contact with chlorine bleach can cause chemical burns, and the fumes can burn the delicate tissues of our eyes.[35]

- **It is absorbed through the skin.** This is not good because chlorine is a poison, straight up. Due to its propensity for bioaccumulation, even minute amounts can add up to dangerous levels over the course of a lifetime.

- **It is a respiratory irritant that viciously attacks the mucous membranes.** The fumes that come off of chlorine bleach are toxic and dangerous, especially for anyone with a heart condition or a chronic respiratory problem like asthma. Inhaling chlorine is almost guaranteed to happen because the washing machine is generally housed in enclosed quarters.

- **It is an indoor air pollutant.** Chlorine bleach contributes to overall indoor air pollution, which, according to the US Environmental Protection Agency, ranks among the top five chronic hazards we deal with on a daily basis.[36]

- **It is dangerously reactive with organic matter.** While most of the horrendous environmental effects of chlorine take place at large in the ecosystem, some can take place right in your laundry room when dirty clothes are soiled with stuff that causes volatile results. Chlorine residue left on clothing can also cause low-grade toxic reactions. But it all adds up, and what goes on in the laundry room doesn't stay there.

Chronic (indirect) hazards from chlorine bleach include the following.

- **It is reactive.** Chlorine causes dangerous and deadly reactions in the environment.
- **You will end up eating it.** Literally. Because at their worst, chlorine and chlorine compounds create dangerous and carcinogenic compounds that persist and accumulate in the environment, traveling up the food chain and ending up in the food we eat.
- **It has serious health effects.** Virtually all chlorinated compounds that have been studied have been linked with a wide range of serious health effects—including reproductive disorders, endocrine system disruption, birth defects, developmental impairment, immunosuppression, and cancer.[37]

## Green Solution: Oxygen Bleach

Oxygen bleach is a green, nontoxic, highly effective option for disinfecting, bleaching, brightening, and removing stains. It's safe for humans, clothing, and the environment.

How does it work?

Oxygen bleach releases oxygen to clean. Like chlorine bleach, it oxidizes, getting between the dirt and the fiber to lift stains and grime. Unlike chlorine, oxygen bleach is environmentally friendly and not hazardous to your health. It breaks down into oxygen, water, and natural soda ash (sodium carbonate).

Oxygen bleach has antiseptic and disinfectant properties, is safe to use on colored fabrics, and can be mixed with other cleaning products without chemical danger. As an added bonus for laundry and stain removal, oxygen bleach naturally benefits the pH of washing water by removing minerals, effectively softening the water. Softer water cleans clothes and removes stains better and boosts the power of the laundry detergent. It's an all-around winner!

There are three types of oxygen bleach products on the market, and they all work the same way.

- Sodium percarbonate: A powder, it is 13 to 14 percent oxygen
- Sodium perborate: A component in powdered laundry and dishwashing detergents, it is 10 to 15 percent oxygen
- Hydrogen peroxide: A liquid, it is typically sold in grocery and drug stores as a 3 percent solution for use as an antiseptic, as a 6 percent solution for use as a laundry bleach, and as a 35 percent food-grade solution (to be handled with extreme care!). There is also a 90 per-

# Oxygen Bleach Profile

*Synonyms:* Sodium percarbonate, sodium perborate, hydrogen peroxide
*Active chemical:* Oxygen
*Human hazards:* None
*Household hazards:* None; can safely be mixed with other cleaning and laundry products
*Environmental hazards:* None; beneficial to agriculture and aquaculture
*Fabric safety:* Safe for use with colors; it brightens colors and does not weaken fibers or fabrics

cent solution that is used for rocket propulsion by the military and for space exploration, but it is unlikely you'll be able to get your hands on any (nor should you want to!).

*Note:* Powdered oxygen bleach is more stable and has a longer shelf life than liquid oxygen bleach. The powders are made from natural soda ash or borax that is treated with hydrogen peroxide, which absorbs the oxygen and remains a free-flowing solid. Though liquid products sometimes seem less expensive, because water is a main ingredient they can be less potent and won't go as far as powders.

## Benefits of Oxygen Bleach

Oxygen bleach offers a number of important benefits over chlorine bleach. It:

- Is nontoxic to humans and wildlife
- Biodegrades—breaks down into oxygen, water, and natural soda ash (sodium carbonate)
- Disinfects and deodorizes. Its natural antiseptic properties make oxygen

bleach effective against odors, bacteria, and viruses

- Boosts the power of laundry detergent by reducing the minerals in washing water to soften the water, making the detergent more effective
- Brightens colors and whitens whites—it doesn't get better than that!
- Prevents yellowing and graying of fabrics and can be used repeatedly
- Is safe for use with all washable fabrics and does not weaken fibers and fabrics
- Is a superb stain remover that has no dangerous side effects
- Is safe when mixed with other cleaning and laundry products
- Is environmentally friendly because the oxygen it releases is actually beneficial for agriculture and aquaculture

## Tips for Using Powdered Oxygen Bleach

To use powdered oxygen bleach, dissolve it in water first, then add clothes. Presoak the clothes before washing for best results. The solution will stay active for 5 to 6 hours, so mix up small amounts at a time.

*To sidestep the ecological and human hazards of chlorine, look to any of these oxygen bleach products for clean, green action.*

## BIOKLEEN

### Chlorine Free Oxygen Bleach Plus
32-ounce and 50-pound containers

This powder is sodium percarbonate based and contains other natural, biodegradable ingredients, including fabric and water conditioning agents; detergent boosters; and stain-, mildew-, and corrosion-fighting additives.

*Available:* online at www.biokleenhome.com

## BIO-PAC

### Non-Chlorine Bleach Powder
10- and 50-pound boxes

This oxygen bleach is powdered sodium percarbonate. It also contains sodium carbonate and sodium chloride.

*Available:* online at www.bio-pac.com

## CHURCH AND DWIGHT

### OxiClean Versatile Stain Remover
This powder has 50 to 60 percent active oxygen ingredients (sodium percarbonate) and is sold in 3.5- and 6-pound tubs.

### OxiClean Free Versatile Stain Remover
This powder is the same as OxiClean Versatile Stain Remover, but it has no dyes or fragrances. It comes in a 3.5-pound tub.

### OxiClean Laundry Stain Remover
This premixed OxiClean bleach comes in a handy 31.5-ounce spray bottle.

### OxiClean Spray-A-Way Instant Stain Remover
OxiClean's stain-removing power has been packed into a convenient 0.47-ounce spray bottle for on-the-spot treating.

*Available:* at most grocery stores and natural markets, large retailers, and retail chains

www.oxiclean.com

## CLEAN ENVIRONMENT COMPANY

### Color Safe Powdered Bleach
This powder has 29 percent active oxygen ingredients (sodium perborate), as well as other natural cleaning agents.

### Liquid Bleach
This nonchlorine bleach is hydrogen peroxide.

The packaging for these products may contain recycled plastic, and the labels include postconsumer recycled paper and are printed with nontoxic ink. The shipping boxes may contain postconsumer recycled cardboard—bravo!

*Available:* online at www.cleanenvironmentco.com

## CLOROX

### Oxi Magic Multi-Purpose Stain Remover Powder
A powdered bleach with 50 to 60 percent active oxygen ingredients, this product is sodium percarbonate based. It is very similar to OxiClean (see Church and Dwight, at left).

### Oxi Magic Multi-Purpose Stain Remover Spray
This liquid formulation of Oxi Magic powder comes in a convenient spray bottle.

*Available:* at most grocery stores and retail chains

www.cloroxoxygen.com

## COUNTRY SAVE

### Non-Chlorine Bleach
2.5-pound box

This product is powdered sodium perborate, plus other natural ingredients such as washing soda.

*Available:* at natural markets

www.countrysave.com

## EARTH FRIENDLY PRODUCTS

**Oxo Brite Non-Chlorine Bleach**
2- and 3.6-pound containers

This powder contains sodium percarbonate and sodium carbonate.

*Available:* at natural markets and online

www.ecos.com

## ECOVER

**Non-Chlorine Bleach**
This powder is 100 percent sodium percarbonate and comes in a 14-ounce carton made with 95 percent recycled cardboard.

**Liquid Non-Chlorine Bleach**
This bleach contains hydrogen peroxide and comes in a 64-ounce jug.

*Available:* at natural markets

www.ecover.com

## MRS. MEYER'S CLEAN DAY

**Oxygen Bleach Stain Remover**
20-ounce container

This powder contains sodium percarbonate and pure essential oils for a great, garden-fresh smell.

*Available:* at natural markets and online

www.mrsmeyers.com

## NATURAL CHOICES OXY-BOOST

**Destainer and Deodorizer Oxygen Bleach**
18-ounce and 2.5-, 6, and 20-pound containers

With 80 to 90 percent active sodium percarbonate, this powder is among the most active oxygen bleach products on the market. And, it goes for a reasonable price.

*Available:* at natural markets and online

www.oxyboost.com

## SEVENTH GENERATION

**Free and Clear Chlorine-Free Bleach**
64-ounce bottle

This liquid contains hydrogen peroxide and an oxygen bleach stabilizer.

*Available:* at many grocery stores and natural markets and online

www.seventhgeneration.com

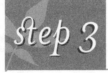

## step 3 — Nontoxic Stain Removal

Removing unsightly stains can be a cinch when you use nontoxic products and savvy know-how.

A lot of stain-removal products would have you think they work like magic: Now you see it, now you don't! While this might be a good trick for stains, in terms of product labeling it is terribly deceptive. What you see on most conventional products is a very vague list of ingredients, and what you don't see is just how hazardous they are to humans, wildlife, and the environment. We're talking about a slew of chemicals and

### COMMON INGREDIENT HAZARDS: STAIN-REMOVAL PRODUCTS

*These chemicals are all found in conventional stain-removal products.*

**Dipropylene glycol methyl ether.** This highly toxic compound is a severe irritant of the eyes, nose, and throat[38] and is neurotoxic.[39] It may have reproductive and developmental effects,[40] as well as damaging the central nervous system.[41] It is hazardous in the environment.[42]

**Ethoxylated alcohol.** An irritant of the eyes, skin, and lungs.[43] Repeated contact may cause defatting of the skin.[44] It may also be contaminated with 1,4-dioxane,[45] a known carcinogen.[46]

**Sodium dodecylbenzene sulfonate.** A severe irritant of the skin, eyes, and lungs,[47] prolonged contact with this chemical may damage tissues.[48] It is corrosive and can burn the lungs.[49] It also has long-term adverse ecological effects.[50]

**Glycol ether.** This highly toxic compound is an irritant of the skin and lungs[51] and a severe irritant of the eyes.[52] It's very harmful to inhale it.[53] It is also a reproductive hazard[54] and a hazard to the environment.[55]

**Nonoxynol-4 and -9.** This severe irritant to lungs and eyes[56] can be absorbed through the skin in potentially harmful amounts[57] and may cause genetic changes, adverse reproductive effects, and birth defects.[58] It is toxic to aquatic life.[59]

**Petroleum solvents.** These toxic compounds are irritants of the eyes, skin, and lungs.[60] They may damage the central and peripheral nervous systems and the respiratory system.[61] Very harmful to inhale, they may cause dizziness and loss of coordination and act as a narcotic.[62] Repeated skin contact may cause defatting, or removal of the skin's natural oils.[63]

**Sodium hydroxide.** This toxic compound is severely caustic and severely corrosive, burning the skin, eyes, and lungs.[64] A severe irritant of the eyes, skin, and lungs,[65] it's very dangerous to inhale it.[66] It may cause chronic damage to tissues.[67]

solvents you don't want to touch with a 10-foot pole, let alone breathe in their fumes or flush them into the ecosystem. But have no fear, nontoxic stain removal is here!

The simply great news is that a number of effective green products can do the dirty work, and you can also brew up simple homemade formulas that will foil all kinds of spots and stains. First, take a look at some ingredients you're likely to find in conventional stain removers.

## Homemade Stain Remedies

Check out these simple, eco-friendly tips for do-it-yourself stain removal.

### GREEN TIPS for Stains

- **TREAT STAINS AS SOON AS POSSIBLE.** The longer they set, the harder it is to get them out.
- **SOFTEN UP OLD STAINS WITH VEGETABLE GLYCERIN** (available at natural markets and online). Rub the glycerin into the stain with your finger or an old toothbrush until the spot is softened. Then, spot treat or soak before washing.
- **WASH IN COLD WATER ONLY.** Hot water sets stains, as does the dryer's heat. If a stain doesn't come clean the first time you treat it, hang dry the item and try treating it again.

- **PRESOAK THE ITEM BEFORE WASHING IT.** Fill the washing machine with water and detergent (add an oxygen bleach product to boost the stain-fighting action). Add the clothes and let them soak for 20 minutes to 1 hour before starting the wash cycle.

## Stain Specifics

These tricks will help you tackle and do away with specific stains. B'bye!

- **Blood.** Blot a fresh stain with club soda (don't rub or the stain will spread), then rub it with a paste of baking soda (1 tablespoon baking soda + 1 tablespoon water). If any pigment remains, spray with All-Purpose Oxygen Bleach Concentrate Stain Remover (see page 250). Blot a dried stain with vegetable glycerin to soften, then spot treat it with hydrogen peroxide, an ecological stain-removal product (see the "Green Thumb Guide" on page 252), or All-Purpose Oxygen Bleach Concentrate Stain Remover.
- **Coffee, black tea.** Treat ASAP because both are stubborn when they've dried and set. Spot wash with castile soap and water, blot dry, then spray with All-Purpose Oxygen Bleach Concentrate Stain Remover (see recipe on page 250) or spot treat with an ecological stain-removal product (see the "Green Thumb Guide" on page 252).
- **Cooking oil.** Liquid dish soaps work well because they're designed to cut oil

(use an eco-friendly variety, of course! See page 82 for some choices).

- **Gum.** Put the garment in the freezer. When the gum is hard, lay the garment on a flat surface and chip the gum off (using an old knife works well). Blot the spot with undiluted Citra-Solv Cleaner and Degreaser concentrate (see page 56 and scrub with an old toothbrush. Citra-Solv is strong enough to dissolve gum, so test it on an inconspicuous patch of fabric before using it.

- **Ink** (ballpoint or nonpermanent felt-tip pen). Use vodka to blot the spot or scrub it with an old toothbrush. If any pigment remains, try spraying it with All-Purpose Oxygen Bleach Concentrate Stain Remover or spot treating with an ecological stain-removal product.

- **Makeup.** Blot the stain with vodka (don't rub or the stain will spread). Then blot it with hydrogen peroxide, spray it with All-Purpose Oxygen Bleach Concentrate Stain Remover, or

# All-Purpose Oxygen Bleach Concentrate Stain Remover

*A solution of oxygen bleach in a spray bottle is super-convenient and works wonders for spot treating stains. It's safe for colors, though you should always test it on a concealed patch of fabric just to be sure.*

3 tablespoons powdered oxygen bleach
(4 tablespoons for heavy-duty jobs)
2 cups room-temperature water

Combine the oxygen bleach and water in a spray bottle. Leaving the top off of the bottle, swish and swirl until the powder has dissolved. Screw the top on the bottle and you are ready to go! If you shake the bottle vigorously with the top screwed on, the oxygen will expand and crack or break the bottle. It's powerful stuff!

Spray the liquid generously on the stain to saturate it. Let it stand for at least 15 minutes before washing.

Note: *Oxygen bleach becomes inactive over time. Make enough stain remover to last no more than 1 week. The recipe can be halved—you can always make more!*

spot treat it with an ecological stain-removal product.

- **Mustard.** If it's a fresh blob, scrape off the excess with a spoon or knife (wiping will make it worse). If it has dried, rub it with vegetable glycerin to soften it. Blot it with hydrogen peroxide and/or spray it with All-Purpose Oxygen Bleach Concentrate Stain Remover. Never use acidic cleansers on mustard because they set the color permanently.

- **Pencil.** Rub the stain gently with a clean, soft eraser. If you have one, an artist's eraser (which is like very dense putty) will work wonders; press the eraser on the pencil mark and lift (don't rub), then repeat until the mark is gone.

- **Ring around the collar.** Shampoo works great because it's designed to remove this type of oil and grime.

- **Rust.** Never use chlorine bleach because it will permanently set the stain. Make a paste of cream of tartar (1 teaspoon cream of tartar + 1 teaspoon water). Coat the stain and let it sit for at least 15 minutes. Scrub it with an old toothbrush. If any pigment remains, try scrubbing it with castile soap.

- **Tomato** (including ketchup and tomato sauce). If it's a fresh blob, scrape off the excess with a spoon or knife (wiping will make it worse). If it has dried, rub it with vegetable glycerin to soften it. Treat with castile soap and scrub, then soak it in a vinegar solution ($1/3$ cup white distilled vinegar + $2/3$ cup water). If all else fails, spray with All-Purpose Oxygen Bleach Con-centrate Stain Remover (see page 250) or spot treat with an ecological stain-removal product (see "the Green Thumb Guide" on page 252).

- **Wax.** Put the garment in the freezer. When the wax is hard, lay the garment on a flat surface and chip the wax off (using an old knife works well). Another trick (especially if wax remains after chipping) is to iron the wax off. Place an old towel on the ironing board, then place the garment, with the wax facedown, on the towel. Iron over the spot and the wax will melt off onto the towel. If there is a stain from oil in the wax, wash the spot with castile soap. If there is a stain from pigment in the wax, spray it with All-Purpose Oxygen Bleach Concentrate Stain Remover or spot treat it with an ecological stain-removal product (see the "Green Thumb Guide" on page 252).

- **Wine** (as well as berries and berry juices). Treat ASAP! If you are in a restaurant, order a glass of club soda and immediately blot the stain with it. Otherwise, take the garment off and cover the stain with salt to absorb the wine. Another age-old trick works well, but it requires caution and should not be used on delicates like silk, rayon, or wool: Stretch the fabric over a wide bowl in the sink and secure it by tucking its edges under the bowl. Pour boiling water on the stain from a height of 2 to 3 feet above it. I am not sure why it works but it does, especially if the stain is fresh.

*When you are in the market for an effective stain remover that is safe for humans and the environment, look for these products for clean, green results.*

## BEGLEY'S BEST

### Household Cleaner and Carpet Spot Remover

This is one of the ultimate all-purpose cleaners, including for removing all types of stains from clothing! From actor Ed Begley Jr.'s company (Thank you, Ed!), this product is biodegradable, plant based, and nontoxic. It contains no soap, detergent, or solvent. And it works well on whites and colors.

*Available:* at some natural markets and online

www.begleysbest.com

## BIOKLEEN

### Bac-Out Stain and Odor Eliminator

Biodegradable, plant based, and nontoxic, this product is excellent for removing the toughest stains and odors. Made of enzyme cultures and botanical extracts, it's gentle enough to use around babies.

*Available:* at natural markets and online

www.biokleenhome.com

## CALDREA

### Sweet Pea Stain Remover

Biodegradable, plant based, and nontoxic; great-smelling Sweet Pea fragrance derived from an essential oil blend of geranium, orange, jasmine, coriander, rose, and bergamot. Highly effective for all types of organic stains, especially for garments and linens of kids and babies.

*Available:* in select home stores such as Sur la Table, Smith & Hawkin, and online

www.caldrea.com

## CITRA-SOLV

### Citra-Spot Natural Enzymatics

Biodegradable, plant based, and nontoxic, Citra-Spot uses natural enzymes and bacterial cultures to break down organic stains and odors (including blood, pet stains, grass stains, and more).

*Available:* at natural markets and online

www.citra-solv.com

## EARTH FRIENDLY PRODUCTS

### Zainz! Laundry Pre-Wash

This prewash concentrate is biodegradable, plant based, and nontoxic. It's good for whites and colors and works on food, coffee, blood, dirt, and oil stains.

*Available:* at natural markets and online

www.ecos.com

## ECOVER

### Stain Remover

This biodegradable, plant based, nontoxic stain remover is good for using on both whites and colors (though it's not recommended for delicates). It removes all kinds of stains, such as grass, blood, mud, oil, and food. It also has a handy built-in brush applicator.

*Available:* at natural markets and online

www.ecover.com

## NATURALLY YOURS

### All-Purpose Fabric Spotter

It removes almost all water-based stains but has no harsh ingredients. It's safe for use on laundry, upholstery, and carpeting.

### Natural Solvent Spotter

It removes tough, non-water-based stains like grease, tar, oil, lipstick, makeup, and crayons from clothing, walls, carpeting, and upholstery.

*Available:* at select natural markets and online

www.naturallyyoursclean.com

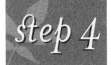

## Step 4

# Eco-Friendly Dry Cleaning and Laundering Delicates

We love our delicate clothing, but laundering those items leaves a lot to be desired. Dropping off and picking up the dry cleaning is a regular errand for a lot of Americans. Lest our fine garments and delicate fabrics be shrunk, mauled, and maimed by an agitating washing machine, off we send them to the dry cleaner's for professional processing. But most of us have little or no idea of what goes into the process of dry cleaning, or the health and environmental hazards attached to it.

## The "Dry-Clean Only" Tag

The dreaded tag. The question is, is this an unavoidable command or is there an easy out? Garments with "Dry-Clean Only" tags have one thing in common—they are too finicky to be thrown in the washing machine with everything else. However, a lot of these choice threads can avoid the fate of being hauled off for professional attention if you know how to handle them with the right care (see "Do-It-Yourself Delicates" on page 257). That being said, if you don't have the time or inclination to do the deed yourself, "green" dry cleaning and "wet cleaning" services are emerging everywhere as eco-safe alternatives to the toxic hazards of conventional dry cleaning.

## The Deadly Deal with Dry Cleaning

Despite its name, dry cleaning is not entirely dry. Though conventional dry cleaning doesn't use water to clean, it does use liquid chemical solvents. Solvents?! Solvents aren't by nature bad—after all, water is a solvent—but the solvents commonly used in dry cleaning are indeed *very* bad. How bad? Bad enough that since 1992, the US Environmental Protection Agency (EPA) has taken a keen interest in a program, called Design for the Environment: Garment and Textile Care Partnership, to reduce exposure to the chemical solvents used by most dry cleaners (namely, perchloroethylene, or perc).[68] Thank you, EPA!

## A Brief History of Dry Cleaning

In the mid-1800s, a French dye works owner, Jean Baptiste Jolly, stumbled upon the idea of using petroleum-based solvents instead of water to effectively "dry clean." This came about when kerosene from a lamp was spilled on a treasured tablecloth and, lo and behold, the cloth was cleaner than it had ever been before. This was pretty major because until then, laundering fine materials involved a lot of boiling, caustic materials, and repeated

# Perchloroethylene

Perchloroethylene, or perc, is the most commonly used dry-cleaning solvent. A clear, colorless liquid, it has a sharp, sweet odor and evaporates quickly. Of the 36,000 dry cleaners in the United States, 85 percent use perc,[69] though more and more dry cleaners are using greener, perc-free methods. Perc is a very effective cleaning solvent. It removes stains and dirt from a wide variety of fabrics without shrinking the material or making dyes bleed. So, what's the rest of the story?

Perc is extremely toxic to humans. Inhaling or ingesting it may cause cancer and birth defects.[70] High levels of exposure to perc, for even brief periods of time, can cause serious health problems, like dizziness; liver and kidney damage; fatigue; confusion; skin, lung, eye, and mucous membrane irritation; and respiratory failure.[71][72][73] People who work in dry-cleaning establishments are at the highest risk for adverse health effects, and those who live in close proximity to dry-cleaning shops are also more vulnerable. Low-level exposure from dry-cleaned clothing may also cause these symptoms; the verdict is still out on how much clothes dry-cleaned with perc affect the wearer. While the extent of the health effects from perc depends on how much a person is exposed to and for how long, some level of increased risk is definite, and it isn't something any of us needs to gamble on.

In terms of the environment, perc is a hazardous menace. It pollutes the air, water, and soil, and its disposal is regulated as a hazardous waste. How much perc escapes during processing and how the waste stream is handled are both primarily the responsibility of the dry cleaners themselves. Fortunately, over the last 10 years there have been about 60 percent reductions in perc use and pollution thanks to new machines that reduce the amount of vapor being released and better waste management by dry cleaners. However, more than 57 million pounds of perc are still used every year, with about 12 million pounds subsequently being released into the air.[74]

Here are some facts about perc pollution.

Perc is a POP (persistent organic pollutant; see page 43) that has pervasively contaminated the near and far corners of our planet. It accumulates in fatty tissues and is found in breast milk, cow's milk, meat, fish, eggs, and certain vegetable oils worldwide.[75][76] It is also widely detected in rainwater, groundwater, oceans, rivers, and lakes.[77][78][79] It is everywhere.

*Air pollution.* During processing, perc can escape dry-cleaning facilities through vents, windows, and air conditioners. Some dry cleaners still use older systems that vent perc directly outside, but most now control or stop perc from escaping. Some of it inevitably escapes, however. Once in the air, perc stays intact in the atmosphere for several weeks before breaking down into other toxic chemicals that are suspected of depleting the ozone layer.[80][81]

*Ground and soil pollution.* Perc is highly toxic to plants. Though its disposal is regulated as a hazardous waste by the EPA, perc can escape through spills; leaky pipes, tanks, and machinery; and improperly handled waste. The big problem occurs when it seeps through the ground to contaminate groundwater.

*Water pollution.* A small amount of perc can contaminate a huge amount of water, whether it is surface water, groundwater, or drinking water. Even small amounts are toxic to aquatic life, including fish, which accumulate and store it in their fatty tissues.[82][83] From there, it travels up the food chain.

drying in the sun, or it was not done at all (which is why perfume was so very popular).

Early dry cleaners carried on after M. Jolly, using petroleum solvents, like gasoline and kerosene, quite effectively. The downside was the ferocious flammability of the stuff, which led to a lot of explosions and fires, and the overwhelming lingering stink. It was troublesome.

After World War I, chlorine and chlorinated hydrocarbons became all the rage. For tasks ranging from chemical warfare to disinfection and miraculous bleaching, chlorine was the answer. Soon after, chlorinated solvents were discovered to be the less-flammable, odor-free ideal chemicals for dry cleaning, with superior cleaning power (and far fewer fires). The most effective of these chlorinated solvents, tetrachloroethylene (aka perchloroethylene), became the modern standard in the 1930s and still rules today in the conventional dry-cleaning trade.

It wasn't until the 1970s that a deep concern about the health and environmental hazards of solvents, especially chlorine-based solvents, showed up in the medical and environmental communities. Some solvents are known to cause cancer, and many have been linked with a host of acute and chronic health problems. Today, as many as 5,000 sites worldwide have severe subsurface solvent contamination, which is a major issue when freshwater aquifers are affected.[84]

The good news is that there are nontoxic, eco-friendly options for dry clean-ing. You can save your clothes, your health, and the planet in one fell swoop!

# Green Dry-Cleaning and Wet Cleaning

Green, eco-friendly cleaning has emerged and is blossoming like a wildflower in the spring. (So, you can now run amok in your fine garb and not worry about causing serious health and environmental risks when it gets soiled! Cheers to that.) Some of the ecological cleaning technology is very new, and some has been in use for a while, especially in Europe, where they are hip to the trick.

Here's the lowdown on eco-friendly options for cleaning clothing that requires special care.

## Wet Cleaning

*Solvent used:* Water

*Detergent used:* Small amounts of a biodegradable detergent and conditioner are used (to be sure, ask the dry cleaner if the detergents and conditioners they use are biodegradable.

*Benefits:* It's nontoxic, eco-friendly, nonpolluting, and poses few risks to workers. It's also gentle and effective for most garments. Many dry cleaners offer wet cleaning, so ask!

*Downside:* The machines are expensive and labor intensive to run, which may be reflected in the bill. It is also fairly water intensive.

# Air Out Perc Dry Cleaning!

If you have clothing that has been dry-cleaned using perc, *air it out* before stashing it in your closet. Remove the plastic bag and let the clothes hang in a well-ventilated place for an hour or two to allow any residual perc to dissipate.

Wet cleaning is a nontoxic, green alternative to dry cleaning that is becoming more widely available. More and more traditional dry cleaners are offering wet-cleaning services. Yea!

As its name implies, the solvent used is water instead of toxic chemicals, along with small amounts of detergent and conditioner (hopefully, ones that are biodegradable). Most "dry-clean only" garments can be safely wet cleaned without risk of shrinkage, damage, or colors running out of the fabric, even silk, wool, sweaters, linen, suede, and leather. It all has to do with the specially designed, computer-controlled, state-of-the-art machines, which are really expensive. The process is also more labor intensive than conventional dry cleaning, requiring training and a good understanding of fabrics, which is why not every dry-cleaning shop does wet cleaning. Brilliant! No harm, no foul.

## Silicone-Based Cleaning

*Solvent used:* Silicone-based siloxane (which is nontoxic)

*Detergent used:* None

*Benefits:* It's nontoxic, eco-friendly, nonpolluting, and poses few risks to workers. It's also gentle and effective for most garments, leaves clothes smelling fresh, and is safe for folks who are sensitive to chemicals. Silicone biodegrades harmlessly.

*Downside:* The machines are expensive and labor intensive to run, which may be reflected in the bill. It's a new process, too, so it isn't regulated yet.

Silicone-based cleaning is an eco-friendly, nontoxic process that is fairly new but quickly becoming a widely available option for professional clothing care. It was developed by GreenEarth Cleaning and is becoming big stuff, in part because it is backed by two of the country's biggest corporate names—General Electric and Procter and Gamble. They're onto something good.

Silicone-based cleaning uses a clear, odorless, nontoxic silicone-based solvent. Its performance reviews are great, with no shrinkage or color fading being reported and the finished garments being said to have a clean, fresh smell, as opposed to the chemical-solvent smell perc-based dry cleaning leaves. Even folks with chemical sensitivities are reported to do fine with silicone-cleaned clothing.

Silicone-based cleaning gets the eco thumbs-up because it's biodegradable—silicone breaks down into sand, water, and carbon dioxide—and the process does not involve any volatile organic compounds (VOCs) that deplete the ozone layer. Good stuff all around, and it works great too.

### Liquid Carbon Dioxide

*Solvent used:* Liquid carbon dioxide ($CO_2$)

*Detergent used:* A small amount is used, and usually it's biodegradable (but it's always worth asking about to ensure that it is eco-friendly).

*Benefits:* It's nontoxic, eco-friendly, and nonpolluting, and poses few risks to workers. It's also gentle and effective for most garments. The $CO_2$ used for processing is recovered from existing industrial and agricultural emissions, making use of a waste by-product, so it doesn't further contribute to global warming.

*Downside:* The machines are expensive and labor intensive to run, which may be reflected in the bill.

Liquid $CO_2$ cleaning is one of the newest technologies in the pro clothing-care scene. Carbon dioxide, the same stuff we exhale, works wonders as a solvent and is proving to be a highly effective, nontoxic, and environmentally sensitive option for cleaning clothing.

$CO_2$, a colorless, tasteless gas, is pressurized into liquid form, which easily penetrates fabrics to dissolve and lift grease and oil-based stains. Detergents are added to remove water-based dirt and stains. Although most cleaners using this process use eco-friendly detergents, it is always worth asking about to make sure.

This newfangled application of $CO_2$ is the same technology used to clean a wide variety of materials, including silicone components in computers. It's also used to degrease engines and wick away oils in vitamin manufacturing. Pretty cool, and an eco-smart option for fine fabrics.

## Do-It-Yourself Delicates

While there are a bunch of great eco-friendly options for professional cleaning, reducing the need for professional services is a capital green step that will also save you green—money, that is.

### Silk

Silk is an elegant material that is quite strong, durable, and resistant to tearing. There are two types of silk—cultivated silk (mulberry silk) and raw or wild silk (tussah silk)—both produced by silkworms. Raw silk is noticeably stronger than cultivated silk, but both will benefit from these savvy laundry tricks.

- **Wash by hand.** The agitation of the washing machine causes shrinkage.
- **Wash in warm or cool water**—100°F or cooler, which feels like a lukewarm bath.

# Long-Lived Delicates

Delicate articles of clothing, such as items with decorative trim or lace—like underwear, blouses, and skirts—should be washed with care. A great trick to extend the life of beloved delicates is to wash them inside a pillowcase that's been tied shut.

Place the items in a plain, clean pillowcase; use a white or neutral-color pillowcase to avoid any transfer of color. Tie the pillowcase closed with string or twine.

Wash in cold water on the delicate cycle.

Hang dry—a folding rack is best. Avoid placing clothespins on decorative details.

*Note:* Machine washing is not recommended for silk and rayon because the agitating action causes shrinkage. Wash silk and rayon items by hand for the best results and a long life.

- **Use a gentle soap or detergent.** Use a soap or detergent with a pH as close to neutral as possible. Regular detergent (even the natural, biodegradable stuff) will strip the natural oils out of silk, leaving it stiff, brittle, and fragile. Castile soaps made for babies work great and are as cheap as beans. Woolite also works like a charm (see the "Green Thumb Guide" on page 261 for details).
- **Swirl, swish, and rinse.** Never squeeze or twist while washing.
- **Press between two towels to dry.** Never twist or wring.
- **Never use bleach.** It damages and weakens silk's fibers. Use hydrogen peroxide to whiten safely, naturally, and effectively.

- **Combat dulling residue with vinegar.** Over time, minerals and soap or detergent residue can dull colors. Try adding 2 tablespoons of white distilled vinegar to the rinse water to reverse the dulling trend. To be safe, test an inner seam first to see how the item reacts.
- **Hang dry, but not in direct sunlight.** Silk dries in a jiffy, but does not take to the dryer at all. Use hangers, because clothespins will leave marks (they're not permanent and can be ironed or steamed out, but you might as well avoid them entirely). Excessive sunlight damages silk, so choose a shady spot.
- **Use a cool to medium iron or steam.** A steamy bathroom will often do the trick to remove wrinkles!

## Rayon

Rayon is a delicate man-made fiber that feels like something between cotton and silk. Made from cellulose, it usually requires special care. Washable rayon is a lot easier to care for than dry-clean-only rayon, and it can withstand the agitation of a washing machine (the care label on your garment will let you know if this is the case). All other rayon garments will be said to need dry cleaning, but you can actually do a lot of it yourself with a few good hints. (*BIG NOTE:* I strongly urge you to try out the tips below on less treasured garments before attempting them on your favorite piece. Though these tips are gentle, it is better to be safe than sorry.)

- **Hand wash only.** The agitation of the washing machine will shrink and wreck rayon fabric.
- **Use cool water**—100°F or cooler, like a lukewarm bath.
- **Avoid acidity.** Never use vinegar or lemon to clean or rinse rayon. It will break the fibers into bits over time.
- **Use a gentle detergent.** Castile soap is the best if you ask me, and always rinse thoroughly.
- **Swirl, swish, and rinse.** Don't squeeze or manhandle.
- **Press and hang dry.** Never put rayon in the dryer! Press the item between two dry towels and then hang it to dry. Rayon is a lightweight fiber that dries in a jiffy.
- **Iron using medium-high heat.**

## Wool and Cashmere

Wool is one of the warmest and cashmere one of the most luxurious fibers of all time. Dry cleaning is recommended for both, but for sweaters and scarves, washing by hand can be just as effective if you know what to do, and it's also the best nontoxic choice if green dry-cleaning or wet cleaning is not available in your area. I wash my own for the most part, especially sweaters that I bum around in. I don't recommend you clean wool suits yourself unless you are willing to risk their becoming misshapen.

Here are a few techniques that will yield great results.

- **Hand wash.** Never put wool or cashmere in a washing machine.
- **Use cool water**—less than 100°F; it should feel lukewarm.
- **Use a mild soap or shampoo.** Detergent will strip out the natural oils, which will weaken and damage the fiber.
- **Gently squeeze to wash.** Rubbing or twisting will cause shrinkage and pilling (those little fuzzy pieces that make the sweater look worn).
- **Rinse and squeeze gently.** Wringing will stretch and ruin the weave.
- **Blot dry between two towels.**
- **Dry flat on a towel.** Coax the garment back into its original shape and make sure all the seams are in the correct places. If the garment is a little snug, this is the time to gently stretch it to achieve a better fit (but be aware that it will be permanently stretched!).

# How to Wash a Baseball Cap

Put it in the dishwasher! Place the hat on the top shelf of the dishwasher and let 'er run. Wash the cap, especially a light-colored one, with dishes that have been rinsed or are not littered with food debris.

## Flax or Linen, Ramie, and Hemp

Flax, ramie, and hemp fibers are among the strongest and sturdiest natural fibers. With the right care, they are also among the longest lasting. Though these bark fibers are sometimes stiff when new, they soften up beautifully after repeated washing. Here are a few natural tips for keeping these fibers fit and fabulous.

- **Use the gentle cycle.** The agitation won't shrink or damage the fibers, but use the gentle cycle to avoid beating them up too much.
- **Wash in cold or warm water.** Hot water will cause shrinkage.
- **Use any natural, biodegradable laundry detergent.** Bark fibers are not fussy about detergent.
- **Don't use vinegar to soften.** It damages these fibers.
- **Hang dry, then tumble on cool to soften.** The heat of a dryer is damaging and causes shrinkage. To soften up the stiffness caused by hang drying, tumble in a cool dryer for 5 to 10 minutes.
- **Use a hot iron.** These fibers can handle it, and high heat is necessary to sufficiently smooth the wrinkles.

## Cotton

Ahhh, breathable, soft cotton. Cotton is a fairly strong fiber with excellent staying power when treated well. Here are few natural tips for keeping cotton crisp and comfy.

- **Wash in cold water.** Cold water prevents shrinkage. Preshrunk garments can be washed in warm water, but cold works just as well and uses less energy.
- **Use any natural, biodegradable laundry detergent.** Cotton isn't picky.
- **Fix the dye on the first wash.** Dye in cotton tends to bleed the first time it is washed. To fix the dye, soak a new garment in a few inches of cool water mixed with $1/4$ cup salt and 1 tablespoon white distilled vinegar. The vinegar might smell strong, but it will wash away with no lingering aroma. Be absolutely sure you don't put any light or white clothing in with colored items on the first go-around.
- **Don't use vinegar or lemon as a fabric softener.** The acids will weaken the fiber over time.
- **Hang dry, then tumble on cool to fluff.** Cotton dries quickly; dryer heat wears the fiber and colors quickly, so go natural! Tumble items on a cool setting for 5 to 10 minutes for fluffy, soft results.

*Taking care of delicate clothing at home requires extra care. These plant–based, biodegradable detergents are designed for delicates to ensure the longest life for your favorite, special threads.*

## DR. BRONNER'S MAGIC SOAPS

### Pure-Castile Baby-Mild Soap

Dr. Bronner's Magic Soaps makes the highest-quality castile soaps on the market from 100 percent vegetable oils—olive, hemp, coconut, and palm kernel. It's ideal for washing silk, rayon, and cashmere. Their use of saponified coconut oil allows for excellent lathering and less soap residue, even in extremely hard water. Dr. Bronner's products are highly concentrated (so a little goes a long way) and 100 percent biodegradable. Big eco-kudos to the company for their new cylinder bottles, which are made with 100 percent postconsumer recycled plastic—bravo!

*Available:* at natural markets and online

www.drbronner.com

## EARTH FRIENDLY PRODUCTS

### Baby Laundry Soap

This gentle, nontoxic detergent made with plant-based, biodegradable ingredients is suitable for hand washing silk, wool, and delicates. It is hypoallergenic and good for sensitive skin. Its pure fragrance comes from the essential oils of chamomile and lavender.

*Available:* at natural markets and online

www.ecos.com

## ECOVER

### Delicate Wash

Made from biodegradable plant ingredients, this product is ideally suited for washing fine fabrics like silk, cashmere, and wool. Its nice, fresh fragrance is also derived from plant-based ingredients. I highly recommend it!

*Available:* at natural markets and online

www.ecover.com

## GEYERMAN'S MERCANTILE COMPANY

### Forever New Fabric Care Wash

This pure, organic, biodegradable fabric care wash is formulated to gently clean, brighten, and promote longer life in all fine washables—lingerie, hosiery, silks, woolens, and colorfast delicates. Its natural base of citrus and sodas does not leave a residue on clothing.

*Available:* online

www.dakotamainstreet.com

## SEVENTH GENERATION

### Delicate Care Laundry Liquid

This detergent is formulated to gently and effectively clean without leaving residue on clothing, so it's good for those with sensitive skin and for washing delicate clothing. It has no fragrances, dyes, optical brighteners, or enzymes. All of Seventh Generation's products are nontoxic, plant based, and biodegradable.

*Available:* at natural markets and online

www.seventhgeneration.com

## WOOLITE

### Delicate laundry detergent

Woolite is a detergent for delicates that has been around for a long time. It's designed to gently clean silk and wool without stripping the natural oils from the fiber or leaving residue. It uses biodegradable surfactants and contains no phosphates.

*Available:* at most grocery stores

www.woolite.com

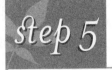

# Fabric Softeners

Fabric softeners do just what their name implies, but much less innocently than cuddly marketing ploys would like you to believe.

Fabric softeners work by coating fabrics with a thin layer of chemicals, which makes them feel softer (almost slick because they become somewhat water resistant) and neutralizes the charge of static cling. The coatings are designed to stay on the fabric for a long time, where they slowly and constantly release chemicals that are inhaled and absorbed through the skin.

There are three main concerns with fabric softening products.

- **Health exposure.** The most common health risks are allergic reactions, rashes, respiratory tract irritation, and constant low-grade exposure to neurotoxic and carcinogenic compounds.
- **Flammability.** They make fabrics more flammable—especially cotton and terrycloth, like towels and bathrobes—and therefore should *never* be used on children's sleepwear.
- **Environmental exposure.** Most chemicals in fabric softeners are not easily biodegradable and are hazardous to the ecosystem. Dryer sheets are particularly insidious because the chemicals are heated up and released inside the laundry room and through the dryer vent.

## Cheap and Easy Homemade Fabric Softeners

Instead of using conventional fabric softener products, which are full of chemicals that can leave residues on fabrics, try these inexpensive, easy-green homemade formulas for soft, cuddly results.

### Vinegar

Vinegar is a good fabric softener, especially for absorbent materials like towels and diapers, as well as for heavy fabrics like blue jeans. It's not recommended for delicate fabrics or linen. It dissolves detergent residue and softens fabrics. It's also cheap and nontoxic, and don't worry, the smell rinses away. Excellent.

Add ½ cup white distilled vinegar to the rinse cycle.

### Vegetable Glycerin

Vegetable glycerin works wonders as a fabric softener. It yields silky, soft results like traditional fabric softeners. It's available at natural markets and online at www.amazon.com and www.nowfoods.com. Brilliant.

Mix 1 cup (8 ounces) vegetable glycerin with 1 gallon of water. Add ½ cup of the mixture to the rinse cycle.

*If you like to use a fabric softener to keep your clothes cushy, look for these natural products that are free from dangerous chemicals.*

## CALDREA

### Fabric Softener

This product contains plant-derived softening elements and a special formulation of essential oils for extra soft, fresh-smelling clothes and linens. Choose from five enticing fragrances such as Ginger Pomelo, Basil Blue Sage, and Green Tea Patchouli.

*Available:* in select home stores such as Sur la Table, Smith & Hawkin, and online

www.caldrea.com

## ECOVER

### Fabric Softener

This liquid is completely biodegradable, nontoxic, and made with plant-based ingredients. It also has a natural, plant-based lavender fragrance.

*Available:* at natural markets and online

www.ecover.com

## METHOD

### Fabric Softener

This liquid is biodegradable, nontoxic, and plant based. Its two fragrances—Morning Bloom and Fresh Air—come from natural and (well-researched) synthetic sources

*Available:* at grocery stores and online

www.methodhome.com

## MOUNTAIN GREEN

### Fabric Softener

This liquid is biodegradable, nontoxic, and made with plant-based ingredients. The Free and Clear variety is unscented. The Lavender variety gets its fragrance from essential oils.

### Dryer Sheets

These sheets use a vegetable-derived softening agent. The Free and Clear variety is unscented. The Lavender variety gets its fragrance from essential oils.

*Available:* at natural markets and online

www.mountaingreen.biz

## MRS. MEYER'S CLEAN DAY

### Fabric Softener

This liquid is biodegradable, nontoxic, and made with plant-based ingredients. Its natural fragrances are derived from plants and the essential oils of lavender, lemon verbena, and geranium.

### Dryer Sheets

They use a vegetable-derived softening agent and natural fragrances from plants and essential oils.

*Available:* at natural markets and online

www.mrsmeyers.com

## PROCTER AND GAMBLE

### Bounce Free Fabric Softener Sheets

These sheets release biodegradable fabric softening agents. They contain no dyes or perfumes.

*Available:* at most grocery and retail chain stores

## SEVENTH GENERATION

### Fabric Softener

A liquid, it's biodegradable, nontoxic, and made with plant-based ingredients. It's also hypoallergenic. Its natural lavender scent comes from lavender oil.

*Available:* at natural markets, grocery stores, and retail chains and online

www.seventhgeneration.com

*Here's a look at some of the hazardous chemical ingredients commonly found in conventional fabric softeners and their possible harmful effects for humans.*

**A-terpineol.** An irritant of the eyes, skin, and lungs, it causes respiratory problems and may cause central nervous system depression and disorders.[85]

**Benzyl acetate.** This carcinogenic compound has been linked to pancreatic cancer.[86] It's an irritant of the eyes, skin, and lungs and may affect the central nervous system.[87]

**Benzyl alcohol.** An irritant of the eyes, skin, and lungs, it is poisonous if ingested[88] and moderately toxic when inhaled or absorbed through the skin.[89]

**Chloroform.** This skin irritant may dry or defat the skin with repeated contact.[90] It may be absorbed through the lungs. It may cause central nervous system effects[91] and is a possible cancer hazard.[92] It may also have adverse reproductive and fetal effects and may be mutagenic.[93]

**Dimethyl sulfate.** This compound may cause skin sensitization and allergic reactions.[94] It may be fatal if inhaled, but the effect may be delayed.[95] It may damage the liver and kidneys[96] and may cause cancer in humans.[97] It may also have adverse reproductive and fetal effects.[98]

**Fragrances, synthetic.** Ninety-five percent of synthetic fragrances are petroleum based and may contain benzene derivatives and other toxic sensitizers that may cause cancer, birth defects, central nervous system disorders, and allergies.[99]

**Isopropyl alcohol.** This irritant of the eyes, skin, and lungs may cause defatting of the skin and dermatitis with chronic exposure.[100] It may also cause lung damage[101] and central nervous system depression.[102]

**Limonene.** An irritant of the eyes, skin, and lungs, it may cause allergic skin reactions.[103]

**Quaternary ammonium compounds (aka n-alkyl dimethylbenzyl ammonium chloride).** These irritate the eyes, skin, and lungs. Prolonged inhalation may cause loss of motor skills and disorientation.[104]

Energy-efficient appliances have come a long way, baby! Because they use loads less water and energy and are high-performance machines, energy-efficient washing machines and dryers will save you time and money (in the long run).

I am not suggesting that you haul a good machine off to the dump (that's not very green, now is it?). I *am* strongly campaigning for getting an energy-efficient model when the time comes to buy a new washer or dryer. You will feel good.

An energy-efficient washing machine or dryer usually comes with a heftier price tag, *but* it saves quite a lot of money in the long run and will pay for itself by lowering your monthly utility bills. An energy-efficient washing machine saves an average of $100 a year in electricity alone (add in the cost of the water it saves and you're rockin'). Do the math: It pays to buy an energy-efficient appliance, period.

## Think Long Term: The Life-Cycle Cost

When you buy a major appliance, there are two costs to consider: the cost of the initial purchase and the cost to run the machine over its lifetime. A washing machine has a 10- to 20-year lifespan, and the cost of the energy needed to run the thing can exceed the initial purchase cost many times over.

## It Pays to Go Green!

Being eco-smart with laundry is green in more ways than one—it's green for the environment and greenback savings for your wallet. A washing machine is a major appliance with a heavy draw of both energy and water. An energy-efficient machine uses less energy and water, so it not only saves you money on utility bills, it also saves the environment, because less energy drawn from power plants means less pollution.

### SAVING THE PLANET
### ONE LOAD OF LAUNDRY AT A TIME

If every American home used the most energy-efficient washing machine, we would conserve 40 million barrels of oil a year. An energy-efficient washing machine can save more than $100 a year in utility costs.[105]

## Energy-Efficient Washing Machines

Energy-efficient washing machines save loads of energy and water. Not only are they better for the environment, they are better for your pocketbook in the long run, and the high-performance capacity of these smart machines will even save you time. That's good green sense all around.

### Features to Look for in a Washer

When you are in the market for a washing machine, you should consider the following if you want to be greener and select the right machine for your needs.

- Choose the right-size machine. Smaller-capacity machines are a better choice for small households; larger families call for larger machines.
- Look for a fast spin cycle, which will reduce drying time by as much as half.
- Look at the ENERGYguide label, the sticker that shows how much energy the machine uses.

## Energy-Efficient Dryers

The most energy-efficient dryer is a piece of rope suspended head-high between two fixed objects. It's called a clothesline, and it is practically free. However, using a clothesline is not always feasible, whether that's due to logistical constraints, weather, or your town's not allowing them for aesthetic reasons (a sad but true trend in some areas).

## Energy Star Appliances

Energy Star appliances must meet strict energy-efficiency standards set by the EPA and the US Department of Energy.

To qualify for an Energy Star, washing machines must:

Use at least 50 percent less energy

Use less water. A full-size machine uses only 18 to 25 gallons of water (as opposed to the 40-gallon average of a standard washing machine), which means an average household can save about 16,000 gallons of water a year!

Have a faster spin cycle to extract more water from fabrics, which saves an average of about half the drying time needed for laundry done in conventional washing machines.

# Front-Loading Washing Machines

In Europe, 90 percent of the washing machines are front loaders, but these machines are just catching on in the United States. They work a little differently than top loaders, but they are highly efficient and save loads of energy and water.

What's so good about them? They:

Use 40 to 60 percent less water

Use 30 to 50 percent less energy

Use 50 to 70 percent less detergent

Have faster spin cycles that reduce drying time.

Energy efficiency in dryers is not as advanced as it is in washing machines. Dryers simply require a lot of juice to heat up and run.

Unfortunately, unlike all other major appliances, dryers are not required to display the ENERGYguide label. Bummer, because without it, figuring out how much energy they use is not possible.

There are a few features to look for that will save you energy, time, and money.

- **Gas-heated dryers.** Gas is a more efficient source of power for dryers than electricity is, and they're a lot less expensive to operate.
- **Moisture sensor.** A moisture sensor tells the dryer to shut off when the clothes are dry. This can save 10 to 15 percent of the energy used by dryers that don't have a sensor. The best models have sensors in the drum.

For a comprehensive list of energy-efficient Energy Star appliances, go to www.energystar.gov.

# CHAPTER 7

# 4 Corners of a Green Bedroom

**Natural** *adjective*

1: based on an inherent sense of right and wrong
2: having an essential relation with someone
or something (*Merriam-Webster's Collegiate Dictionary*)

**Eco-friendly** *adjective*

1. not harmful to the environment (*Oxford English Dictionary*)

The bedroom is one of the most intimate parts of a home. There are lots of ways to be green and create a safe haven in the bedroom, primarily by choosing natural materials over synthetic. Bedding made from natural and organic fabrics and other materials—sheets, mattresses, pillows, comforters—feel good, look good, and don't emit indoor air pollutants. Whether you start with small steps or dare to dream big, creating a greener bedroom with clean, natural materials is a comforting prescription for sound sleep and rejuvenating rest.

# All about Cotton

Cotton is one of the most versatile natural fibers of all time, and it evokes thoughts of white, fluffy, natural purity. The fiber of cotton is almost entirely cellulose—a natural polymer—which makes it strong, durable, and absorbent. Cotton is widely used in textiles of all sorts—40 to 47 percent of all textiles produced worldwide are made with cotton.[1] T-shirts, socks, underwear, bedsheets, terrycloth towels and robes, denim blue jeans, chambray work shirts, corduroy, seersucker, and cotton twill, even gunpowder manufacture and bookbinding all use cotton, and the demand for it grows surely and steadily every year.

Cultivated for millennia worldwide, cotton requires a long growing season, plenty of sunshine, and massive amounts of water. This is one thirsty plant! Conventional cotton growing is so water intensive that it is causing vast desertification in some areas of the world, whereas organic cotton growing practices are known to more responsibly manage water use to ensure the long-term sustainability of farmland.

Though most of us think of cotton as a pure, natural fiber, these days, cotton cultivation is incredibly chemically intensive (to the tune of $2.6 billion in chemical inputs annually worldwide[2]) and riddled with literally tons of the most toxic fertilizers and insecticides known to man. Therefore, choosing organic cotton is an essential eco-move for all of your household cotton products.

## Long-Lasting Impact

It's not just the amount of pesticides and insecticides used on cotton that all the fuss is about, it's the depth of the impact those chemicals have on human and environmental health. Although, compared to many synthetic textiles, the life cycle of cotton—cultivating, processing, and manufacturing—has a lower ecological impact, causing less harm and damage to humans and the environment, conventional cotton exacts a heavy toll on people and the planet.

- Cotton consumes about 25 percent of worldwide insecticides and more than 10 percent of pesticides, even though it occupies only about 3 percent of farmland.[3]
- The US Environmental Protection Agency (EPA) classifies 7 of the top 15 pesticides used on cotton as human carcinogens. In fact, all seven are classified as Class I or II chemicals by the EPA (the most toxic of all chemicals).[4]
- It takes about a quarter of a pound of chemicals to produce one single cotton T-shirt.[5]
- More than 2 billion pounds of synthetic fertilizers are used annually on conventional cotton in the United States.[6]
- An estimated 14 million people in the United States are drinking water contaminated with toxic chemicals used in conventional cotton growing.[7]

## Be Green: Organic Cotton to the Rescue!

If you love cotton *and* uncontaminated health and clean drinking water, organic cotton is for you. If conventional cotton growing is so horrendous, is organic cotton that much better? Yes, yes, yes!

Consider these green benefits of organic cotton.

- It's grown using methods and materials that have a lower impact on the environment and on us humans, both directly and indirectly.
- It's grown using production methods that replenish and maintain soil fertility.
- It's free of toxic and persistent chemical pesticides, insecticides, and processing chemicals.
- It's GMO free (it contains no genetically modified organisms) and supports agricultural diversity.
- There's no chemical residue on the finished materials.

## After-Harvest Chemical Bath

I am truly sorry to lay all of this on you, but the chemical barrage doesn't stop after cotton is harvested. Cotton is typically bleached and scoured with chlorine and other chemicals (see "Dioxins" on page 42 for details about chlorine bleaching), dyed with more chemicals, then treated with formaldehyde finish, a chemical flameproofing substance, and sometimes mothproofing chemicals. All of this adds up to serious trouble for the health of people who use or wear the cotton.

## Waste Not, Want Not

Cotton "gin trash"—leaves, stems, and short fibers—is a bulky by-product that's left over after high-quality cotton is stripped in production. Typically, this type of agricultural waste is valued as bulk fodder for cattle—each milk and beef cow

### WHAT COTTON LABELS MEAN

| | |
|---|---|
| *All cotton is not created equal. Here are four different designations you may find on the labels of cotton products.* | |
| **100% COTTON** | Yes, this is 100% cotton, but that's not all. It's cotton laden with pesticides and insecticides, processed with chemical softeners, bleached or dyed, and possibly treated with formaldehyde finishes. |
| **ORGANIC COTTON** | The cotton was grown on land farmed in accordance with United States Department of Agriculture (USDA) organic standards for more than 3 years: no chemical pesticides, defoliants, or insecticides could be used; only natural fertilizers, beneficial insects, and crop rotation were employed. The cotton was also processed without chemical treatment. |
| **TRANSITIONAL COTTON** | The cotton was grown organically, but on land farmed in accordance with USDA organic standards for less than 3 years |
| **GREEN COTTON** | The cotton was processed without bleaches, dyes, or chemicals such as formaldehyde finishes, but not necessarily organically grown. |

# Cotton Finishing Chemicals

Most cotton textile goods are treated with a bath of chemicals for finishing. The two most popular finishing chemicals in the textile industry are:

1. Formaldehyde for wrinkle resistance and stain proofing—at the cost of serious health effects. Formaldehyde is very toxic and it's readily absorbed through the skin.[8] It's a probable human carcinogen[9] as well as a mutagen,[10] which means that it may cause genetic changes and increase the occurrence of mutations (many mutations cause cancer and therefore the substance that caused them is a carcinogen). Formaldehyde also may damage the kidneys, and may cause heritable genetic damage.[11]

2. Really nasty flame-retardant chemicals for fire resistance—though the jury is still out on how well a flameproof shirt protects you in a burning building.

## Healthy Green Tip

Wash all new (nonorganic) cotton goods—clothing, sheets, towels—at least once before wearing or using to slough off and wash out some of the chemical finishes.

in the United States eats about 6 to 8 pounds of cottonseed a day.[12] Waste not, want not. However, in California, conventional cotton gin trash is so contaminated with concentrated levels of pesticides that it is illegal to feed it to cows.[13] Instead, it is used to make mattresses, pillows, tampons, cotton balls, swabs, and the like. That kind of waste, no one really wants.

Cotton is treated with chemicals throughout its life cycle—from planting and growing through harvest, processing, and manufacture. Here's what goes into conventionally grown cotton.

1. Planting
   Seed: Treated with insecticides
   Soil: Fumigated and treated with chemical fungicides, herbicides, and synthetic fertilizers
   Sprouts: Treated with fungicide
2. Growing
   Soil: Treated with synthetic fertilizer
   Plant: Treated with multiple heavy applications of pesticides, herbicides, and insecticides
3. Harvesting
   Plant: Treated with a defoliant from a crop duster so the leaves drop off the plant and do not stain the cotton

# GMO Cotton

Eighty percent of the cotton now produced in the United States is genetically engineered for increased yield and pest and disease resistance.[14] GMO crops bred for pest resistance have had pesticides genetically spliced into their DNA so they literally "grow" in the plant. Although it might seem that GMO crops would require less intensive application of pesticides in the field, the opposite is true—these crops are designed to withstand greater amounts of pesticides without being killed by them.

Organically grown cotton, by definition, has not been genetically manipulated.

4. After-harvest processing
    Cotton: Washed and scoured with bleach and toxic scouring chemicals to soften the fibers

5. Manufacturing
    Cotton: Treated with finishing chemicals like formaldehyde and flame retardants

## Natural Mattresses and Accoutrements

We humans spend about a third of our lives snoozing. Restful, sound sleep is essential for recuperation, regeneration, and a generally good attitude for beholding the world.

Resting your precious head on a pillow made of synthetic materials that are emitting chemicals is not exactly a relaxing path to peaceful sleep and good dreams. Yet most Americans are unwittingly exposed to some nasty stuff right in their very own beds. Fortunately, well-crafted natural bedding goods are widely available and varied, with options that don't require sacrificing luxurious comfort or personal taste.

Making the move to natural bedding materials is a worthwhile investment.

Quality goods can be a little costly, but they last a long time and can be acquired in steps and stages to ease the fiscal burden.

### Mattresses and Pillows: What's in Them?!

Here's a rundown of what's likely to be in conventional mattresses and pillows.

### *Conventional Cotton*

Conventional cotton can be heavily laden with the residues of pesticides and insecticides. It's typically scoured and bleached with compounds that release dioxins (some of the most dangerous carcinogenic substances) to whiten it or prepare it for dyeing. It is also treated with dyes and fixers, which include heavy metals and chemicals that are harmful to humans and contaminate the water and soil.

## Synthetic Fillings and Fabrics

Synthetic fabrics used for bedding are made from petroleum products and treated with toxic chemicals that emit harmful materials. The big three are nylon, polyester, and polyurethane.

Nylon is a polyamide plastic made from petroleum. Though generally considered safe, nylon may cause skin irritation, rashes, and dermatitis.

Polyester is another synthetic fiber made from petroleum. It emits minute amounts of plastic vapors that can cause respiratory irritation. Contact may cause acute irritating skin reactions.

Polyurethane foam, yet another synthetic material, is used to make the majority of mattresses. Even if you have an innerspring mattress, it is likely wrapped with this stuff. Polyurethane foam may be treated with PBDEs (polybrominated diphenyl ethers), which accumulate in human tissues and may cause serious health problems. This foam emits VOCs (volatile organic compounds), which have been linked to respiratory problems and skin reactions.[15] It also emits toluene diisocyanate, a compound known to cause severe lung problems.[16]

## Flame Retardants: Fire "Safety" with Serious Concerns

As less-combustible natural materials have been supplanted by highly flammable synthetic materials in this day and age, chemical fire retardants have invaded our most private quarters—namely, our beds. Conventional mattresses and pads are doused with fire retardants, usually more than once during production, to comply with federal regulations, but at what cost to our health?

A big cause for alarm about bedding is the materials themselves. Mattresses made with polyurethane foam are the most heavily treated with fire retardants because they are basically like solid gasoline and are extremely flammable. Hence, the material requires exorbitant treatment with chemical fire retardants to neutralize the danger. Other synthetic materials like nylon and polyester also combust with ease.

There are three types of flame-resistant fabric.

- Materials that are inherently fire resistant, such as wool and natural latex rubber
- Synthetic materials that are treated with flame-retardant chemicals during manufacture
- Synthetic materials that are treated with flame-retardant chemicals during and after manufacture

PBDEs are the most common flame retardants, and the most persistent in the environment. PBDEs are classified as

## That "New" Smell

The distinctive olfactory signature of new cars, mattresses, carpets, and other creature comforts is more than you bargained for. That synthetic aroma is plastic vaporizing. Yikes!

Reducing synthetic materials at home in favor of natural fibers for bedroom essentials like mattresses will improve the indoor air quality and help reduce the amount of VOCs—like vaporizing plastics—you breathe in. Another way to improve indoor air quality when it's not possible to reduce or remove synthetic materials is by populating your home with houseplants, which purify the air by absorbing chemicals and producing fresh oxygen day and night.

persistent organic pollutants (POPs),[17] a category in which they cavort with the most sinister carcinogenic materials, including the banned pesticide DDT and PCBs (polychlorinated biphenyls).

Like all POPs, flame-retardant PBDEs accumulate in our fatty tissues and never go away.

PBDEs have a nasty proclivity for migrating in the environment and in our bodies. They are found in increasing concentrations in remote Arctic lakes[18] as well as in breast milk,[19] blood samples,[20] and food, particularly animal products.[21] These chemicals may cause birth defects and harm developing brains.[22] They also may cause deficits in motor skills,[23] learning,[24] and memory,[25] and decrease sperm counts.[26]

## Natural Mattresses and Bedding to the Rescue!

Scouting for the right mattress hinges on personal preference. Well, your pocketbook influences your choices a bit, but knowing what's available is helpful for making a wise, sensibly priced choice that will please you in the long-term.

There are two main camps in the mattress kingdom—innerspring and non-innerspring—both of which have unique characteristics to support the body. A mattress can be customized with mattress pads and mattress toppers to create the ultimate heavenly nest for you.

### Innerspring Mattresses

Innerspring mattresses are the classic type of mattresses that kids long to bounce on. The core of a mattress is what supports the weight of your body, and in the case of innerspring mattresses, the core is constructed of steel coil springs. Hence, they feel springy. The number of coils and their gauge determine how firm the bed is. The more coils and the thicker their gauge, the firmer the mattress is. How firm you want it is up to you.

Surrounding the coils, or springs— and here is where the roads begin to diverge—are either synthetic or natural materials used for the insulation and upholstery. In conventional mattresses, the coils are topped with polyurethane foam (a carcinogen) and sprayed with fire retardant. That layer is then topped with synthetic materials and sprayed with fire retardant again. All of these materials give off toxic fumes. The springs of natural mattresses are topped with natural fibers like cotton and wool that don't vent noxious fumes—a big plus. Wool is favored because it is naturally fire retardant and does not have to be treated with chemicals. Yea! Ideally, the cotton is organically grown and the wool is Pure Grow Wool (check out page 278 for the full scoop).

Most conventional mattresses are covered and quilted with synthetic fibers like polyester (which is a type of plastic that also emits gasses), then treated with formaldehyde-based finishes for easy, no-stain care. Sometimes they are treated with fire retardant again. That's a lot of fire retardant. Does this sound like a chemical nightmare or what? Fortunately, natural mattresses are covered and quilted with natural materials that simply don't emit gases. I feel like I can breathe better already; how about you?

## Non-Innerspring Mattresses

As their name reveals, non-innerspring mattresses don't have springs for a core. Conventional non-innerspring mattresses, sometimes called memory foam mattresses, are most commonly made from polyurethane foam, which is not such nice stuff. Polyurethane foam is a carcinogen made from petroleum. Firefighters call it "solid gasoline" because it burns fast and furiously. To combat the hazardously combustible nature of polyurethane foam, these mattresses are doused with an extravagant amount of fire retardants, namely PBDEs, which are classified among the worst of the worst nasty chemicals (please read page 273 carefully!) . However, there is a dignified, celebrated alternative for non-innerspring lovers: natural latex.

## Natural Latex Mattresses

Natural latex foam mattresses are a lot like polyurethane foam mattresses, except the foam is blown from natural rubber, which is naturally fire resistant—no chemicals or noxious gases emitted! Natural latex is made from sap tapped from rubber trees, which hail from subtropical climates. The tapped rubber used to make foam for mattresses is stabilized to yield a durable, flexible, resilient block of really comfy stuff in a nice range of thicknesses. Europeans have favored natural latex foam as a metal-free mattress option for a good long time, though it is new to a lot of us. A bonus of this kind of latex foam is that it contours nicely to support bodies of all shapes and sizes, and springs back to its original form again and again without becoming compacted. These mattresses aren't for everyone, but they are nonallergenic and antibacterial, resist moisture buildup, and naturally fend off mold and dust.

Latex mattresses come in a slew of densities for different firmnesses. Because they don't have innersprings, they work best on a nice firm foundation like a platform bed with or without slats.

Additionally, latex mattresses are impressively durable and long lasting. Because of their super resilience, they don't have to be turned or flipped like innerspring mattresses, and they have been known to last for up to 30 years.

*Note:* If you are among the 6 percent of Americans with latex allergies, consider that pure natural latex has not been linked to latex sensitivity. However, although your skin will not contact a latex mattress because it will be covered by a sheet, you should consult your doctor before making a purchase.

## *Futons*

A futon is a simple non-innerspring mattress loosely based on the Japanese invention. Lacking coils and synthetic casing, futons naturally lean in the green direction at an affordable range of prices. Most often, they are constructed of cotton, though the more posh, modern varieties are sometimes layered with cushy wool as well. Organic cotton and Pure Grow Wool are ideal materials to look for (see the "Green Thumb Guide: Mattresses," opposite, for good leads). Ranging from just a pious few inches to a foot of padding, futons are on the firmer side of mattresses, though adding a comfy mattress topper can make a futon lovely and plush. A huge plus of futons is that they are pretty inexpensive compared to innerspring or latex mattresses. They can also save a lot of space in a small apartment, because many covert into a couch during the day.

Some futons layer foam with the batting, but be mindful of what the foam is made of. Some nifty natural latex hybrids made with cotton and/or wool layered with latex foam are softer and more resilient than straight-up cotton futons.

## Mattress Toppers and Mattress Pads

Oh, lovely, cushy beds. Mattress toppers are a simple way to soften a bed. To step up to a luxurious natural bed, buying a high-quality topper made from pure, clean materials is more affordable than buying an entirely new mattress.

The best mattress toppers are made of pure cotton and/or wool and are 1 to 3 inches thick. For extra-plush softness, feather down is an option, though it is less breathable and, if not constructed with quilting to keep it evenly distributed, it can clump and end up lumpy. Down is also prone to harboring dust mites, mold, and mildew, and it may aggravate allergies and asthma.

Wool toppers are from 1 to 3 inches thick and add a resilient, breathable layer of softness atop any mattress. Wool naturally insulates without overheating and helps regulate body heat during rest. In addition, wool is naturally fire retardant and does not require chemical treatment; it wicks moisture and dries quickly; and it is naturally mold-, mildew-, and dust-mite-resistant. Some wool toppers tend to "nest"—leave a body impression where you sleep—so consider before buying whether you prefer that kind of mattress topper.

*While some mattress stores do carry them, many online retailers sell a great selection of natural mattresses that may not be available at stores in your area. Take a look at these companies to see the best of the natural mattress world.*

## ABUNDANT EARTH

Abundant Earth offers a wide variety of environmentally sensitive products for people who want to make a difference in the world. The company has organic cotton mattresses, futons, mattress pads, toppers, covers, barrier cloth covers, children's bedding, pillows, blankets, comforters, and sheets.

www.abundantearth.com

## ECOCHOICES ECOBEDROOM

Offering a full selection of innerspring and non-innerspring choices and combinations, EcoChoices EcoBedroom also makes custom natural mattresses in almost any size, shape, and style. They carry the works as well—futons, baby mattresses, bed frames and furniture, pillows, mattress pads, toppers and barrier cloths, sheets, duvets, and comforters.

www.ecobedroom.com

## LIFEKIND

Lifekind is the only independently certified organic mattress and bedding manufacturer in North America. All of its products are hand-made in its "Eco-Factory," and the company is dedicated to manufacturing without chemicals. Absolutely no synthetic materials, products derived from petroleum, natural gas, or chemicals are used in the production process.

www.lifekind.com

## NIRVANA SAFE HAVEN

Nirvana Safe Haven sells high-quality mattresses made from natural, organic fibers that provide correct orthopedic support. With chemical- and fire-retardant-free materials, they claim to beat competitors' prices for products of the same quality. They specialize in Royal-Pedic organic mattresses, which contain organic, handpicked Peruvian and US cotton and organic French wool, and natural latex mattresses with box springs. You can also find everything for a safe nursery as well as bedding, mattress covers and cloths, and organic cotton and wool bedding.

www.nontoxic.com

## PURE-REST

Pure-Rest guarantees that their products are 100 percent natural and meet federal flammability standards without using chemicals. They stock an ample selection of mattresses—innerspring, organic cotton, Pure Grow Wool, natural rubber, vegan rubber, pocket coil, and latex futons—as well as slat and box spring foundations, toppers, mattress pads, pillows, comforters, and sheets. Pure-Rest also makes custom split mattresses, allowing bed partners to custom-ize their side to their liking. That's very cool, and it may even save a relationship.

www.purerest.com

## THE ORGANIC MATTRESS STORE

The Organic Mattress Store was the first and is the largest organic mattress store in the United States. They carry a select line of premium natural and organic mattresses—innerspring, non-innerspring, and hybrid—made from organic cotton, Pure Grow Wool, and natural latex rubber. Specializing in the Vivètique and Royal-Pedic lines, the Organic Mattress Store also stocks bed frames, mattress toppers, and organic pillows and bedding.

www.theorganicmattressstore.com

# Wool, the Regulating Insulator

Wool is a natural fiber that has long been favored as the perfect insulator in both hot and cold climates. Fiber and air combine to make wool one of the most comfortable, breathable, and healthful materials for bedding.

- Wool is a regulating insulator. It does not make your body overheated or too cool. Wool contains tiny pockets of air that excellently insulate naturally in both warm and cool climates.
- Wool is resilient. Wool fibers are naturally springy; wool batting is especially springy because its structure cushions with a lot of air, providing soft, supportive comfort that doesn't compact like other natural fibers and bounces back from pressure.
- Wool wicks moisture. It has a superior ability to wick moisture without losing its insulating properties (wool can absorb up to 30 percent of its weight in moisture and still feel dry. Brilliant.) Wool's fibers are uniquely spiral and hold little chambers of insulating air that absorb moisture masterfully. Because wool breathes, it dries quickly and does not retain the moisture it wicks.
- It regulates the humidity of the body, maintaining steady comfort as the body's generation of heat changes during sleep.
- Wool is mold and mildew resistant. Because it "breathes," it naturally and effectively resists mold and mildew, helping us breathe more deeply.
- Wool is dust mite resistant. Because wool breathes and dries quickly, it is naturally inhospitable to dust mites, which thrive in moist environments.
- Wool is soft, yet supportive. Its long, strong fibers provide the ultimate balance for comfort.
- It is a natural fire retardant.[27]
- Wool is long lasting. Its strong fibers keep it flexible and resilient for years.
- Ultimately, it's biodegradable, unlike synthetic materials, which stay around forever.

## Pure Grow Wool or Premium Eco Wool

The quality, purity, and humane sustainability of wool vary greatly from product to product depending on how the sheep are reared and how the wool is cleaned and processed.

Pure Grow Wool, also known as Premium Eco Wool, is a program for producing wool under conditions requiring extremely high standards. The program was established in Sonoma County, California, and more than 200 wool ranchers in that state now adhere to the strict regimen that requires responsible and healthful farming practices. Pure Grow Wool products are not only clean, pure, and chemical free, they are of a superior quality and last longer because only long fibers are used. The result is material that is markedly more resilient and better than the industry standard.

## Pure Grow Wool Standards

- **Pesticide free.** No pesticides can be used in pastures and no chemicals can be in the feed.
- **Scrupulously washed.** The wool is washed five times in hot water (two of the times include a biodegradable detergent).
- **Not chemically cleaned.** The wool is not cleaned using the toxic chemical carbonization process that is standard for regular wool.
- **Chemical free.** It's not treated with formaldehyde or carbonic acid.
- **Fibers are carefully inspected.** Fibers are inspected for their length and strength. Only 1- to 1½-inch fibers are used. Wool made with long, strong fibers is of a fine character that is loftier and more resilient and therefore lasts longer than wool of a lesser quality.
- **Not treated during processing.** The wool is not treated in any way during processing.
- **Sheep are treated humanely.** The sheep are fed a natural, complete diet, never tattooed or dyed, kept on 1½ to 2 acres of free-range land per animal, and never denied medical attention when ill.
- **Farmers and sustainable business practices are supported.** The wool is purchased at fair prices and farmers are empowered to care for the land by providing value-added products that are healthy for the consumer and the environment.

## Wool versus Cotton

Wool and cotton are both natural, breathable fibers. Wool has more resilient spring than cotton due to the structure of its fibers, and it does not compact as much as other natural fibers, even after you've been laying on it for a long time. For clothing, cotton is a lighter material that is excellent when the temperature is warm. However, Bedouin tribes in the Sahara Desert have long used wool to keep them cool—the tiny pockets of air held by wool fibers wick moisture and heat away from the body.

## Wool versus Down

Wool and down are both insulating natural fibers, though there are significant differences between them.

When it comes to items like mattress toppers, wool is firmer and more resilient than down and it distributes body weight nicely, which relieves pressure points with support. Though down is luxuriously soft, it tends to sink and bottom out under body weight, especially at pressure points.

Down is very fluffy because it is made

# Bamboo and Legna:
## A New Generation of Sustainable Natural Fibers

Bamboo and Legna are both incredibly soft and cozy natural materials that are gaining in popularity for bedding and clothing. Here's a look at what they are made of and their inviting attributes.

## BAMBOO

Bamboo, a giant plant in the grass family, grows prolifically without the use of pesticides or extensive agricultural tending. It can be made into a lusciously soft yet strong fabric that feels softer than the softest cotton and has a natural luster similar to that of cashmere. Some varieties of bamboo grow several inches to several feet per day and have a root system that, after the plant is cut, sends out new shoots to replenish growth without being replanted. Therefore, bamboo is considered to be a renewable resource in a league of its own.

Bamboo fabric is easy to care for in a washing machine and dryer and naturally wrinkle resistant. It's extremely breathable, more absorbent than cotton, and keeps you cooler in hot weather and warmer in cool weather. Proponents say that it has antimicrobial, hypoallergenic, and deodorizing properties due to a bacteriostatic agent called *bamboo kun* or *kunh*, that helps the fiber resist odors and bacteria. Bamboo fabric is soft, supple, and comfortable.

Bamboo cultivation gets high marks for being eco-friendly. It grows rapidly, improves soil quality, and shores up eroding soil, and it has an impressive ability to absorb carbon dioxide and produce oxygen. But processing bamboo into fabric can raise environmental concerns because of the harsh chemical solvents used by some manufacturers to "cook" the bamboo fiber down into a form that can be woven into yarn to make fabric. There are new, more eco-friendly technologies and chemical processes being used to process bamboo, such as the Lyocell process (which is also used to process Lyocell, aka Tencel, a rayonlike fabric made of wood). These methods dissolve the wood pulp using less toxic and nontoxic chemicals in a closed-loop system that captures and recycles the chemicals to be used again and again during processing. When you buy bamboo fabric products, look for the stamp of approval from an international body such as the Soil Association, the International Association of Travel and Tourism Professionals (SKAL), Demeter-International, KRAV, or the International Öko-Tex Association. If you don't see the insignia of any of these groups, you can always contact the company or manufacturer to ask how the fabric was processed. It's worth seeking out eco-friendly bamboo fabrics.

## LEGNA

Legna (pronounced LANE-ya) is a luxurious natural fabric with the supple feel of silk, but the ease of care of cotton. Created by an Italian company called SDH, Legna is made entirely of wood harvested from sustainably managed forests. Legna's eco-friendly manufacture has won sustainable-development-technology awards in Europe. More than 99 percent of the water and chlorine-free solvents used during manufacturing are continuously recycled, and low-impact, fiber-reactive dyes are used to process the fabric. It's long lasting and sensuously soft, drapes beautifully, and gets softer with washing. For more information on Legna, visit www.sdhonline.com.

from the small feathers that are under the outer plumage of ducks and geese. Generally, down is taken from the bird's breast. Therefore, it is not a humane product. Though down originally was harvested as a by-product of the meat industry, the worldwide demand for down has created a separate industry with very cruel standards. Feathers are ripped from live birds and grown back four or five times before the birds are slaughtered. In addition, countries with humane-treatment standards drastically different from ours produce most of the down we use, providing grounds to evaluate if it is an industry sufficiently humane for you to support with your dollars. There are exceptions to these cruel practices; in general, European producers have a better reputation.

Though wool is also an animal product, sheep grow a coat of wool annually, and it can be humanely sheared without causing the animal to suffer (especially when Pure Grow Wool standards are used; see page 278).

Like wool, down must be washed during processing, though usually much more extensively because feathers host tons of grime, dust, and odor. Down products labeled *hypoallergenic* are usually treated with ozone to remove impurities, a process that is safe and does not require chemicals. However, hypoallergenic down usually is also treated with antimicrobial chemicals to kill anything living in the feathers. Though the practice has been approved by the Food and Drug Administration, the chemical treatment raises concerns about health and safety. Hypoallergenic down is as clean as a whistle when it's new, but the nature of the material makes it susceptible to dust mites, mold, and mildew over time. Cleaning down generally requires a professional to use chemical cleaning solutions (though in some areas, specialty ecological dry cleaners use biodegradable and nontoxic chemical washes; see "Step 4: Eco-Friendly Dry Cleaning and Laundering Delicates" on page 253).

Whereas wool wicks moisture and dries quickly, down absorbs moisture and holds it. This makes down a perfect environment for breeding dust mites, mold, and mildew. Eeww. An alternative to chemically cleaning down is regularly giving down materials a sunbath to naturally sanitize them and keep everything fresh. Simply lay down pillows and comforters in full sun for a few hours once a month, or every other month, for great-smelling, naturally clean results.

## Wool versus Synthetic Fibers

Synthetic fibers and materials obviously are not natural because they are made from nonrenewable resources, which comes with certain consequences. The manufacturing process is toxic and pollutes the environment, and ultimately, when these materials are discarded, they do not biodegrade. Synthetic materials such as polyurethane foam, which is commonly found in mattresses, also have a nasty habit of emitting VOCs,[28] which are not good to breathe. And as far as breathing goes, synthetic materials do not "breathe." Since synthetic materials don't allow air to pass through them the way natural fibers do, they trap hot air and moisture instead of venting them into the air. Therefore, they do not regulate your body's temperature the way wool does.

Synthetic fibers tend to be smooth and straight, rather than springy like wool, and therefore they don't always provide great support for the body. Conversely, wool's spiral fibers keep it springy and resilient. For comfort items such as mattress toppers, synthetic fibers can't evenly support the body and they tend to give way, especially at the body's pressure points, making them less comfortable for the joints.

Synthetic fibers don't absorb moisture. Though fake fibers are not hospitable to mold, mildew, and dust mites, they also don't wick moisture away from the body like wool does. The result can be a clammy, sweaty night, and that's not fun.

See "Do-It-Yourself Delicates" on page 257 for some easy tips on how to green-clean wool at home.

# Pillows

Pillows are such a pleasant part of snuggling into bed, and we have a more intimate relationship with few other home furnishings. After all, we spend about a third of our time in cozy, personal contact with them. When I think of my pillow, I exhale with a deep sense of comfort. When I inhale, I wonder what kind of material my face is pressed against, and just what that material is doing for me and to me.

A majority of pillows are made from either a synthetic material, like polyester, or down. Like the synthetic materials used for mattresses, synthetic pillows emit gases constantly. Given the intimate situation, choosing a comfy pillow made from natural fibers is a top priority for creating a green, nontoxic bedroom.

## All Kinds of Natural-Fill Pillows!

For cushy green comfort, consider the great range of natural, eco-friendly materials available for all kinds of pillows.

### Kapok Pillows

These are amazing! Kapok is a remarkable natural fiber made from the flower seeds of a tall rain-forest fruit tree. It has a downy quality that is as soft as silk. It is delightfully cushy and eight times lighter than cotton. Much like silk, kapok feels extremely soft, yet it is a wonderfully supportive fill in a pillow, and it's nonallergenic. It is a very durable fiber that does not compress or mat together over time like cotton or wool. Kapok grows wild in the rain forest, and harvesting the renewable seedpods for fiber provides sustainable employment for indigenous peoples and revenue to help maintain that vanishing ecosystem.

## Organic Cotton Pillows

Pillows filled with organic cotton offer firm support and are good props for reading in bed. Although cotton starts out fluffy, it compresses by about one-third over time (more than wool), so unfortunately, it isn't great for pillows unless you like putting your head on a brick.

## Down Pillows

Down is certainly fluffy, though it tends to attract dust mites and comes with a host of other humane considerations (see "Wool versus Down" on page 279). Down pillows have a tendency to trap moisture, and considering how much heat and moisture your head gives off while you sleep, a down pillow can become dank and musty over time. Kapok is a much better, healthier, greener choice if you are like me and like fluffy pillows.

## Wool Pillows

Wool is an ideal natural fiber for pillows because its springy resilience keeps it comfy night after night. Available with soft, medium, and firm support, wool pillows don't feel quite like a traditional pillow and will compress a bit over time. However, wool "breathes" beautifully and naturally absorbs moisture from your head, nurturing comfy, sound sleep. (Check out page 278 for more on the benefits of wool.)

## Natural Latex Foam Pillows

Natural latex foam pillows feel strangely different—like a squishy foam—to the average bear, but they offer excellent support and superior flexibility for contouring to the shape of your neck.

## Shredded Natural Latex Foam Pillows

These things are very cool. They are soft, super supportive, and a bit like a cross between a natural latex foam pillow and a buckwheat pillow. Made from shredded natural latex, these pillows are loftier than simple natural latex pillows and are fully washable. The shredded rubber molds to the contour of your neck for ideal spinal alignment.

## Buckwheat Hull Pillows

Buckwheat pillows are very firm and supportive, and they contour well. They are filled with the hulls of buckwheat, the seeds of an herb also used as a grain, and they are hypoallergenic. To me, they feel a little like sleeping on a beanbag, but some people love them. They shape and shift to support the head and neck while keeping the spine straight. Buckwheat also stays nice and cool, never becoming warmer than the body. Some people consider these pillows to be very healthy for those reasons, but I like a little more fluff.

## Pillow Protectors

For long-lived pillows, protect them with pillow protectors! A pillow protector, or barrier cloth, is a simple pillowcase with a zipper closure. These covers offer an added layer of protection from dust, dirt, and the oil naturally produced by our skin, and they can easily be removed and washed.

Choose natural or organic cotton pillow protectors. Most of the conventional cotton used for these pillowcases is treated with a formaldehyde-based finish for easy, wrinkle-free care. Avoid fabric blends that include synthetic fibers like polyester, because they quietly emit gases. If you are in the market for an organic pillow protector, check out Lifekind (www.lifekind.com), Gaiam (www.gaiam.com), Janice's (www.janices.com), and Rawganique (www.rawganique.com) for a great selection.

## Green Cleaning for Pillows

Pillows harbor dust, dust mites, sloughed skin cells, mold, and mildew to varying degrees. Pillow protectors are a good barrier against dirt, dust, and oil, but pillows still need a good cleaning now and again

to have a long, healthy life. To keep pillows healthy and hygienic, clean them at least every 6 months. In damp climates or seasons, cleaning them every few months is a good idea. How the heck do you clean a pillow? Depends on what it's made of. Here are some tips.

### Cotton Pillows

- Machine wash on the gentle cycle with cold water.
- Dilute the detergent (natural and biodegradable, by all means!) in water first to prevent detergent residue. A small amount of detergent will do the trick. Put the detergent in the machine and let the water run for a few minutes, then add the pillow.
- Don't overfill the machine. One large pillow or two small pillows is the maximum per load.
- Squeeze the pillow first to let out some of the air. Then squish it down into the soapy water and squeeze it again to let out any remaining air, so it'll stay submerged.
- Giving it an extra rinse cycle is a good idea. If your machine doesn't have an extra rinse setting, simply put the pillow through the final rinse cycle manually a second time to rinse out any residue.
- Add $\frac{1}{4}$ teaspoon of white distilled vinegar to the final rinse cycle to thoroughly remove excess residue.
- Add two tennis balls to the spin cycle to prevent the batting from bunching up (don't use brand-new tennis balls,

To pick the perfect pillow made with luxuriously green materials, check out the offerings from these companies.

## A HAPPY PLANET

Shop here for organic wool, organic cotton, organic buckwheat, and natural rubber pillows.

www.ahappyplanet.com

## ECOCHOICES ECOBEDROOM

EcoChoices EcoBedroom stocks pillows made of Pure Grow Wool, natural latex, organic buckwheat, organic cotton, and kapok.

www.ecobedroom.com

## GAIAM

This site offers organic cotton, Cleandown, kapok, organic hemp, and organic cotton and wool pillows.

www.gaiam.com

## JANICE'S

Janice's has organic cotton, organic wool, organic wool contour, and throw pillows.

www.janices.com

## PURE-REST

Check here for organic cotton, kapok, natural wool, natural shredded rubber, and molded natural rubber pillows.

www.purerest.com

## RAWGANIQUE

Rawganique offers organic cotton, hemp, and wool pillows, as well as organic cotton pillow protectors.

www.rawganique.com

## THE NATURAL SLEEP STORE

Organic cotton, organic wool, shredded natural rubber, natural latex, and kapok pillows are available here.

www.thenaturalsleepstore.com

## THE ORGANIC MATTRESS STORE

Here, you'll find pillows made of natural wool, organic cotton, Pure Grow Wool, buckwheat hull, kapok, natural rubber, and shredded natural rubber, as well as organic cotton pillow covers.

www.theorganicmattressstore.com

because the neon dye might transfer). Racquetballs work well, too.

- Run the spin cycle twice to remove as much water as possible for quicker drying.
- Tumble dry on medium heat, or air dry.
- Thorough drying may require several drying cycles.
- Air drying takes a long time and is best done in the sun.

### Natural Latex Foam Pillows

- Dilute a small amount of detergent in warm water and wash the pillow gently by hand. For the best results, squeeze and press the pillow to wash and rinse it; don't wring or twist it too much. Rinse it well in cold water.

- Press the pillow firmly between two towels to squeeze out excess water.
- Air dry away from direct sunlight.
- Do not expose to heat. *Never* tumble dry latex pillows.

### Wool Pillows

- Expose it to sunlight or use an ecological dry-cleaning method.
- Expose it to direct sunlight or open air for an hour every month to evaporate any moisture that's built up inside.
- Do not machine wash.
- If you dry-clean it, opt for chemical- and solvent-free cleaning only.
- To boost the loft of a wool pillow, place it and two tennis balls in the dryer on the lowest possible heat setting for 20 minutes.

## Comforters and Eco-Friendly Linens

Even the name "comforter" induces fuzzy feelings of safety, comfort, and joy. Who can argue with the pleasure of nestling beneath a delicious comforter? Like other bedding goods, comforters and blankets can be made of natural or synthetic materials. Cotton, wool, and down are the most popular natural materials for comfy covers, all of which are available in a variety of weights to suit the season and personal preference. Cotton and wool are great natural choices for breathable comfort when it comes to comforters and blankets. Down comforters are often equated with cushy luxury, but they may leave a lot to be desired when it comes to harboring mold and mildew, as well as for humane standards (see "Wool versus Down" on page 279). Bamboo and Legna (a wood-pulp fiber made from the trees in sustainably managed forests) are a new generation of natural and sustainable materials that are becoming more widely available for incredibly soft and sensational bedding goods. (See page 280 for more.) No matter what material gets you through the night, make it natural and green—the most comforting material of all.

*For greener snuggles, check out the wide selection of eco-friendly comforters and blankets fit for every season.*

## EARTHSAKE

This retailer sells Pure Grow Wool comforters—cozy Pure Grow wool fleece covered in soft, hand-tufted organic cotton. The natural color comforters are available in regular and tropical weights (tropical being lighter than regular) and in twin, queen, oversize queen, king, and oversize king sizes.

www.earthsake.com

## GOOD NIGHT NATURALS

This outlet stocks Pure Grow Wool comforters and natural blankets made of bamboo, cotton, and Legna; all are available in twin, queen, and king sizes. It also offers a bamboo coverlet (with 2 percent polyester fill) in eight different solid colors and a "brick" quilting pattern.

www.goodnightnaturals.com

## LIFEKIND

Lifekind has an organic wool and cotton comforter in natural color (twin, queen, and king sizes); an organic wool blanket, an organic cotton thermal blanket, and an organic Egyptian cotton blanket (all available in twin, queen, king, and crib sizes); and ivory and camel organic chenille throws (one size).

www.lifekind.com

## PURE-REST

Pure-Rest's comforters are 100 percent certified organic cotton and available in twin, queen, king, and crib sizes. Its circle quilted wool comforters are covered in organic cotton and available in twin, queen, and king sizes. Eco Wool–filled organic comforters come in regular and tropical weights and are available in twin, full, queen, and king sizes.

www.purerest.com

## SATARA

The tufted Pure Grow Wool comforter has an organic cotton cover and is available in twin, full/queen, and king sizes. A quilted Pure Grow Wool comforter is also offered in the same sizes. The blanket selection includes a Legna blanket in four colors and throw, twin, queen, and king sizes; a 100 percent organic merino wool blanket in natural color only, but throw, twin, queen, and king sizes; an organic cotton jacquard blanket in five colors and throw, twin, full/queen, and king sizes; and a brushed organic cotton blanket in white in twin, full/queen, and king sizes; and a bamboo blanket in three colors and throw, queen, and king sizes.

www.satara-inc.com

## TOMORROW'S WORLD

Go here for an organic cotton quilted coverlet in crib, twin, queen, and king sizes; an organic wool blanket in throw, twin, full/queen, and king sizes; and an organic wool quilted comforter covered in organic cotton sateen in regular and light weights and crib size.

www.tomorrowsworld.com

## WILDFLOWER ORGANICS

This outlet offers bamboo comforter covers in three colors and full/queen and king sizes. A handstitched Habotai silk coverlet has a soft and luscious texture on the outside and pure cotton filling; it comes in two colors (one reversible) and throw, queen, and king sizes.

www.wildflowerorganics.com

*To be green even while you sleep, check out the spectrum of eco-friendly, luxurious linens offered by these companies.*

## COYUCHI

Coyuchi makes 100 percent organic cotton sheets and duvet covers. Options include percale, sateen, flannel, and lace (available in twin, full/queen, and king) and damask stripe, damask check, and a jacquard print (available in full/queen and king).

www.coyuchi.com

## EARTHSAKE

Look here for 100 percent organic cotton sheets and duvet covers in sateen and percale in twin, full/queen and king; the Purist Collection's Classic Sateen (unbleached and undyed), Jasmine, Marrakesh, Hibiscus, Linen Plus, and Windowpane Damask in twin, full, queen, king, supreme queen, and supreme king; and bamboo (sheets only) in twin, full/queen, and king. Also available are Legna Seville linens in seven jacquard patterns in twin, full/queen, king, and California king.

www.earthsake.com

## GOOD NIGHT NATURALS

Here, you can find 100 percent bamboo sheets in a 250 thread count twill in queen and king sizes; the Purists Collection's Classic Sateen, Flannel, Jasmine, Linen Plus, Marrakesh, and Windowpane Damask in twin, full, queen, king, supreme queen, and supreme king; Haven Organic Linens' Aspen Collection (100 percent certified organic cotton quilted coverlet and sheet sets) in twin, full, queen, and king; Legna sheets and duvets from their Classic, Seville, and Portofino Collections in twin, full/queen, king, and California king; and baby bedding (Purist organic sateen and flannel and Legna).

www.goodnightnaturals.com

## INDIKA ORGANICS

This manufacturer offers products made with 100 percent certified organic Peruvian cotton and vegetable dyes. Their designs are inspired by ancient wooden block patterns. Look here for environmental sheeting in twin, standard, queen, king, California king, and baby sizes; Malabar in twin, standard, queen, king, and California king; and Otago for a selection of accent pillowcases.

www.indikaorganics.com

## JANICE'S

Janice's has 100 percent organic cotton single sheets, pillowcases, and sheet sets in sateen, available in twin, full, queen, and king sizes, as well as damask stripe and check available in full, queen, and king.

www.janices.com

## LIFEKIND

Look here for 100 percent organic cotton sheets and duvet covers in sateen and flannel whitened with only hydrogen peroxide in twin, full/queen, and king sizes, and for organic baby bedding also whitened only with hydrogen peroxide.

www.lifekind.com

## NATIVE ORGANIC COTTON

These 100 percent United States–grown and certified organic cotton sheets come in four colors in twin, full, queen, and king.

www.nativeorganic.com

## PURE-REST

These 100 percent certified organic sheets come in nine varieties, one undyed and another dioxin free. All are available in twin, full/queen, and king, and some also in California king.

www.purerest.com

## SATARA

Go here for 100 percent certified organic sheets and duvets in sateen, linen/cotton, and classic linen in twin, full, queen, and king sizes; printed design duvet covers in queen and king; 100 percent bamboo sheets in full/queen and king; and Legna sheets and duvets in five varieties, available in twin, full, queen, and king.

www.satara-inc.com

## WILDFLOWER ORGANICS

Wildflower Organics offers Purist sheets and duvet covers in natural color only (twin, full/queen, king, and California king), printed design organic duvet covers (queen and king), 100 percent bamboo sheet sets in a 250 thread count that are extremely soft and breathable (twin, queen, and king), Cluny sheets made with 100 percent natural linen milled in Italy and sewn with crochet trim detail (queen and king), a hand-stitched silk coverlette (queen and king), and a Hammock linen and lace duvet and shams made with 100 percent Italian milled linen and detailed with crochet trim and reverse French seams (queen and king).

www.wildflowerorganics.com

# CHAPTER 8

# Energy-Efficient Lightbulbs: Save Energy and Money

**Energy** *noun*

**1a**: dynamic quality; **4**: usable power: the resources for producing such power (*Merriam-Webster's Collegiate Dictionary*)

**Efficient** *adjective*

**2**: productive of desired effects; especially: productive without waste (*Merriam-Webster's Collegiate Dictionary*)

Where would we be without lightbulbs? In the dark, obviously. Ha. But seriously, the vast majority of lightbulbs in use today are practically from the Dark Ages—well, from 1879, when Thomas Edison invented the first long-lasting, practical incandescent bulb that illuminated the world. It was big stuff. At the time, and for a long time after, incandescent bulbs were the best things going, despite their massive mismanagement of electricity. Lightbulbs by design produce light, but incandescent bulbs give off only 10 percent of the electricity they consume as light and hemorrhage the other 90 percent as heat. This is why it was possible to bake cookies in older models of the Easy-Bake Oven, which were heated by a lightbulb (now they have a heating element).

More than 20 percent of the energy used nationwide goes for lighting.[1] Billions of dollars in energy costs and millions of tons of pollution result from producing this much energy. It's time to make the switch that will let us have our cake and eat it too by enjoying the same amount of light while using drastically less energy. It's simple.

Energy-efficient bulbs, like compact fluorescent lightbulbs (CFLs) and light-emitting diode (LED) bulbs, have come a long way, baby! They are green, clean, and ready to light up the world. Once upon a time, CFLs were only available in space-age-looking spiral bulbs. Now, they're available in a wide selection of shapes and sizes and a spectrum of brightnesses to fit any range of needs. A-shape CFLs look the most like traditional incandescent bulbs, globe-shape CFLs are round, and candle-shape CFLs are shaped like, well, a candle's flame. All are suitable for use in lamps, ceiling fixtures and fans, wall sconces, and hanging pendants, and globe-shape bulbs are also great for vanity lighting. Floodlight CFLs, suitable for both recessed cans and track lighting, are available for indoor and outdoor use, and some are even tinted to discourage bugs from hanging around. Look for three-way bulbs if you like having the option of low, medium, and high brightnesses with lamps designed to accommodate them. For lighting that you can dim, be sure to choose CFLs that are dimmable.

## Compact Fluorescent Lightbulbs

CFLs are a brilliant green choice across the board. We're not talking about those horrible flickering fluorescent tubes that cast a cold, harsh light and give you an unflattering pallor. The new generation of fluorescent bulbs has a full spectrum of wavelengths that look more like natural daylight. These lights are a bright idea for saving energy, saving money, and reducing pollution. It just makes sense across the spectrum.

CFLs come in a wide variety of shapes and wattages, including A-shape, globe-shape, candle-shape, floodlight, tube, and spiral. Here are some stats on CFLs.

- CFLs use about a quarter of the energy standard incandescent bulbs do (for example, a 26-watt CFL gives off as much light as a 100-watt incandescent bulb).
- CFLs last about 10 times longer than incandescent bulbs (a CFL will last an average of 6,000 to 15,000 hours, whereas an incandescent bulb has an average life of 750 to 1,500 hours). That means you use fewer lightbulbs.
- Though CFLs cost more to purchase than standard incandescent bulbs, an energy-efficient bulb will pay for itself

many times over in savings on your electric bill and replacement bulbs (on average, a CFL bulb pays for itself after 500 hours of use, so the rest of the savings is gravy).

- A very small amount of mercury is sealed inside the glass tubing of a CFL. The mercury is an essential part of what allows CFLs to be so efficent. The mercury is harmless while the bulb is in use, and manufacturers are collectively taking steps to reduce its use. Nonetheless,

CFLs should be disposed of properly. Contact your recycling center to see if it will accept used CFLs, or visit www.epa.gov/bulbrecycling or www.earth911.org to identify recycling options in your area. If you really just want to throw away a used CFL and your state allows it, you should seal the used bulb in two plastic bags for trash collection. If there is an IKEA store near you, they will accept used bulbs and do the recyling for you. Thanks, IKEA, that's nice.

# Light-Emitting Diode Bulbs

This is the next generation of lighting, beyond brilliant and ultra-efficient. The only caveat is that you might need to rewrite your will because these bulbs will likely outlast you—no kidding. The average life expectancy for Americans is 77 years. An LED bulb can last as long as 92 years.

Here are some stats on LED bulbs:

- LEDs use one-tenth the energy of incandescent bulbs.
- They last 100 times longer (LEDs average 60,000 to 150,000 hours, compared to 750 to 1,500 hours for incandescent bulbs!).
- Though LEDs are expensive to purchase, they literally last a lifetime (and likely longer) and reduce energy costs dramatically.
- LEDs are the ultimate durable choice for battery-powered and rechargeable gear like flashlights, lanterns, and

emergency lights. A green bonus: LEDs' low energy draw significantly extends battery life.

## An Energy-Efficient Success Story

Here's a great example of how LED lights can save money.

In 2001 the city of Portland, Oregon, in cooperation with its utility companies, Portland General Electric (PGE) and Pacific Power, replaced 13,300 incandescent traffic lights with highly efficient LED bulbs. For an investment of $2.2 million, which was funded with no capital budget, the city got a net return of 37 percent in energy savings and a total savings of 44 percent.

Savvy planning and financial management are saving the city more than

$400,000 every year in energy and maintenance costs, with the initial cost being paid back in less than 3 years. The rest is gravy. $$$!

## Highly Efficient, Reliable, and Long Lasting

LED traffic signals use 90 percent less energy than conventional traffic signals.

LED signals can last up to 10 years (even though they're used continuously), compared to less than 2 years for conventional signal lights, which saves money on maintenance costs, too!

LED lights rarely fail, lowering the risk of accidents at intersections and therefore lowering liability costs.[2]

The city offset the $2.2 million cost of changing the signals to LEDS by spreading out payments to match the savings in energy and maintenance. Contract laborers were used to complete the project quickly so rebates from PGE and Pacific Power could be claimed, for a total savings of $715,000.

The city also took advantage of Oregon's Business Energy Tax Credit, worth 35 percent of the higher cost of energy-efficient equipment compared to standard equipment. This move saved the city a cool half-million bucks. Can you imagine the savings of energy and money if every city and town made the switch to energy-efficient bulbs? It would be magnificent.

# How Many Lightbulbs Does It Take to Change the World?

*One*—but everyone has to get on board!

Here are some pretty amazing facts:

If every American changed just *one lightbulb* to an energy-efficient CFL, it would prevent pollution equivalent to taking *1 million cars off the road* and save us $600 million in energy costs per year.[3]

If every American household changed just five of their most frequently used lightbulbs to CFLs, we would save *$8 billion* a year in energy costs and prevent greenhouse gas pollution equivalent to taking more than *10 million* cars off the road.[5]

If *every* lightbulb in America were replaced with an energy-efficient bulb, we would save *$18 billion* a year on electricity—the total amount of power produced by *30 nuclear reactors* or as many as *80 coal-fired power plants*, which would prevent *158 million tons* of carbon dioxide from being released every year (as well as significant amounts of mercury emitted from burning coal, which is poisoning everyone, especially the fish).[6]

> *One CFL saves 700 pounds of carbon dioxide emmisions.*[4]

## How Many Leaders Does It Take to Change a Lightbulb?

*One,* and the rest will follow.

Here's the first leader: On February 20, 2007, Australia's prime minister, John Howard, and environment minister Malcom Turnbull announced that, effective immediately, inefficient incandescent lightbulbs would begin to be phased out for the entire country, with a complete ban in place by 2010.

And the rest will follow. Gearing up to make the switch are:

- **The European Union.** The European Commission is considering banning the least energy-efficient bulbs, namely incandescent bulbs, throughout the European Union.[7]
- **Canada.** The provinces of Ontario and Nova Scotia are moving toward phasing out and eventually banning incandescent bulbs altogether.[8][9]
- **New Zealand.** The country plans to ban incandescent bulbs with legislation similar to Australia's.[10]
- **California.** In April 2007, California Assembly member Lloyd Levine intro-duced a bill that would ban the sale of incandescent bulbs by 2012.[11]
- **Connecticut.** In January 2007, Connecticut General Assembly members James A. O'Rourke and three others proposed an initiative to ban all incandescent bulbs deemed inefficient by the state's commissioner of environmental protection. A surcharge of 10¢ would be applied to all incandescent bulbs sold in the state, and retailers and wholesalers could be fined $100 for each inefficient incandescent bulb they sold.[12]

> *The average American house has 28 light sockets, and about 10 to 20 percent of your electricity bill is the cost of lighting. Choosing energy-efficient bulbs really adds up![13]*

## Lightbulbs at a Glance

**Type of Bulb: Incandescent**

*How it works:* Electricity passing through a filament makes the filament glow.

*Life span:* 750 to 1,500 hours; a bulb lit for 4 hours a day will last for 6 to 8 months. This is the shortest life span of all types of bulbs.

*Energy use:* The most inefficient type of bulb, incandescents lose 90 percent of the energy they draw as heat.

*Bonus features:* It provides the warm-looking light we are used to. Bulbs are inexpensive to purchase, but more expensive to run and have to be replaced more often.

*Best uses:* If you must use them, restrict them to where you most want a warm, familiar glow.

*Downsides:* They're a massive waste of electricity.

## Type of Bulb: Long-Life Incandescent

*How it works:* Electricity passing through a filament makes the filament glow.

*Life span:* 10,000 to 20,000 hours; a bulb lit for 4 hours a day will last for 7 to 14 years. A long-life incandescent lasts 6 to 10 times longer than a standard incandescent.

*Energy use:* They're inefficient, but longer lasting than standard incandescents. A long-life bulb uses the same amount of energy as a standard incandescent bulb, but may produce less light per watt.

*Bonus features:* Infrequent replacement means you put less waste in the landfill.

*Best uses:* These bulbs are intended for use in areas where the electrical voltage tends to fluctuate, such as in rural areas.

*Downsides:* Long-life incandescent bulbs are inefficient. They require the same amount of energy to run as standard incandescent bulbs, but may produce a little less light. They're also more expensive to purchase than standard incandescents.

## Type of Bulb: Halogen

*How it works:* Electricity passing through a capsule filled with halogen gas and a tungsten filament makes the filament glow.

*Life span:* 2,000 to 3,000 hours; a bulb lit for 4 hours a day will last 22 to 36 months. That's two or three times longer than a standard incandescent bulb.

*Energy use:* Halogens produce more light using less energy—about 10 to 15 percent less energy than standard incandescent bulbs.

*Bonus features:* The light is of a high quality with excellent color rendering.

*Best uses:* These bulbs are great in track lighting and specialty lighting fixtures, such as those illuminating artwork.

*Downsides:* Halogen bulbs run at very high temperatures and can pose a fire hazard.

## Type of Bulb: Compact Fluorescent

*How it works:* An electrical current illuminates the gas filling the tube.

*Life span:* 6,000 to 15,000 hours; a bulb lit for 4 hours a day will last 5½ to 14 years; that's 10 to 15 times longer than a standard incandescent bulb.

*Energy use:* They're very efficient, using one-quarter of the energy a standard incandescent does to create the same amount of light.

*Bonus features:* They come in many shapes, sizes, and wattages. And, their initial cost is recouped after 500 hours of use.

*Best uses:* There are models that will fit your every need indoors and outdoors (including dimmable and three-way lights).

*Downsides:* Some models flicker when they come on and take a minute to reach full light. The bulb also contains a minute amount of mercury (which is harmless while the bulb is in use) and should be disposed of properly. Do not put CFLs in your household garbage if better disposal options exist. To find out, check www.earth911.org (where you can find disposal sites by entering your zip code) or call 877-EARTH911. Another option is to check with your local waste management agency for recycling options and disposal guidelines in your community. Additional information is available at www.lamprecycle.org. Finally, IKEA stores take back used CFLs. If your local waste management agency offers no other disposal options except your household garbage, place the CFL in two plastic bags and seal them before putting it in the trash. If your waste agency incinerates its garbage, you should search a wider geographic area for proper disposal options. Never send a CFL or other mercury-containing product to an incinerator.

### Type of Bulb: Light-Emitting Diode

*How it works:* Electricity passing through a semiconductor chip makes the chip emit light.

*Life span:* 100,000 or more hours; a bulb lit for 4 hours a day will last more than 92 years. That's 100 times longer than a standard incandescent bulb.

*Energy use:* The bulbs are ultra-efficient, using one-tenth the energy a standard incandescent bulb does to create the same amount of light.

*Bonus features:* They're very durable, because there's no filament to break. They have a longer life expectancy than the average American does.

*Best uses:* They're good for task-specific lighting, track lighting, reading lights, refrigerator lights, spa or pool lights, flashlights, nightlights, and Christmas lights, for example.

*Downsides:* They're expensive, and not as bright as some other bulbs of an equivalent wattage (though new technology is changing that).

## What's a Watt? Brightness Guide for Energy-Efficient Bulbs

The brightness of a lightbulb makes or breaks how pleasing the light is. Brightness is measured in lumens, which in lightbulbs translates into watts—the higher the wattage, the brighter the light.

With incandescent bulbs, measuring brightness by a bulb's wattage is pretty misleading because 90 percent of the wattage is wasted as heat instead of light. CFLs and other energy-efficient bulbs use about a quarter of the energy incandescent bulbs do to make the same amount of light, and all of it goes to make light, not heat. That's the purpose of a lightbulb, right?

The brightness of energy-efficient lightbulbs is characterized in both watts and lumens. Energy-efficient bulbs need a lot less wattage to generate the same amount of light as incandescent bulbs, and the "Brightness Guide" below will help you translate the difference so you'll get the right fit when replacing an incandescent bulb. The guide also tells you how much you'll save in cost and carbon dioxide emissions. For example, a traditional 60-watt bulb can be replaced by a CFL of about 15 watts. Illuminating, isn't it?

**Notes:**

- Calculations for cost savings and carbon dioxide savings are based on the average life of 10,000 hours for CFLs.
- Electricity usage is measured in kilowatt-hours.
- The cost of electricity per kilowatt-hour varies among states and utility providers.

Ten cents per kilowatt-hour is at the low end of typical costs. Twenty cents per kilowatt-hour is at the high end of typical costs. Your electric bill should tell you how much you pay per kilowatt-hour, so you can figure your savings accordingly.

- Given that the average American family spends close to $2,000 a year on electricity,[14] and that lighting accounts for up to 20 percent of home energy use,[15] it's likely that going green with energy-efficient lightbulbs will really add up!

## GREEN TIP Turn It Off!

According to the US Naval Engineering Laboratory, *1 extra hour* a day of unnecessary lighting (such as a light left on in a room that no one is in, or an extra light turned on in a well-lit room) can increase a family or business's electricity costs by 5 to 10 percent a month.[16]

## BRIGHTNESS GUIDE

| INCANDESCENT LIGHTBULB (WATTS) | COMPACT FLUORESCENT LIGHTBULB (WATTS) | LUMENS | COST SAVINGS AT 10¢ PER KILOWATT-HOUR ($) | COST SAVINGS AT 20¢ PER KILOWATT-HOUR ($) | CARBON DIOXIDE SAVINGS (LB) |
|---|---|---|---|---|---|
| 40 | 11–14 | > 490 | 26–29 | 52–59 | 338–381 |
| 60 | 15–19 | > 900 | 41–45 | 83–91 | 537–589 |
| 75 | 20–25 | > 1,200 | 51–55 | 101–111 | 659–719 |
| 100 | 26–29 | > 1,750 | 71–75 | 143–149 | 927–970 |
| 150 | 38–42 | > 2,600 | 109–113 | 217–225 | 1,413–1,461 |

*Source:* Based on figures calculated by Environmental Defense, www.environmentaldefense.org/page.cfm?tagid=630&campaign=480.

## Will the United States Pledge Allegiance to Energy-Efficient Lighting?

A coalition of major-player advocates for energy efficiency announced a call to action in spring 2007, proposing an industrywide initiative and legislative action to shift the nation toward using energy-efficient lighting technology. Lightbulb giant Philips Lighting Company is leading the coalition, which includes Senator Mark Pryor (D-Arkansas), Congressman Don Manzillo (R-Illinois), the Natural Resources Defense Council, and two other energy-efficiency organizations. The plan proposes public policies that would provide incentives for consumers and businesses and set standards for phasing out the least efficient products, such as incandescent bulbs.

Philips Lighting announced its plan to become the first lighting manufacturer in North America to stop manufacturing inefficient incandescent bulbs by 2016.

By switching to energy-efficient lighting, Americans can make a significant economic and environmentally responsible impact on the ecological footprint of the world.

## Where to Buy Lightbulbs

Energy-efficient lightbulbs are widely available. Look for them at big box stores such as Home Depot, Lowe's, Target, IKEA, and Wal-Mart; hardware stores such as Ace Hardware; and discount chains such as Costco and Sam's Club. It's never been easier to make the switch to using energy-efficent bulbs to light up your life while saving energy, money, and peace of mind.

Online sources of energy-efficient lightbulbs include www.bulbs.com, www.appliancepartscompany.com, www.blackenergy.com, www.americanlight.com, and www.servicelighting.com, www.efi.org.

Just one CFL can save 700 pounds of carbon dioxide emissions. Once upon a time, CFLs were only available in space-age-looking spiral bulbs. Now, they're available in a wide selection of shapes and sizes and a spectrum of brightnesses. Check out any of these bulbs to fit any range of needs for feel-good ambience and lighting up your life.

## A-SHAPE BULBS

A-shape CFL bulbs look the most like standard incandescent lightbulbs and come in wide range of brightnesses and a few sizes, some a little smaller and others larger. They are most suitable for lamps, ceiling fixtures and fans, recessed can fixtures, wall sconces, track lighting fixtures, and hanging pendants.

### GENERAL ELECTRIC

#### 11-watt Soft White A17
4.4 inches long

This bulb has a warm white light and is for home use. Its low brightness suits it for ambient lighting (400 lumens, equivalent to a 40-watt incandescent bulb).

#### 15-watt Soft White A19 and A21
4.7 inches and 5.4 inches long, respectively

This bulb has a warm white light and is for home use. Its medium brightness suits it for hallway and room lighting (825 lumens, equivalent to a 60-watt incandescent bulb).

#### 20-watt Soft White Biax A23
6.1 inches long

This bulb has a warm white light and is for home use. Its medium brightness suits it for hallway and room lighting (1,125 lumens, equivalent to a 75-watt incandescent bulb).

**Life expectancy:** 10,000 hours

None are dimmable or three-way. All are Energy Star rated.

### MAXLITE

#### 13-watt A-Style
4.3 inches long

This bulb has a warm white light and is for home use. Its medium brightness suits it for hallway and room lighting (800 lumens, equivalent to a 60-watt incandescent bulb).

**Life expectancy:** 15,000 hours

It is not dimmable, three-way, or Energy Star rated.

### WESTINGHOUSE

#### 20-watt A-Shape Soft White
6.58 inches long

This bulb has a warm white light and is for home use. Its high brightness suits it for reading (1,000 lumens, equivalent to an 80-watt incandescent bulb).

**Life expectancy:** 6,000 hours

It is not dimmable, three-way, or Energy Star rated.

## CANDLE AND TORPEDO BULBS

Candle and torpedo CFLs are shaped like their name and available in a lower brightness spectrum that is ideal for gentle ambient lighting. They are recommended for use in such lighting fixtures as ceiling fans, hanging pendants, wall sconces, and table lamps.

### GENERAL ELECTRIC

#### 5-watt Soft White Candle
4.8 inches long

This bulb has a warm white light and is for home use. Its low brightness suits it for ambient lighting (200 lumens, equivalent to a 25-watt incandescent bulb).

*(continued)*

### 7-watt Soft White Candle

5.2 inches long

This bulb has a warm white light and is for home use. Its low brightness suits it for ambient lighting (370 lumens, equivalent to a 32-watt incandescent bulb).

### 9-watt Soft White Candle

5.4 inches long

This bulb has a warm white light and is for home use. Its low brightness suits it for ambient lighting (430 lumens, equivalent to a 40-watt incandescent bulb).

*Life expectancy:* 6,000 hours

None are dimmable or three-way. All are Energy Star rated.

## MAXLITE

### 3-watt MiniCandle

4.4 inches long

This bulb has a warm white light and is for home use. Its low brightness suits it for ambient lighting (135 lumens, equivalent to a 20-watt incandescent bulb).

### 5-watt MiniCandle Bulb

4.9 inches long

This bulb has a warm white light and is for home use. Its low brightness suits it for ambient lighting (220 lumens, equivalent to a 25-watt incandescent bulb).

*Life expectancy:* 6,000 hours

Neither is dimmable or three-way. Neither is Energy Star rated.

## SYLVANIA

### 4-watt Delux Candle

4.4 inches long

This bulb has a warm white light and is for home use. Its low brightness suits it for ambient lighting (195 lumens, equivalent to a 16-watt incandescent bulb).

### 5-watt Delux Candle

4.4 inches long

This bulb has a warm white light and is for home use. Its low brightness suits it for ambient lighting (425 lumens, equivalent to a 40-watt incandescent bulb).

*Life expectancy:* 10,000 hours

Neither is dimmable or three-way. Both are Energy Star rated.

## TCP (TECHNICAL CONSUMER PRODUCTS)

### 4-watt Torpedo

4.4 inches long

This bulb has a warm white light and is for home use. Its low brightness suits it for ambient lighting (195 lumens, equivalent to a 16-watt incandescent bulb).

### 9-watt Torpedo

4.4 inches long

This bulb has a warm white light and is for home use. Its low brightness suits it for ambient lighting (425 lumens, equivalent to a 40-watt incandescent bulb).

*Life expectancy:* 8,000 hours

Neither is dimmable, three-way, or Energy Star rated.

# FLOODLIGHT BULBS

Floodlight CFLs are available in a wide range of brightnesses for both indoor and outdoor use. Excellent for recessed can and track lighting fixtures, floodlight bulbs spread light throughout a room. Some floodlights have a reflective coating that directs light forward and a few have parabolic aluminized reflectors, which control and concentrate the light. Not only will CFL floodlight bulbs save you money on your electric bill, they will save you time and effort because they don't need to be changed as frequently as incandescent bulbs.

## GENERAL ELECTRIC

### 11-watt R20 Soft White Genura Flood
4.7 inches long, reflector

This bulb has a warm white light and is for home use. Its low brightness suits it for ambient lighting (400 lumens, equivalent to a 40-watt incandescent bulb).

### 15-watt R30 Soft White Genura Flood
5.5 inches long, reflector

This bulb has a warm white light and is for home use. Its medium brightness suits it for hallway and room lighting (700 lumens, equivalent to a 60-watt incandescent bulb).

### 23-watt R25 Soft White Genura Flood
4.9 inches long, reflector

This bulb has a warm white light and is for home use. Its high brightness suits it for reading (1,100 lumens, equivalent to a 90-watt incandescent bulb).

### 26-watt R40 Soft White Genura Flood
6.5 inches long, reflector

This bulb has a warm white light and is for home use. Its high brightness suits it for reading (1,200 lumens, equivalent to a 100-watt incandescent bulb).

### 26-watt PAR38 Soft White Genura Flood
6.5 inches long, parabolic aluminized reflector

This bulb has a warm white light and is for home use. Its high brightness suits it for reading (1,200 lumens, equivalent to a 100-watt incandescent bulb).

**Life expectancy:** 6,000 hours for R40 and PAR38, 10,000 hours for R20 and R30, 15,000 hours for R25

None are dimmable or three-way. All but R25 are Energy Star rated.

## PHILIPS

### 16-watt R-30 Dimmable Flood
5.7 inches long

This bulb has a warm white light and is for home use. Its medium brightness suits it for hallway and room lighting (630 lumens, equivalent to an 80-watt incandescent bulb).

**Life expectancy:** 8,000 hours

It is dimmable, but not three-way or Energy Star rated.

## TCP (TECHNICAL CONSUMER PRODUCTS)

### 14-watt Indoor/Outdoor R-30 Flood
5.4 inches long

This bulb has a warm white light and is for home use. Its medium brightness suits it for hallway and room lighting (650 lumens, equivalent to a 65-watt incandescent bulb).

### 16-watt Indoor/Outdoor R-30 Flood
5.7 inches long

This bulb has a warm white light and is for home use. Its medium brightness suits it for hallway and room lighting (750 lumens, equivalent to a 75-watt incandescent bulb).

**Life expectancy:** 8,000 hours

Neither is dimmable or three-way. The 14-watt bulb is Energy Star rated, but the 16-watt bulb is not.

*(continued)*

## WESTINGHOUSE

### 14-watt R30 Dimmable Flood

5.1 inches long

This bulb has a warm white light and is for home use. Its medium brightness suits it for hallway and room lighting (600 lumens, equivalent to a 60-watt incandescent bulb).

*Life expectancy:* 6,000 hours

It is dimmable, but isn't three-way or Energy Star rated.

# GLOBE BULBS

Globe CFLs are round spheres available in an array of brightnesses for indoor lighting. The best uses for globe-shape bulbs are in vanity fixtures, floor and table lamps, hanging pendants, and wall sconces. Choosing CFL globe lightbulbs is a gift to our globe, saving energy and preventing pollution.

## FEIT ELECTRIC

### 11-watt G25 Globe

5.3 inches long

This bulb has a warm white light and is for home use. Its medium brightness suits it for hallway and room lighting (550 lumens, equivalent to a 40-watt incandescent bulb).

*Life expectancy:* 8,000 hours

It is not dimmable or three-way, but it is Energy Star rated.

## GENERAL ELECTRIC

### 11-watt Soft White G25 Globe

4.8 inches long

This bulb has a warm white light and is for home use. Its low brightness suits it for ambient lighting (550 lumens, equivalent to a 40-watt incandescent bulb).

### 15-watt Soft White G29 Globe

5.8 inches long

This bulb has a warm white light and is for home use. Its medium brightness suits it for hallway and room lighting (750 lumens, equivalent to a 60-watt incandescent bulb).

*Life expectancy:* 10,000 hours for G25 and 12,000 hours for G29

Neither is dimmable or three-way, but they are Energy Star rated.

## MAXLITE

### 14-watt G30 Globe Lamp

5.2 inches long

This bulb has a warm white light and is for home use. Its medium brightness suits it for hallway and room lighting (900 lumens, equivalent to a 60-watt incandescent bulb).

*Life expectancy:* 8,000 hours

It is not dimmable or three-way, but it is Energy Star rated.

## PHILIPS

### 12-watt Marathon Classic Globe

4.58 inches long

This bulb has a warm white light and is for home use. Its low brightness suits it for ambient lighting (525 lumens, equivalent to a 48-watt incandescent bulb).

*Life expectancy:* 8,000 hours

It is not dimmable or three-way, but it is Energy Star rated.

## SYLVANIA

### 9-watt Warm White Deluxe Globe 40 Bulb
4.6 inches long

This bulb has a warm white light and is for home use. Its medium brightness suits it for hallway and room lighting (450 lumens, equivalent to a 40-watt incandescent bulb).

*Life expectancy:* 8,000 hours

It is not dimmable or three-way, but is Energy Star rated.

## TCP (TECHNICAL CONSUMER PRODUCTS)

### 19-watt G40 Globe
6.87 inches long

This bulb has a warm white light and is for home use. Its medium brightness suits it for hallway and room lighting (925 lumens, equivalent to a 75-watt incandescent bulb).

*Life expectancy:* 8,000 hours

It is not dimmable, three-way, or Energy Star rated.

# OUTDOOR BULBS

Using CFLs for outdoor lighting is a smart green move. Not only do they save energy, consequently saving you money on your electric bill, their long life expectancy means they don't need to be changed very often, which is especially great for hard-to-reach places. Use these bulbs in flush-mounted outdoor ceiling fixtures, hanging pendants, and lamps.

## PHILIPS

### 15-watt Marathon Outdoor
5.37 inches long, dome shape

This bulb has a warm white light and is for home use. Its medium light suits it for outdoor use (800 lumens, equivalent to a 40- or 60-watt incandescent bulb).

### 18-watt Marathon Outdoor
5.7 inches long, dome shape

This bulb has a warm white light and is for home use. Its medium light suits it for outdoor use (1,100 lumens, equivalent to a 75-watt incandescent bulb).

### 16-watt Marathon Bug-A-Way Classic 60 Globe
4.5 inches long, A-shape

This bulb has a medium light and is for outdoor use to repel mosquitos (600 lumens, equivalent to a 60-watt incandescent bulb).

*Life expectancy:* 10,000 hours for the Marathon Outdoor bulbs and 8,000 hours for the Marathon Bug-A-Way bulb

These bulbs are not dimmable or three-way. The Marathon Outdoor bulbs are Energy Star rated, but the Marathon Bug-A-Way bulb is not.

# SPIRAL BULBS

Spiral CFLs are what come to mind when most of us think of energy-efficient lightbulbs. With a wide range of uses for indoors and out, spiral bulbs are available in a broad spectrum of brightnesses that use a fraction of the energy of incandescent bulbs and have an impressively long life expectancy. There are spiral bulbs for use in ceiling fans and flush-mounted ceiling fixtures; recessed lighting, track lighting, and outdoor fixtures; floor and table lamps; hanging pendants; and wall sconces.

## FEIT ELECTRIC

### 18-watt Spiral
4.6 inches long

This bulb has a warm white light and is for home use. Its medium brightness suits it for hallway and room lighting (1,100 lumens, equivalent to a 75-watt incandescent bulb).

*(continued)*

### 23-watt Spiral

5 inches long

This bulb has a warm white light and is for home use. Its medium brightness suits it for hallway and room lighting (1,600 lumens, equivalent to a 100-watt incandescent bulb).

### 13–20–25-watt 3-Way Eco-Twist

6.2 inches long

This bulb has a warm white light and is for home use. Its low brightness suits it for ambient lighting (13 watts: 700 lumens, equivalent to a 40-watt incandescent bulb; 20 watts: 1,150 lumens, equivalent to a 75-watt incandescent bulb; 25 watts: 1,700 lumens, equivalent to a 100-watt incandescent bulb.).

### 20-watt 3-Way Eco-Twist

6.2 inches long

This bulb has a warm white light and is for home use. Its medium brightness suits it for hallway and room lighting (1,150 lumens, equivalent to a 75-watt incandescent bulb).

### 23-watt 3-Way Eco-Twist

6.2 inches long

This bulb has a warm white light and is for home use. Its high brightness suits it for hallway, room, and task lighting (1,600 lumens, equivalent to a 100-watt incandescent bulb).

*Life expectancy:* 8,000 hours

None are dimmable. The 18- and 23-watt spiral bulbs are not three-way, but the 13-, 20-, and 23-watt Eco-Twist bulbs are. All are Energy Star rated.

## GENERAL ELECTRIC

### 10-watt Soft White T2 Spiral

3.7 inches long

This bulb has a warm white light and is for home use. Its low brightness suits it for ambient lighting (580 lumens, equivalent to a 40-watt incandescent bulb).

### 13-watt Soft White T2 Spiral

3.9 inches long

This bulb has a warm white light and is for home use. Its medium brightness suits it for hallway and room lighting (870 lumens, equivalent to a 60-watt incandescent bulb).

### 10-watt Soft White T3 Spiral

4.4 inches long

This bulb has a warm white light and is for home use. Its medium brightness suits it for ambient lighting (520 lumens, equivalent to a 40-watt incandescent bulb).

### 15-watt Soft White T3 Spiral

4.8 inches long

This bulb has a warm white light and is for home use. Its medium brightness suits it for hallway and room lighting (950 lumens, equivalent to a 60-watt incandescent bulb).

### 20-watt Soft White T3 Spiral

4.7 inches long

This bulb has a warm white light and is for home use. Its high brightness suits it for task lighting (1,200 lumens, equivalent to a 75-watt incandescent bulb).

### 26-watt Soft White T3 Spiral

5.2 inches long

This bulb has a warm white light and is for home use. Its high brightness suits it for hallway, room, and task lighting (1,700 lumens, equivalent to a 100-watt incandescent bulb).

*Life expectancy:* 8,000 hours for all but the 26-watt model, which will last for 10,000 hours

None are dimmable or three-way, but all are Energy Star rated.

# GREENLITE

### 15-watt MiniSpiral
4.25 inches long

This bulb has a warm white light and is for home use. Its medium brightness suits it for hallway and room lighting (1,100 lumens, equivalent to a 60-watt incandescent bulb).

### 18-watt MiniSpiral
5.25 inches long

This bulb has a warm white light and is for home use. Its medium brightness suits it for hallway and room lighting (1,200 lumens, equivalent to a 75-watt incandescent bulb).

### 23-watt Spiral
5.75 inches long

This bulb has a warm white light and is for home use. Its high brightness suits it for hallway, room, and task lighting (1,600 lumens, equivalent to a 100-watt incandescent bulb).

### 23-watt Dimmable Spiral
3.9 inches long

This bulb has a warm white light and is for home use. Its high brightness suits it for hallway, room, and task lighting (1,380 lumens, equivalent to a 90-watt incandescent bulb).

*Life expectancy:* 8,000 hours for all but the Dimmable Spiral, which will last for 10,000 hours

None are three-way. Only the Dimmable Spiral is dimmable. All are Energy Star rated.

# HARMONY LIGHTWIZ (LITETRONICS)

### 11-watt 3-Way Spiral
6.2 inches long

This bulb has a warm white light and is for home use. Its low brightness suits it for ambient lighting (960 lumens, equivalent to a 40-watt incandescent bulb).

### 23-watt 3-Way Spiral
6.2 inches long

This bulb has a warm white light and is for home use. Its medium brightness suits it for hallway and room lighting (1,380 lumens, equivalent to a 90-watt incandescent bulb).

### 30-watt 3-Way Spiral
6.2 inches long

This bulb has a warm white light and is for home use. Its high brightness suits it for hallway, room, and task lighting (1,600 lumens, equivalent to a 100-watt incandescent bulb).

### 15-watt Mini-Spiral
4.1 inches long

This bulb has a warm white light and is for home use. Its medium brightness suits it for hallway and room lighting (675 lumens, equivalent to a 60-watt incandescent bulb).

*Life expectancy:* 6,000 hours for the 3-Way bulbs, 10,000 hours for the Mini-Spiral bulb

None are dimmable. The 11-, 23-, and 30-watt 3-Way Spiral bulbs are three-way. All are Energy Star rated.

# MAXLITE

### 15-watt MaxLite Dimmable Spiral
5 inches long

This bulb has a warm white light and is for home use. Its medium brightness suits it for hallway and room lighting (900 lumens, equivalent to a 60-watt incandescent bulb).

### 20-watt MaxLite Dimmable Spiral
5.6 inches long

This bulb has a warm white light and is for home use. Its medium brightness suits it for hallway and room lighting (1,380 lumens, equivalent to a 90-watt incandescent bulb).

*Life expectancy:* 6,000 hours

Both bulbs are dimmable, but neither is three-way or Energy Star rated.

*(continued)*

## N:VISION

### 23-watt Suave Blanco Spiral
5 inches long

This bulb has a warm white light and is for home use. Its high brightness suits it for hallway, room, and task lighting (1,300 lumens, equivalent to a 100-watt incandescent bulb).

### 27-watt Daylight Spiral
5.6 inches long

This bulb has a bright white light (simulating daylight) and is for home use. Its high brightness suits it for hallway, room, and task lighting (1,600 lumens, equivalent to a 100-watt incandescent bulb).

**Life expectancy:** 10,000 hours

They are not dimmable or three-way. Only the Suave Blanco bulb is Energy Star rated.

## SATCO

### 13-watt Energy Saving Spiral
5.5 inches long

This bulb has a cool white light and is for offices and stores. Its medium brightness suits it for hallway and room lighting (800 lumens, equivalent to a 60-watt incandescent bulb).

### 26-watt Energy Saving Spiral
5.6 inches long

This bulb has a warm white light and is for home use. Its high brightness suits it for hallway, room, and task lighting (1,600 lumens, equivalent to a 100-watt incandescent bulb).

**Life expectancy:** 10,000 hours

They are not dimmable or three-way, but they are Energy Star rated.

## SYLVANIA

### 12-watt Delux EL 3-Way Twist
5.1 inches long

This bulb has a soft white light and is for home use. Its medium brightness suits it for hallway and room lighting (600 lumens, equivalent to a 60-watt incandescent bulb).

### 19-watt Delux EL 3-Way Twist
5.5 inches long

This bulb has a soft white light and is for home use. Its medium brightness suits it for hallway and room lighting (1,100 lumens, equivalent to a 75-watt incandescent bulb).

### 28-watt Delux EL 3-Way Twist
6.1 inches long

This bulb has a soft white light and is for home use. Its high brightness suits it for hallway, room, and task lighting (1,800 lumens, equivalent to a 100-watt incandescent bulb).

### 30-watt Delux EL 3-Way Twist
5.13 inches long

This bulb has a soft white light and is for home use. Its high brightness suits it for hallway, room, and task lighting (1,800 lumens, equivalent to a 100-watt incandescent bulb).

### 7-watt Delux EL Mini Twist
4.4 inches long

This bulb has a cool white light and is for offices and stores. Its low brightness suits it for ambient lighting (300 lumens, equivalent to a 32-watt incandescent bulb).

### 11-watt Delux EL Mini Twist
4.5 inches long

This bulb has a cool white light and is for offices and stores. Its low brightness suits it for ambient lighting (400 lumens, equivalent to a 40-watt incandescent bulb).

### 13-watt Delux EL Mini Twist

4.6 inches long

This bulb has a cool white light and is for offices and stores. Its low brightness suits it for ambient lighting (800 lumens, equivalent to a 60-watt incandescent bulb).

### 19-watt Delux EL Mini Twist

5.5 inches long

This bulb has a cool white light and is for offices and stores. Its medium brightness suits it for hallway and room lighting (900 lumens, equivalent to a 75-watt incandescent bulb).

### 23-watt Delux EL Mini Twist

5.75 inches long

This bulb has a cool white light and is for offices and stores. Its high brightness suits it for hallway, room, and task lighting (1,100 lumens, equivalent to a 90-watt incandescent bulb).

*Life expectancy:* 6,000 hours

None are dimmable. The 3-Way Twist bulbs are three-way, but the Mini Twist bulbs are not. All are Energy Star rated.

## TCP SPRINGLAMPS (TECHNICAL CONSUMER PRODUCTS)

### 15-watt Dimmable

5.3 inches long

This bulb has a warm white light and is for home use. Its medium brightness suits it for hallway and room lighting (600 lumens, equivalent to a 60-watt incandescent bulb).

### 20-watt Dimmable

5.6 inches long

This bulb has a warm white light and is for home use. Its medium brightness suits it for hallway and room lighting (1,200 lumens, equivalent to a 75-watt incandescent bulb).

*Life expectancy:* 10,000 hours

Both are dimmable, but neither is three-way or Energy Star rated.

# CHAPTER 9

# Sustainable, Ecological Home Furnishings and Materials

**Sustainable** *adjective*

**2a:** of, relating to, or being a method of harvesting or using a
resource so that the resource is not depleted or permanently damaged;
**b:** of or relating to a lifestyle involving the use of sustainable
methods (*Merriam-Webster's Collegiate Dictionary*)

The life cycles of the materials that furnish and
appoint our homes play a big role in the quality of
our environment inside and out. The broad
strokes of those life cycles include the effects on
humans and the environment of the materials they are
made of and how they are made, used, and disposed of.
Choosing greener materials for home furnishings isn't just
about preserving the environment in the great outdoors,
it's about immediately improving the environment in your
home, and particularly about improving the indoor air

quality with paints, flooring materials, carpets, counters, cabinets, and candles that will not harm your health or the planet. Synthetic materials used in conventional home furnishings—whether functional, decorative, or both—can be major causes of indoor air pollution. They quietly, constantly emit volatile organic compounds (VOCs) while they're in your home. And the impact of what happens before and after their stay in our homes (during their manufacture and disposal) is something we all have a responsibility to think about. The good news is that there is a new generation of eco-friendly options when it comes to walls, floors, and decorative items like candles that serve both form and function in eco-style.

This chapter opens the door to a new green horizon of eco-smart home decorating and furnishing products. So, place a bookmark here for great ideas and savvy ecological options for your next green home improvement or decorating project.

# Green, Nontoxic Paints

Paint usually doesn't get much attention unless it's exquisite—or horribly uncouth—in a room. However, if you've ever walked into a freshly painted room that is rank with fumes, it's hard to ignore. Conventional paint is noxious stuff—to manufacture, to use, and to dispose of. The slew of nasty chemicals, heavy metals, and VOCs in run-of-the-mill paints are seriously harmful to humans and the environment. Those putrid fumes? They're VOCs, baby, and that's just part of the problem. The good news is that due to consumer demand and tighter federal regulations, there are new options in nontoxic paints, stains, and strippers (no, not the dancing kind, silly). Whether you want simple tones of white or bold splashes of color, choosing nontoxic paint gives you a green winning hand—functional, beautiful, and safe for all living things.

## What's in Paint

Paint can be used to protect and decorate just about any surface—walls, wood, metal, concrete, masonry, furniture, floors—after all, it's been around in one form or another since cavemen and cavewomen decorated the walls of their caves. Of course, today, paint comes in a wide variety of sheens and a broad palette of colors. The materials used to make paint are equally diverse, but three basic components make paint what it is: a binder, a vehicle or solvent, and pigments. There are two ways to go when choosing paint: toxic and nontoxic. What do you think is worth putting on your walls and breathing in? If you are in the market for paint, be sure to read labels carefully. Here's some information that will help you choose paint wisely.

**Binder.** The binder, or resin, is the solid part, or body, of the paint—it's the substance that holds it all together. The binder adheres to the pigment and is responsible for the paint's sheen (flat, satin, semigloss) and durability (making it appropriate for indoor or outdoor application). Paint binder can be made from synthetic or natural materials, and it may be toxic or nontoxic depending on the material used.

- Toxic binders can be synthetic oil (which is petroleum based), polyure-thane (a plastic), melamine resin (a plastic that is also called *melamine formaldehyde*), polyester (a plastic), or epoxy (which may contain the hardening additive bisphenol A, an endocrine disrupter[1] that is linked to reproductive problems, especially in men.[2]
- Nontoxic binders can be acrylic, latex, natural oils, milk, or clay.

Binders are categorized according to how they dry, which is determined by how the paint's vehicle, or solvent, evaporates. This is where VOCs come into play.

**Vehicle or solvent.** The vehicle, or solvent, is responsible for the viscosity of the paint, affecting how it goes on and dries. As a vehicle, it carries the body of the paint, and as a solvent, it evaporates rather than becoming one with the paint. It's volatile, meaning that it doesn't stick around, and it's the main source of paint fumes. Conventional paints are loaded with toxic solvents, many of which are VOCs, but water works as a vehicle too, and that's what nontoxic paints rely on. Paints marketed as "fast drying" may contain greater amounts of VOCs and solvents.

- Toxic vehicles or solvents in conventional solvent- and oil-based paints may include, but are not limited to:
  - *Petroleum distillates.* These toxic irritants of the eyes, skin, and lungs[3] may damage the central and peripheral nervous systems and the respiratory system.[4] They are very harmful to inhale, may cause dizziness and loss of coordination, and act as narcotics.[5]
  - *Esters such as butyl acetate or n-butyl ester.* Esters are very harmful to inhale;[6] can severely irritate the eyes, skin, and lungs;[7] cause skin reactions, discoloration, allergies, and damage;[8] and affect the central nervous system.[9] Repeated inhalation may damage the lining of the nose and may temporarily blur the vision.[10] Chronic exposure may cause liver and kidney damage.[11]
  - *Ketones, such as 2-butanone, aka methyl ethyl ketone.* Ketones are severe irritants of the eyes, nose, and throat[12] that may cause birth defects and developmental effects,[13] nervous system damage,[14] neurological and behavioral effects,[15] and liver and kidney effects.[16] Another interesting property is that when ketones are inhaled along with other chemicals that damage health, increased damage can occur.[17]

# Reading Labels: Tips for Choosing Green Paint

*VOC content.* VOCs are measured in grams per liter (g/l), and the lower, the better. Low-VOC paints should have less than 50 g/l, but some contain considerably less, in the range of 25 g/l. Zero-VOC paints must contain less than 5 g/l, but many actually contain zero.

*Solids content.* Solids are the body and pigment of paint and should range from 25 to 45 percent. The higher the percentage of solids is, the lower the percentages of other volatile substances like solvents and VOCs there are.

*EPA, OSHA, or DOT registration number.* Registration of a product with the US Environmental Protection Agency, Occupational Safety and Health Administration, or Department of Transportation indicates that it contains toxic ingredients that must be monitored by law. Products that are safe for you and the environment will not be registered with these agencies, so they won't have a registration number.

*Coverage information.* Paints differ in how many square feet they cover per gallon, how many coats are necessary, and whether a primer coat is required. Information on the coverage per gallon can be found on most paints' label, as can how many coats are advised for the job and whether a primer is recommended. Use these figures to calculate how much paint you'll need for the job before you buy it.

---

- *Glycol ethers* are highly toxic irritants of the skin and lungs[18] that are very harmful to inhale,[19] pose a reproductive hazard,[20] and are hazardous in the environment.[21]

**Pigments for color.** Historically, toxic heavy metals, like lead, have been used as pigments. Though lead is no longer allowed in house paints (it is still used in artist's paints), other toxic metals like cadmium and chromium and petroleum-derived chemicals *are* used to make pigments for a spectrum of colors. Deep colors, like reds and blues, and bright colors, like yellows, are most likely to contain more of these toxic pigment compounds. The good green news is that less toxic materials are being more widely used to create pigments, especially in low-VOC and zero-VOC paints. Natural paints contain the least harmful pigments of all, substituting materials such as clay and silica to create a rainbow palette and nontoxic beauty.

**Additives.** Okay, additives are the fourth component of paint. Employed to improve the characteristics of paint, additives may include foam-controlling agents, mold inhibitors, fungicides, biocides, insulators, fire retardants, and more. You can bet your bottom dollar that these additives are toxic and anything but natural.

## VOCs in Conventional Paints

VOCs have become a cause for concern in paints in particular, and with good reason.

*(continued on page 314)*

# 4 Green Standards to Look For
# in Sustainable Products and Services

## 1. Environmentally Preferable Purchasing (EPP) Program

The EPP program was established by the US Environmental Protection Agency in 1993 to identify and promote the purchase by federal agencies of products that have minimized environmental impacts. According to the executive order that set up the program, *environmentally preferable* means "products or services that have a lesser or reduced effect on human health and the environment when compared with competing products or services that serve the same purpose." The comparison applies throughout the life cycle of a product, including the raw materials' sourcing, manufacturing, packaging, distribution, use, reuse, maintenance, and disposal. For more information, visit www.epa.gov/epp.

The guiding principles for EPP dictate:

- Consideration of a product's environmental impact should be part of normal purchasing decision making, just as traditional factors such as safety, price, and performance are.
- Measures to reduce and eliminate waste should be considered throughout the life cycle of a product, from its sourcing through its manufacture and use to its disposal.
- The life cycle impact of a product should be compared to that of competitive products and services on a local, regional, national, and global scale.

## 2. Leadership in Energy and Environmental Design (LEED) Green Building Rating System

LEED is a nationally accepted benchmark established by the US Green Building Council for designing, building, and operating green buildings. It views sustainability as a whole-building endeavor with five key aspects affecting human and environmental health: sustainable site development, water conservation, energy conservation, materials selection, and indoor environmental quality. The LEED Green Building Rating System gives building owners a way to improve their buildings' ecological performance. The materials used in a building, such as paint, carpeting, and flooring, are awarded points according to performance-based requirements, particularly relating to indoor environmental quality. Products that have been used in constructing or furnishing LEED-certified buildings are generally notable for their high green standards. For more information, visit www.usgbc.org.

## 3. Cradle to Cradle Design Protocol

Cradle to Cradle is a new design paradigm dedicated to creating products whose materials can be continuously recycled in closed loops to maximize their material value without damaging ecosystems (as opposed to the cradle-to-grave cycle in place since the Industrial Revolution). Developed by William McDonough and Michael Braungart of "product and process design firm" MBDC (McDonough Braungart Design Chemistry) to create products and systems that contribute to economic, social, and environmental prosperity, Cradle to Cradle certification provides a company with a means for tangibly, credibly measuring its achievement in environmentally intelligent design and helps consumers purchase products that have a broader definition of quality. This means using environmentally safe and healthy materials; designing for reutilization, such as recycling or composting; using renewable energy and improving energy efficiency; efficiently using water and maximizing water quality associated with production; and instituting strategies for social responsibility. For more information, visit www.mbdc.com.

## 4.   Green Seal Certification

The Green Seal is a mark recognizing environmental responsibility that is given to products and services by Green Seal, an independent, nonprofit organization operating under the international guideline for environmental labeling programs set by the International Organization for Standardization (ISO 14020 and 14024—for more on these standards, visit www.iso.org) and the EPA's criteria for third-party certification, which includes peer review, data verification, testing protocols, and authority to ensure compliance. Products that get the Green Seal stamp of approval are in the major league for environmental integrity and lofty standards that must meet rigorous, science-based environmental standards. To obtain Green Seal certification, products are reviewed and evaluated on the basis of a life cycle approach, including raw material extraction and sourcing, manufacturing, use and application, and disposal.

Each candidate in the more than two dozen categories of products (like paper, cleaning products, windows, and paints) and services (like cleaning services, vehicle maintenance, and lodging) that can apply for the Green Seal is evaluated on a categorical basis. For instance, a Green Seal certified cleaning product cannot contain ingredients that would require it to be labeled toxic (as defined by US Consumer Product Safety Commission regulations; for more information, visit www.cpsc.gov); that are carcinogens, mutagens, or reproductive toxins; that are corrosive to the skin or eyes (as tested by the Organisation for Economic Co-operation and Development Guidelines for Testing Chemicals; for more information, visit www.oecd.org); that are toxic to aquatic life; or that significantly contribute to smog, damage the ozone layer, or create poor indoor air quality. In addition, no phthalate fragrances may be used, and the primary packaging must be recyclable. I must say, Green Seal standards are impressively thorough.

Paints certified by Green Seal must meet standards for VOCs. For Green Seal certified interior paints, flat paints cannot contain VOCs of more than 50 grams per liter, and nonflat paints (like gloss) cannot contain more than 150 grams per liter. For exterior paints, flat paints cannot contain VOCs of more than 100 grams per liter, and nonflat paints cannot contain more than 200 grams per liter.

See "What Labels Really Mean" (page 21) for more details, or visit www.greenseal.org.

VOCs are the fumes from fresh paint, which you can smell sometimes even days after it's been applied. They are pungently mischievous and cause serious problems for humans and the atmosphere. According to the US Environmental Protection Agency (EPA), the concentration of VOCs in indoor air is consistently higher than it is outdoors—concentrations 2 to 10 times higher are common.[22] Aggressive activities like paint stripping can boost indoor VOC pollution to 1,000 times[23] that of any level found outside. Have mercy! The deal is that VOCs are volatile, and they escape from paint in the form of a gas. It's their job. VOCs in a paint's solvent function as the vehicle that carries the paint, and then they evaporate so the paint will dry. The trouble is, they are seriously bad to breathe and put us at serious risk. Some effects associated with VOCs include:

- Major irritation of the eyes, nose, throat, and lungs[24]
- Headaches, loss of coordination, and nausea[25]
- Liver, kidney, and central nervous system damage[26]
- Cancer in animals (some VOCs)[27]
- Atmospheric and biospheric harm[28]
- Harm from ground-level smog and pollution caused by VOC-induced chemical and photochemical reactions[29]

See "Volatile Organic Compounds" on page 46 for more details.

## TYPES OF NONTOXIC PAINTS AND FINISHES

| TYPE OF PAINT OR FINISH | VOC CONTENT (G/L*) | INGREDIENTS | ADDITIONAL INFORMATION |
|---|---|---|---|
| LOW VOC | Paints and stains: less than 250; varnishes: less than 300 | Latex and acrylic paints use a water-based carrier instead of a petrochemical vehicle | Emits much lower levels of harmful emissions, but will emit fumes until dry |
| ZERO VOC | 0 to less than 5** | Most are water-based latex or acrylic enamels and have very low to no VOCs | Adding color may increase the VOC level to 10 g/L, which is still very low and harmless when dry |
| NATURAL | 0 | Water-based, with natural plant and mineral ingredients like plant oils and resins, plant dyes, mineral pigments, and milk casein | Has very little smell unless essential oils are added |

* g/L = grams per liter

** According to the EPA Reference Test Method 24, paints with VOCs of 5 g/L or less can be called zero-VOC paints.

# Why Are California's Standards Higher?

In 1986, California residents overwhelmingly approved an initiative to address the growing concerns about exposure to toxic chemicals. Passed as the Safe Water and Toxic Enforcement Act of 1986, it is better known by the name *Proposition 65*.

Proposition 65 publishes a list of chemicals deemed by the State of California to cause cancer, birth defects, or reproductive harm—many of the more than 550 chemicals that have been listed since 1986 can be found in paint and cleaning products! Ever fill up a car at a gas station in California? Ever notice the sticker on the pump that says the fuel contains stuff that is known to cause cancer and birth defects? It's the truth, and thanks to Proposition 65, consumers are more informed about just what the chemicals in the products they use are capable of.

| STANDARDS FOR LOW-VOC CONTENT | FLAT (G/L) | SATIN (G/L) | EGGSHELL (G/L) | SEMIGLOSS (G/L) | PRIMER OR SEALER (G/L) |
|---|---|---|---|---|---|
| Environmental Protection Agency (federal) | 250 | 380 | 380 | 380 | 350 |
| California | 50 | 50 | 50 | 50 | 100 |

## Why Green Paints Are Better

Green paints are better for humans and the planet. They are less toxic to manufacture, contain less toxic materials, and produce less harmful fumes.

- **Healthier for humans.** Nontoxic paints are better for adults and kids, especially those with allergies, asthma, or chemical sensitivities.
- **Kinder to the environment.** Conventional paint made with petrochemicals doesn't do the planet any good. Manufacturing paint can create 10 times the paint's weight in toxic waste.[30] Low-VOC and zero-VOC paints contain fewer chemicals that can escape to damage the atmosphere and biosphere and cause ground-level smog.
- **Effective.** They have coverage, versatility, and a color palette par excellence, as well as convenient washability and long-lived durability.
- **Easy cleanup.** Brushes and rollers can be cleaned with soap and water, as can surfaces painted with eco-friendly paints.
- **Low or no fume production.** The fewer VOCs in a paint, the quicker it will be safe to occupy freshly painted spaces.

*Green is the way to go. Check out the palette of products on the market today.*

## LOW-VOC PAINTS

### BENJAMIN MOORE

#### Aura

One coat with this interior paint line is enough to cover most surfaces. It is washable in all sheens, which include matte, eggshell, and satin. And it's available in all 3,300 Benjamin Moore colors.

www.myaurapaints.com

#### Eco Spec

This interior paint comes in a full range of colors. Sheens include flat, eggshell, and semigloss.

*Available:* at most hardware, home supply, and paint stores and online

www.benjaminmoore.com

### CLOVERDALE

#### EcoLogic

This enamel paint has lower levels of VOCs. It's for both interior (does not require primer) and exterior use. It comes in flat, eggshell, semigloss, gloss, epoxy, primer, and sealer.

*Available:* at select hardware and paint stores and online

www.cloverdalepaint.com

### KELLY-MOORE PAINT

#### Enviro-Cote

This very low VOC (less than 10 g/l) paint comes in a full range of colors. For interior use, it's available in flat, eggshell, semigloss, and primer/sealer (with less than 20 g/l VOCs).

*Available:* at Kelly-Moore paint stores, select hardware and paint stores, and online

www.kellymoore.com

### MAB PAINTS

#### Fresh Kote

This paint is available as an interior paint in flat, eggshell, semigloss and primer and in white, medium, and deep bases (with 140 g/l VOCs). For exterior use, it comes in flat and satin white (with 40 g/l).

*Available:* at MAB paint stores and online

www.mabpaints.com

### MILLER PAINT

#### Evolution

The interior Evolution ceramic matte finish has 80 g/l VOCs and comes in a full range of colors. In bases, it is available in white, medium, neutral, and accent. The exterior Evolution paint also comes in a full range of colors, has 133 g/l VOCs, and is available in flat and velvet satin.

*Available:* at select paint stores and online

www.millerpaint.com

### SHERWIN-WILLIAMS

#### Duration Home Interior Latex

This paint exceeds GS-11 criteria—the national standard for low-VOC paints—with less than 50 g/l VOCs. It comes in a full range of colors, and it's washable.

*Available:* at hardware and paint stores and online

www.sherwin-williams.com

### VISTA PAINT

#### Carefree Earth Coat

These low-VOC (some very low VOC) paints are Green Seal certified. Interior sheens include velva sheen (with 8 g/l VOCs), eggshell (49 g/l), flat (90 g/l), semigloss (44 g/l), and gloss (119 g/l).

*Available:* at Vista Paint stores, select paint and hardware stores, and online

www.vistapaint.com

# ZERO-VOC PAINTS AND FINISHES

## AFM

### Safecoat

This product line is available in a full range of colors and an extensive range of products. For interior use, choose from flat, eggshell, semigloss, and trim and door enamel. Its color palette now includes the new Ayurveda Essence, a specific range of 108 colors designed to suit the customer's Ayurvedic constitution; an interactive Web page (www.afmsafecoat.com/ayurveda) that shows these highly distinctive colors is worth visiting! The primer is available in wallboard, transitional, and metal varieties. The exterior products include stain, concrete and floor paint, and trim and door enamel. The finishes available include clear, clear gloss, and high gloss. The stains and sealers are nontoxic and contain natural pigments. They include interior and exterior wood stain; WaterShield for painted or unpainted surfaces; WaterStop, for use on brick, stone, tile, and concrete; Hard Seal clear gloss; medium gloss; multiuse Safe Seal; and grout sealer.

*Available:* at select paint, home supply, and hardware stores and online

www.afmsafecoat.com

## AMERICAN PRIDE

This line is Green Seal certified. Interior paints come in a full range of colors and toned whites and in flat, eggshell, and semigloss. Bases are available in pastel, medium, deep, and accent. The ceiling paint is standard sheen. The primer/sealer is flat (drywall) in white and toned whites or interior/exterior multiuse primer in a full range of colors.

*Available:* at select home supply, design, and hardware stores and online

www.americanpridepaint.com

## BEST PAINT

### Microsol, Duracryl, Universal

A full range of colors—1,000 varieties as well as a match for any color you can find—is available for this paint. Microsol interior comes in primer/sealer, flat, eggshell, satin, semigloss, gloss, and floor paint. Duracryl exterior comes in primer, eggshell, semi-gloss, and floor paint. Universal primer is for interior or exterior use.

*Available:* at select paint and hardware stores and online

www.bestpaintco.com

## DEVOE PAINT

### Wonder-Pure

Wonder-Pure is available in a full range of colors. For interior use, choose from flat, eggshell, and semi-gloss sheens.

*Available:* at select paint and hardware stores and online

www.devoepaint.com

## ECOS ORGANIC PAINTS

There's a full range of 108 colors to be had, or you can match any custom color. The interior paint comes in matte, soft sheen, and masonry. The company's specialty interior varieties include Super Chalky, Eggshell, Feng Shui, Stainblock, Atmosphere Purifying, Anti-EMR (which shields against electrical radiation and mobile phone bands), Cover Up, Insulating Wall Paint, Radiator Paint (in satin and gloss), and Anti-Formaldehyde Radiator Paint (in white satin only). Ecos's paints for wood include, for interior applications, satin-gloss and Feng Shui, and, for interior or exterior use, undercoat and primer. Its interior varnishes for floors and other surfaces are available in clear and wood stain with matte, satin, and gloss sheens. Exterior wood stains are satin-gloss. Floor paints are

*(continued)*

satin and gloss for wood and concrete floors. Stone and Tile Floor Sealer and M22 Concrete Sealer are also available. Specialty products include wood glue, M23 paint sealer, Stormseal, Eco-Friendly Paint Stripper, Shed and Fence Treatment, and Woodwash.

*Available:* online

www.ecospaints.com

## FRAZEE PAINT

### EnviroKote

This paint, with very low to zero VOCs (less than 10 g/l), is available in a full range of 1,400 colors. For interior use, choose from flat, eggshell, semigloss, gloss, and primer/sealer.

*Available:* at Frazee paint stores and online

www.frazee.com

## ICI DULUX PAINTS

### Lifemaster

This highly washable line comes in a full range of colors for interior use in flat, eggshell, and semigloss.

*Available:* through architects and builders, at ICI Dulux stores, and online

www.duluxpaints.com

## MAB PAINTS

### Enviro Pure Interior Latex

This Green Seal certified line comes in interior sheens flat, eggshell, and semigloss and in white/pastel and medium bases.

*Available:* at MAB paint stores and online

www.mabpaints.com

## MILLER PAINT

### Acro Pure, Super Acro Pure

These two lines are Green Seal certified. Both are for interior use in flat, eggshell, satin, and semigloss sheens.

Acro Pure comes in a full range of colors.

Super Acro Pure has more titanium dioxide and resin for one-coat coverage with white and light colors.

*Available:* at select paint, home supply, and hardware stores and online

www.millerpaint.com

## OLYMPIC

### Premium Interior Paint

A full range of colors is available for interior use in flat, flat enamel, eggshell, satin, and semigloss sheens; for ceilings in flat; and for kitchens and baths in semigloss.

*Available:* at most paint, home supply, and hardware stores and online

www.olympic.com

## PITTSBURGH PAINTS

### Pure Performance

This is a Green Seal certified line available in a full range of more than 1,800 colors. Interior products include flat, eggshell, semigloss, and primer/sealer.

*Available:* at select paint stores and online

www.pittsburghpaints.com

## RODDA PAINT

### Horizon

This Green Seal certified brand does not require a primer. Interior products (with VOCs of less than 1 g/l) include flat, eggshell, satin, and primer/sealer. Exterior products are low VOC (with less than 99 g/l unthinned) and available in flat, satin, semigloss, and primer and sealer.

*Available:* at select paint and hardware stores and online

www.roddapaint.com

## SHERWIN-WILLIAMS

### Harmony Interior Latex

Choose primer or topcoat in a full range of colors and flat, eggshell, and semigloss sheens.

*Available:* at most paint, home supply, and hardware stores and online

www.sherwin-williams.com

## YOLO COLORHOUSE

### Inside Paints

This Green Seal certified paint comes in a nice range of colors—40 in the Earth's Color Collection and 40 in the 1st Edition line, as well as special yearly palettes. It's for interior use in flat, satin, semi-gloss, and primer.

*Available:* at select paint and home supply stores and online

www.yolocolorhouse.com

# NATURAL PAINTS AND FINISHES

## AGLAIA NATURAL PAINTS

This complete range of 100 percent natural finishes comes in a full array of colors for interior use. All are made with plant- and mineral-based ingredients. The wall paint is available in primer, Full Color, Economic White, resin, resin bonding, washable, and clay plaster paint. Aglaia's various textures can be applied to new or old painted walls to create depth, then covered with paint or the company's beeswax-based glaze. Wood finishes, which are made with solvent-free, natural oils and a water carrier, come in floor, casework, and exterior varieties. Aquasol natural oil finishes are available as primer, wood glaze, oil sealer, and hard wax.

*Available:* at select home supply stores and online

www.aglaiapaint.com

## ANNA SOVA

### Healthy Wall Finish

Made from 99 percent food-grade ingredients, the interior paint is available in 14 color palettes with seductive names like Ancient Asia, Americas, Europa, Odd Sorbets, Mid Century Modern, Au Naturals, 7/10ths of the Planet, and White to Grey. Organic aromatherapy blends are available for mixing into paints for subtle or stronger, long-lasting scents, and aromatherapy blends exclusively developed for Anna Sova's food-grade wall finish include Fresh Lemons, Vanilla, Orange and Cloves, and Exotics.

*Available:* online

www.annasova.com

## AURO NATURAL PAINTS AND FINISHES

This is a line of completely natural products that come in a full range of colors. Interior paint comes in satin, matte, professional, antimold, white economy, powder, whitewash, and color concentrates and tints (eight shades are available for mixing an unlimited color palette). All products are tintable except the antimold paint. Interior/exterior paint is available in gloss enamel. Primer comes in multisurface and white powder. Also available are a tintable base and a metal primer. For exterior use, the company offers a tintable and weather-resistant masonry paint. Its interior/exterior stain can be used on cabinets, furniture, decks, and more. Interior/exterior finishes are available to prime, seal, varnish, shellac, wax, and preserve, and the adhesives offered are for use with flooring, linoleum, natural fiber carpets, tile, cork, and more.

*Available:* online

www.aurousa.com

*(continued)*

## ECO DESIGN

### Bioshield

These completely natural products are derived from renewable resources and come in a full range of colors. The interior wall paints and finishes offered include clay paint; solvent-free wall paint in matte and satin; color washes in wall glaze and color concentrate; casein milk paint; clay plaster, primer, and stucco; and Kinder paint for nurseries and kids' rooms. BioShield's primers, thinners, and sealers provide a breathable, elastic, waterproof, and stain-resistant coating that enhances the natural beauty of any wood. The company's wood stains are resin and color finishes for wood, and its floor and furniture finishes are available in Hard Oil, Resin Floor Finish, Wax, and Hard Wax. Pigments used for glazes, paints, and finishes are natural water- and oil-soluble powders made from rocks, minerals, and earth. BioShield also offers cork flooring and adhesives.

*Available:* at select paint, hardware, home supply, and design stores and online

www.bioshieldpaint.com

## GREEN PLANET PAINTS

These clay-based paints are made with natural mineral and plant ingredients. The interior paint comes in a matte finish and a nice range of colors. Green Planet's specialty products include glazes for sealing clay paints and soy resin for sealing clay paints.

*Available:* at select home supply, paint, and design stores and online

www.greenplanetpaints.com

## LIVOS

Livos's products are made with totally natural, plant-based ingredients such as hemp, eucalyptus, and citrus oils that are biodegradable, sustainable, and emit no or low VOCs, but come in a limited range of colors. Its wall and ceiling paints are solvent free and washable. Its primer/sealers are for use on walls and wood. Coloring Pastes are pigment mixes for tinting paints. The company's varnishes and stains include interior/exterior wood stain and a weather protection product that can be added to the wood stain or used alone. Wood oils and waxes offered include a clear oil wax, furniture wax, parquet oil, and resin hardening oil.

*Available:* online

www.livos.us

## REAL MILK PAINT

Milk paint has been used for hundreds of years. For its interior paints, this company uses all-natural, nontoxic ingredients and organic raw materials—purified casein, lime, and natural pigments. Its paints require no primer, and they work well on all porous interior surfaces, including walls, wood, concrete, and brick. Iron oxide and earth pigment powders come in 28 colors that can be blended for paint and can also be used to color concrete and plaster. Natural Crackle is a faux paint finish that lends an antique look. Waxes available for wood surfaces, floors, and furniture include Mylands Clear, Antique Pine, Antique Brown, and Antique Mahogany as well as carnauba clear and brown waxes. The company also offers an oxalic acid wood bleach to return stained wood to its natural color (rather than bleaching it white); a milk paint remover powder that removes up to eight layers of old paint; a soy-based paint stripper that removes paint, varnish, and urethane and is safe for use on wood, brick, stone, concrete, and metal; and heavy-duty cleaners for preparing surfaces for painting.

*Available:* at select home supply, paint, hardware, and design stores and online

www.realmilkpaint.com

## SILACOTE

Silacote is a fully tintable, highly durable, inorganic mineral silicate exterior paint for concrete and masonry. It comes in 282 colors and is water-vapor permeable, which means that it will not trap water between the paint and the substrate. It is also light fast, so exposure to ultraviolet (UV) light will not change the color.

*Available:* online

www.silacote.com

## WEATHER-BOS

Weather-Bos makes environmentally friendly and safe stains, finishes, preservatives, coatings, and paints that protect, waterproof, and restore surfaces. The products contain trans-oxides and/or UV light stabilizers to reduce damage from environmental factors. Masonry Boss is a clear, odorless blend of all-natural ingredients for waterproofing and weather-proofing all masonry surfaces. Deck Boss is a wood treatment with natural oils and resins that penetrate wood to create a protective bond. Log Boss is a natural tinted coating for all wood logs, including cedar, pine, fir, and oak. Roof Boss provides durable protection for tile, shake, and composition roofs. Marine Boss stains and finishes provide durable marine protection for wood, fiberglass, metal, fabric, sailcloth, and high-end woods like teak and mahogany.

*Available:* online

www.weatherbos.com

# NONTOXIC PAINT STRIPPERS

*Go easy on the environment and check out these nontoxic paint strippers.*

## AMERISTRIP

This is a nonmethylene chloride paint stripper in gel form that is highly effective for lead abatement and difficult paint removal applications. It is water washable, biodegradable, and nontoxic.

*Available:* by e-mail at ameristrip@10mb.com (no Web site)

## CITRISTRIP

### Safer Paint and Varnish Stripper

Citristrip makes a versatile, biodegradable stripper that has the power of citrus and a fresh orange scent. Available as a gel or an aerosol, it has no methylene chloride, strips multiple layers, and stays active for 24 hours. The all-purpose stripper is suitable for indoor and outdoor use to remove latex, oil-based paints, varnish, lacquer, enamel, polyurethane, shellac, acrylics, and epoxy from walls, wood, metal, and masonry. Also available is Paint Stripper After Wash, which cleans up the residue that's left after stripping, preparing the surface for refinishing.

*Available:* at most hardware and home supply stores, at big box retail chains, and online

www.citristrip.com

*(continued)*

## DUMOND CHEMICALS

### Peel Away

These paint and coating removers are nonhazardous, environmentally friendly, and user safe; some are biodegradable.

Peel Away 1 is a lead paint remover that has zero VOCs. It can remove 30-plus layers of paint in one application. Designed for eco-safe lead paint removal and restoration of historic buildings, it can be used on wood, brick, concrete, stone, stucco, plaster, iron, steel, marble, or fiberglass. It generates no fumes and contains no flammable solvents. It contains lime, which starts to stabilize the lead paint upon applying the paste. Peel Away laminated paper is then applied to the surface to control evaporation while the paint is being dissolved. *Note:* Peel Away 2 contains methylene chloride and Peel Away 4 contains n-methyl-2-pyrrolidone, both of which are regulated chemicals that are considered hazardous.

Peel Away Smart Strip is for removing architectural and industrial coatings. It is 100 percent biodegradable, has zero VOCs, and does not contain methylene chloride. Used with Peel Away paper, it can remove 15-plus layers with one application.

Peel Away 5 is a floor coating and paint remover formulated as a gel for application with Peel Away paper on high-strength, chemically resistant floor coatings such as epoxies and urethanes. It is eco-safe and contains no methylene chloride or flammable solvents.

Peel Away 21 removes paint and industrial coatings from wood, metal, plastic, brick, fiberglass, stone, and more. Peel Away paper is not used with this product. It will remove four to six layers of latex-, oil-, and lead-based paint, as well as industrial coatings such as epoxies, urethanes, and vinyl.

*Available:* at select home supply and paint stores and online

www.dumondchemicals.com

## NAPIER ENVIRONMENTAL TECHNOLOGIES

### RemovALL

This environmentally friendly, user-safe, biodegradable stripper contains no methylene chloride. The product line includes an exterior wood paint stripper, an interior wood and furniture stripper, a concrete and masonry paint stripper, a metal paint stripper, a multipurpose paint stripper, and Rinse or Peel, which removes oil and latex paints from wood, concrete, masonry, and steel. Also available is Organic Strip for stripping varnish, polyurethane, epoxies, enamel, and oil and latex paint from fine wood, cabinets, and furniture without damaging the wood. RemovALL's wood restoration products include a gray wood remover for exterior wood, an exterior wood cleaner and brightener, and a deck and fence stain remover. The company's specialty products include a waste paint hardener that hardens leftover paint for curbside disposal, a rust remover, a graffiti remover, a concrete oil stain remover, and a flooring adhesive remover.

### Bio-Wash

Bio-Wash is an environmentally friendly, user-safe, biodegradable line of products. It includes Stripex and Stripex-L, which remove oil-based wood stains and sealers and are designed for use on decks, fences, railings, siding, cedar shingles, and log homes. Simple Wash cleans and brightens outdoor surfaces, including wood and plastic decks, vinyl siding, gutters, stucco, concrete, and fiberglass. Woodwash restores weathered wood and removes gray wood, water stains, mold, mildew, and discoloration. Mill Glaze Away Stain Prep prepares wood for stain application and extends the life of coatings.

*Available:* at select home supply, hardware, and paint stores and online

www.biowash.com

## Nontoxic Paint Strippers

Traditional paint strippers are absolutely noxious—we're talking super-toxic solvent mixtures that eat through highly durable paints and finishes. This is stuff you don't want to be in the same building—let alone the same room—with, unless you have a gas mask handy. The principal active materials in conventional paint strippers are acutely hazardous and include things like aromatic hydrocarbons, methylene chloride, and dimethylformamide, which are dangerous to inhale,[31] [32] can be absorbed through the skin,[33] [34] are linked with serious health effects like central nervous and cardiovascular system damage[35] [36] [37] [38] and kidney and liver damage,[39] [40] and may cause cancer.[41] Typically, conventional paint strippers are also formulated with other toxic compounds to activate the heavy-duty solvent muscle, like methyl ethyl ketone and phenols, which are equally hazardous, being dangerous to breathe[42] [43] and linked to birth defects,[44] nervous system damage,[45] [46] neurological and behavioral effects,[47] and liver and kidney damage.[48] [49] These are serious effects to incur in the name of paint stripping.

But here's the great news: Stripping the paint off of pretty much anything has never been easier with nontoxic products. See the "Green Thumb Guide" on page 321 for suggestions.

# Green Flooring and Carpeting

Flooring material makes a fundamental contribution to the overall quality of a home's environment, particularly the indoor air quality. Both conventional and green flooring consist of similar types of materials—rugs, carpets, and hard flooring materials—but there are significant differences in their impact on human and environmental health throughout their life cycle. For instance, manufacturing and disposing of conventional synthetic carpets made with petroleum-derived materials are heavily polluting. They also pollute in your home. Have you ever walked into a room where a new carpet has been laid? It smells like chemicals. In your home, conventional synthetic carpets and rugs and the adhesives and backing materials used to affix them all emit VOCs, often throughout their lifetime. Conventional synthetic hard flooring materials like vinyl and laminate flooring pose similar problems over their life cycle: they pollute during manufacture, emit VOCs while in your home, and contain substances that are toxic to dispose of.

The good news is that there are a lot of green options that will give you beautiful, plush, and well-appointed floors. Synthetic carpets made with low-VOC recycled content, available in a wide range of styles, are a great green choice, especially for high-traffic areas. Carpets and rugs made with natural materials like wool and plant fibers such as sisal (agave cactus fiber), sea grass, coir (coconut fiber), and jute offer fantastic form and function for any room. Also widely available are greener synthetic hard flooring choices, such as linoleum and Marmoleum, both of which are made with natural raw materials like linseed oil and are incredibly durable and functional.

When it comes to natural hard flooring materials, ample green options that have a lower impact on the environment are also available for any room. Greener hardwood flooring made with wood from Forest Stewardship Council—certified sustainably managed forests is a classic and durable choice for healthy, long-lived floors. Floors of bamboo and cork are also gorgeous green choices that are made with quickly renewable materials and are available in a beautiful array of colors and styles. Reclaimed wood floors, made from wood recovered from old buildings, is about as green as it gets, and it's some of the most beautiful flooring I have ever seen. My neighbor Tom has wood floors made from materials recovered from an old tobacco warehouse, and the wide planks have a rich, deep color that can't be matched by modern wood.

While some of these green materials cost more money than conventional products, bear in mind that a good floor should last a lifetime and will improve your quality of life and the indoor air significantly (and probably also increase the value of your home!). I'm not suggesting that you rip up a perfectly good floor—

that's not very green, now, is it? But if you are considering renovating or building a home or are simply in the market for an area rug, think green under your feet.

Check out the broad spectrum of green possibilities that are better for you and better for the planet. Then, everybody wins.

## Carpets and Rugs

Carpets made with recycled content (such as plastic water bottles) are a great green choice, especially in high-traffic areas. These carpets help divert a massive amount of landfill waste and usually emit few VOCs into your home. A new green wave taking hold in the carpet industry is to use materials that are designed to be recycled from the start—a "closed-loop" process in which a material can be recycled again and again to maximize value and minimize environmental impact. Many of the manufacturers of recycled-content carpeting have in-house recycling programs that collect old carpets for making into new carpets. They recognize that the value in recycling carpet material is not just because it's eco-friendly, but also because it saves them money! Everybody wins. Some manufacturers are even incorporating bio-based materials, like plastic made from corn, to make durable, lower-impact carpets and carpet backings that don't emit toxic fumes. Good green things are afoot! Check it out in the "Green Thumb Guide" opposite.

*When it comes to gorgeous, durable, eco-friendly flooring, consider the spectrum of long-lasting, low-impact options.*

## RECYCLED-CONTENT CARPETS

### INTERFACEFLOR

InterfaceFlor is the largest modular carpet manufacturer in the world with the goal of providing environmentally responsible products and processes with innovation, performance, and value. Its Mission Zero initiative goes beyond creating green product attributes to making creative, manufacturing, and building decisions that will help the company achieve a "zero environmental footprint" by 2020 by offsetting energy use and waste, using renewable energy, and creating closed-loop recycling processes and products and efficient transportation and carpet recovery programs.

InterfaceFlor's green carpet products include:

Opening Night, a hybrid-yarn carpet made with a blend of nylon and corn-based bioplastic that comes in eight styles; Rawhide, a corn-based bioplastic and rapidly renewable content hybrid fiber with 57 percent total recycled content that comes in five colored patterns; Chenille Warp, which features retro patterns made with 62 to 65 percent recycled content; Cotswold, a carpet with medieval patterns that is made with a hybrid yarn that includes recycled content and corn-based bioplastic; Entropy, which has 62 to 74 percent recycled content; and Pure, a carpet made with 53 to 59 percent recycled content that is available in six styles of natural-world patterns.

*Available:* at most carpet stores and online

www.interfaceflor.com

### INVISTA ANTRON CARPET FIBER

Antron manufactures carpets that third-party certifier Scientific Certification Systems has designated as environmentally preferable products for the US government's Environmentally Preferable Purchasing (EPP) Program (see "4 Green Standards to Look For in Sustainable Products and Services" on page 312 for details). The carpets meet EPA and ISO standards for products that have a lesser impact on the environment throughout their life cycle. Most notable in environmental terms are Antron's Lumena line, which is made with 25 percent preconsumer recycled nylon and is available in 50 colors, and the Legacy line, which contains at least 90 percent postindustrial recycled nylon. Antron also has a carpet reclamation program that diverts carpets from landfills. It accepts any old carpet (not just its own) and processes it into valuable materials that are used for new products, including new carpets, filtration devices, automotive parts, packaging materials, and furniture. To date, Antron has recycled more than 100 million pounds of used carpet!

*Available:* at select carpet stores and online

www.antron.net

### LEES CARPETS

Lees Carpets manufactures a wide range of carpets that meet EPP program standards (see "4 Green Standards to Look For in Sustainable Products and Services" on page 312 for details). The company's green initiatives include using postconsumer and postindustrial recycled content and bio-based and environmentally preferable materials; maintaining manufacturing facilities that meet stringent federal Clean Air Act standards and reduce energy use, water use, emissions, and solid waste; and manufacturing all products to meet low-VOC standards and many products to be recyclable. Lees Carpets is a member of the US Green Building Council and has been involved in the development of the LEED Green Building Rating System.

*Available:* at carpet stores and online

www.leescarpet.com

*(continued)*

## THE MOHAWK GROUP

Mohawk offers a wide range of manmade and natural yarn carpets chosen for their durability, sustainability, and small environmental footprint. The company uses a closed-loop recycling process. Notable green carpets manufactured by the Mohawk Group include Everstrand residential carpeting, a 100 percent postconsumer carpet fiber made from recycled plastic bottles; SmartStrand, residential carpeting made with 37 percent renewable resources (bio-based plastic); Colorstrand Solution Dyed Nylon, a commercial carpet made with 15 percent postconsumer recycled content and 15 percent preconsumer recycled content and manufactured using the most pollution-free, energy-efficient method out there, one that uses no water and no steam; and Ultron, a commercial carpet made with 50 percent preconsumer recycled materials. Mohawk's ReCover program makes it easy for consumers to recycle old carpeting; the company arranges for it to be picked up!

*Available:* at carpet stores and online

www.mohawkgreenworks.com

## SHAW INDUSTRIES

Shaw Industries is one of the largest carpet manufacturers in the world, and it has an impressive number of green initiatives that affect the life cycle of its products. Shaw is dedicated to using a "cradle-to-cradle" approach to production that emphasizes recycling. The company's green initiatives include using materials like Nylon 6, which is designed to be recycled again and again; recovering and recycling resources used during manufacturing, such as water, wastewater heat, and air compressor waste heat, for use as energy; recycling pallets used for storage and transport; using lighter-weight and less packaging for products; using biodiesel in its fleet of trucks; and even recycling its employees' cell phones. Shaw's carpet recovery program, an ambitious initiative to divert carpets from landfills, involves working with carpet collectors across the United States to reclaim old carpets. To date, the company has collected more than 100 million pounds of postconsumer carpeting and 10 million pounds of postindustrial carpeting. Shaw's green carpeting includes:

EcoWorx Tiles, which are 24- by-24-inch carpet tiles that can be pieced together. Made with 40 percent recycled content, the tiles have recyclable backing. They have low VOC emissions, contain no polyvinyl chloride (PVC), and are backed by a lifetime commercial warranty.

Eco Solution Q, a recycled carpet backing made with a minimum of 25 percent recycled content. It can be recycled after use.

Endurance II Cushion, a 100 percent recycled synthetic fiber carpet cushion.

EcoLogix recycled carpet cushioning, which is made with 91 percent postconsumer recycled content from plastic bottles.

*Available:* at most carpet stores and online

www.ecoworx.com

## UNIVERSAL TEXTILE TECHNOLOGIES

This maker of carpet backing manufactures environmentally responsible products including BioCel Cushion and Laminate, which incorporates bioplastic and postindustrial recycled polyurethane.

*Available:* at carpet stores and online

www.universal-textile.net

# NATURAL CARPETS AND RUGS

Natural carpets are available in a wide range of textures, styles, sizes, and colors, and they keep indoor air fresh and clean because they don't emit VOCs like synthetic materials do. You should consider durable and long-lasting materials like wool, sisal (agave fiber), sea grass, jute, coir (coconut fiber), hemp, and silk when you are in the market for rugs and carpets. Here's a look at some gorgeous natural rugs and carpets to get you started.

## FIBREWORKS

Fibreworks offers a huge selection of 250 different natural-fiber broadloom carpets and bordered area rugs—with more than 275 border options—in many shapes and sizes. Available in a wide range of colors and textures, you can choose among indoor and outdoor rugs made from materials like jute, wool, sisal, coir, sea grass, mountain grass, tulip grass, linen blends, bamboo, and straw blends.

*Available:* at select carpet and home stores and online

www.fibreworks.com

## FJ HAKIMIAN

FJ Hakimian has an extensive collection of antique carpets and classic pieces from the world's major weaving regions. You can also design your own carpets by adapting unique period pieces to any color range and size. Vintage kilim carpets from Persia and Turkey, Moroccan tribal weavings, and European and Oriental carpets are among the textiles available.

*Available:* at the FJ Hakimian Gallery in New York City and online

www.fjhakimian.com

## HENDRICKSEN NATÜRLICH FLOORING

Hendricksen Natürlich Flooring specializes in environmentally sound, sustainable flooring, including natural fiber carpets and rugs. Wool carpets are available in a variety of styles, from plush to woven, and can be dyed to almost any color. Area rugs are also available, including an extensive collection of hand-knotted, natural-dyed Tibetan rugs; Axminster, Wilton, kilim, dhurrie, and Belgian machine-made rugs; and sisal, sea grass, coir, and woven paper rugs and carpets. All are available in many patterns, weaves, and colors.

*Available:* at the Hendricksen Natürlich Flooring showroom in Sebastopol, California, and online

www.naturalfloors.net

## JOAN WEISSMAN STUDIO

Joan Weissman offers an incredible range of elegant classic and modern rugs of the highest quality. Among them are Tibetan hand-knotted rugs made with wool, silk, and hemp; American hand-tufted rugs made with pure New Zealand wool and backed with natural latex; and needlepoint tapestries and Soumak rugs made with wool and silk that are hand-spun and naturally dyed by women in Pakistan's Hunza Valley in a fair-trade project that supports the local economy.

*Available:* at select showrooms and online

www.joanweissman.com

## MARLA HENDERSON DESIGNS

Marla Henderson created Babik, a collection of rugs fabricated from patches of vintage Turkish fabrics made with handmade, flat-woven wool by the nomadic tribes of Anatolia, Turkey. The richly colored textiles are hand-dyed using natural materials—roots, flowers, leaves, berries, barks, and

*(continued)*

woods—that are indigenous to the surrounding habitat. Available in a wide range of sizes and colors, each piece is a unique work of art. I have several of them and treasure them for their sensibility and style.

*Available:* at select design stores and online

www.marlahenderson.com

## NATURAL CARPET COMPANY

This manufacturer, importer, and exporter of unique carpets and rugs specializes in natural fibers such as abaca (made with the leafstock of a Philippine banana), raffia (palm fiber), wool, silk, buri (palm leaf fiber), sea grass, cotton, and rattan from around the world. These rugs are available in a wide selection of sizes, styles, and colors.

*Available:* at select carpet stores and online

www.naturalcarpetcompany.com

## NATURE'S CARPET

Nature's Carpet makes 100 percent wool carpets with a natural fiber backing made of jute and natural latex rubber. They are durable, ultra-low-toxicity floor coverings that are available in a variety of colors, textures, and sizes.

*Available:* at select carpet and home stores and online

www.naturescarpet.com

## NEST BY CLAYTON MILLER

Nest makes pure New Zealand wool carpets tufted into beautifully textured patterns ranging from classic to modern. They come in 12 solid colors.

*Available:* at select carpet stores and online

www.nestcarpets.com

## PRESTIGE MILLS

Prestige Mills offers a wide range of natural fiber carpets and rugs, including sisal, jute, coir, papyrus (derived from a grasslike plant), and New Zealand wool and wool blends, and a unique collection of handcrafted rugs from Hungary, the Czech Republic, Holland, Germany, Africa, and other countries.

*Available:* at select carpet stores and online

www.prestigemills.com

## PURE-REST

Pure-Rest offers 100 percent wool carpeting that is untreated, undyed, and chemical free and has a natural backing made with a hemp–cotton blend, jute, and natural adhesive from the rubber tree. Several styles of tufted, textured loop weaves are available in natural colors, as are rug gripper pads made with 100 percent natural rubber and natural wool carpet padding that is free of dyes, fire retardants, glues, mothproofing substances, and adhesives.

*Available:* online at www.purerest.com

## HARD FLOORING

*Choosing green hard flooring will improve your quality of life and probably the value of your home, too! Consider wood harvested from sustainably managed forests; bamboo, which rivals traditional wood in beauty and durability; and reclaimed wood. Cork, another eco-friendly material, is derived from the bark of the cork tree, a variety of oak that regenerates after harvesting, leaving the tree unharmed. Cork is durable, comfortable, naturally fire resistant, antimicrobial, insect repelling, and a great thermal and acoustical insulator. Linoleum and Marmoleum (not to be confused with vinyl), made with natural raw materials like linseed oil, offer eco-friendly durability, especially in high-traffic areas and utility rooms. Check out these products.*

## ARMSTRONG WORLD INDUSTRIES

Armstrong offers genuine linoleum (not to be confused with vinyl), an environmentally preferred product made with natural raw materials, including linseed oil from the flax plant, wood or cork powder, resins, and ground limestone. It's highly durable, though it must be polished to get the shiny protective layer that prevents staining. Linoleum releases a harmless odor (from the linseed oil) when it is first installed, but it will dissipate. It is available in sheets and tiles in a range of colors derived from mineral pigments.

*Available:* at most hardware and flooring stores and online

www.armstrong.com

## CARLISLE WIDE PLANK FLOORS

Carlisle is a leader in reclaimed wood flooring—wood that has been carefully recovered from old buildings, farmhouses, and barns. Available in different grades, widths, and thicknesses, antique woods like Antique Chestnut, Antique Heart Pine, Milled Barn Siding, Antique Oak, Original Surface Barn Siding, and Grandpa's Floor are among your choices.

*Available:* online at www.wideplankflooring.com

## COVERINGS ETC.

Coverings Etc. is a member of the US Green Building Council (see "4 Green Standards to Look For in Sustainable Products and Services" on page 312 for details) and is committed to providing building materials with environmentally friendly and sustainable attributes. The company's ECOverings line is made with naturally occurring elements such as sand, clay, and cement and recycled content and manufactured with processes that conserve natural resources. The line includes Eco-Gres, porcelain sheets available in 23 colors, tiles available in 28 colors, and mosaics available in 24 colors made with 50 percent recycled content; Bio Glass, made with 100 percent recycled glass available in four colors; Eco-Terr, eco-friendly terrazzo tiles available in 36 colors and slabs available in 12 colors made with 75 to 80 percent recycled marble or granite chips; and Eco-Cem, large-format sheets and tiles made with 20 percent postconsumer and 40 percent preconsumer cement strengthened with cellulose fibers, available in seven colors.

*Available:* at select design, flooring, and tile stores and online

www.coveringsetc.com

## DODGE-REGUPOL ECOSURFACES

ECOsurfaces makes 100 percent recycled postconsumer flooring made from rubber tires. It is a low-VOC floor that comes in an extensive array of 70 colors. Choose from styles like ECOstone, which has the classic look of marble chips; ECOearth, which has organic colors inspired by the natural world; ECOrocks, which has a terrazzo look; ECOsand, which has a splash of color; and ECOnights, which has colorful flecks. All are available in rolls or tiles that can be cut to any shape and length.

*Available:* at select design and flooring stores and online

www.ecosurfaces.com

## ECO DESIGN BIOSHIELD PAINT CORK FLOORING

Bioshield Paint offers cork floor tiles that can easily be installed over most subfloor surfaces. The tiles are available in four patterns that can be finished and stained a wide variety of colors.

*Available:* at select design and home stores and online

www.bioshieldpaint.com

*(continued)*

## ECO-FRIENDLY FLOORING

Eco-Friendly Flooring is a woman-owned and -operated business that offers a wide variety of sustainable flooring products, including bamboo; prefinished cork floor planks; 100 percent postconsumer or postindustrial recycled glass tiles in hundreds of variations of color, style and finish; linoleum floor planks in 25 colors; stone tiles from well-managed quarries; wood reclaimed from structural beams and timbers in warehouses; and sustainably harvested wood from sustainably managed forests.

*Available:* online at www.ecofriendlyflooring. com

## ENVIROGLAS ENVIROTRAZ

EnviroTRAZ is a colorful, highly durable, eco-friendly terrazzo made with multicolored glass chips from discarded bottles, mirrors, and plate glass windows and porcelain chips from discarded toilets, sinks, and tubs. More than 100 styles and colors are available.

*Available:* at select flooring and design stores and online

www.enviroglasproducts.com

## FORBO MARMOLEUM

Forbo offers Marmoleum flooring, a highly durable floor covering made with linseed oil, resins, and wood flour that does not emit VOCs and is available in a huge array of colors. Marmoleum's life cycle makes it one of the most environmentally friendly flooring materials available.

*Available:* at select flooring and design stores and online

www.themarmoleumstore.com

## HENDRICKSEN NATÜRLICH FLOORING

Hendricksen Natürlich offers environmentally sound, sustainable flooring materials, including EcoTimber sustainable hardwoods, which are Forest Stewardship Council–certified; bamboo that is processed without formaldehyde and available in a variety of shades; cork tiles and planks that come in many colors and patterns; and linoleum sheets and tiles that are available in more than 100 colors.

*Available:* at the Hendricksen Natürlich Flooring showroom in Sebastopol, California, and online

www.naturalfloors.net

## LAMIN-ART ABACÁ

Lamin-Art is a member of the US Green Building Council (see "4 Green Standards to Look For in Sustainable Products and Services" on page 312 for details). The company offers a wide selection of decorative laminate flooring that contains 40 percent postconsumer recovered paper content in addition to Abacá, a recycled banana fiber flooring with a naturally dimensional surface. It is available in sheets in 10 colors.

*Available:* at design and flooring stores and select showrooms and online

www.laminart.com

## MOUNTAIN LUMBER

Mountain Lumber crafts beautiful antique flooring from materials reclaimed from old buildings and historic sites. The company's solid plank reclaimed woods include Historic Heart Pine, a rich amber heartwood grain available in six grades, authentic distressed, and weathered antique. Other reclaimed hardwoods include Antique American Oak, Antique Chestnut, Antique Hard Maple, Granary Oak, and Ancient Chinese Elm.

*Available:* online at www.mountainlumber.com

## NATURAL CORK AND MORE

Natural Cork offers a wide range of cork and bamboo flooring materials that have unique character and sustainable style. Cork flooring is available in sheets (Classic Series in eight styles and Earth Series in 12 styles) and tiles (Square Tiles in six styles, Parquet Tiles in seven styles, and Eco Cork in 10 styles). Bamboo flooring is available in Traditional Bamboo in four styles, Solid Stained Bamboo in four styles, Solid Scraped Bamboo in four styles, Engineered Stained Bamboo in five styles, Engineered Handscraped Bamboo in five styles, and Engineered Strand Woven Bamboo in three styles.

*Available:* at select flooring and design stores and online

www.naturalcork.com

## NORTH SLOPE SUSTAINABLE WOOD TREADLIGHT

Treadlight flooring is made with Western larch (aka *tamarack*) trees from forest restoration sites in Montana and the Northern Rockies. Trees are harvested with a "greener than green" approach by culling stunted trees from overcrowded forests to allow the largest and healthiest trees to thrive. This honey-and-cinnamon-hued wood is available in several widths.

*Available:* at select design stores and online

www.northslopewood.com

## STRANDWOVEN WOOD BAMBOO

Strandwoven Wood offers a line of bamboo flooring that they process with advanced technology to yield a flooring material that is harder and more stable than traditional hardwoods. The process used to make Strandwoven Bamboo flooring makes better use of the harvested raw material (84 percent of the bamboo harvested is used in their products, compared to traditional bamboo flooring's use of 65 percent of the raw mate-

rial). Using cut bamboo culms and postindustrial bamboo waste from other manufacturers, the raw bamboo is kiln dried, coated with a formaldehyde-free resin, and compressed with heat under pressure to yield a dense log, which is cut into planks and milled. The result is an extremely durable, beautiful product. I have this type of bamboo in the foyer of my home and it can withstand a crowd of people in stiletto heels without damage.

*Available:* at select flooring supply stores and online

www.strandwoven.com

## SUSTAINABLE FLOORING

Sustainable Flooring offers nine styles of bamboo flooring: carbonized natural-, light-, and dark-colored horizontal-grain bamboo flooring; carbonized natural-, light-, and dark-colored vertical-grain bamboo flooring; and light-, dark-, and mocha-colored Strandwoven bamboo flooring. Also available are 10 styles of cork floating floor planks and 10 styles of cork flooring tiles.

*Available:* online at www.sustainableflooring.com

## WE CORK

A family business with five generations in the cork industry, WE Cork offers a wide variety of cork products and flooring. Cork floor tiles are available in five styles and floating floor panels are available in 13 styles. Also offered are a cork underlayment, which controls sound and prevents stress cracks under ceramic tile, marble, and hardwood floors, and 100 percent recycled cork floors.

*Available:* at most floor and carpet stores and online

www.wecork.com

# Carpet America Recovery Effort

In 2002, the carpet industry, government agencies, and nongovernmental groups agreed to work together as the Carpet America Recovery Effort (CARE) to reduce the amount of postconsumer carpeting going to landfills and incinerators by increasing the reuse and recycling of carpeting removed from buildings and homes. At the time that the agreement was made, the amount of waste carpet disposed of annually was estimated to be 4.7 billion pounds, and only 4 percent of that was being reused or recycled. The goal of CARE is to eliminate the disposal of carpets in landfills and incinerators. For more information, visit www.carpetrecovery.org.

# Kitchen and Bath Counters

Green countertops have come a long way in form and function to fit a wide array of kitchen and bathroom styles. To leave a lighter footprint on the planet, green counters are made from recycled, renewable, and nontoxic materials and contribute to a clean indoor environment. Conventional counters made with synthetic, petroleum-based materials like Formica and Corian pollute during their manufacture and typically require toxic adhesives and binders to both make and install them. Granite counters have grown in popularity, but they exact a heavy toll on the environment through quarries that scar the landscape and remove rock that can never be replenished. Granite is also an energy-intensive material to ship around.

The latest in green counters includes gorgeous terrazzo and composite counters made with recycled crushed stone, and postconsumer recycled glass and porcelain offer all of the durable and good-looking benefits of virgin materials like stone, but have a lower impact on the planet. If you like tile counters, look for a growing green selection of recycled-content tiles. Other green counter options include bamboo, recycled aluminum, biocomposite materials made from bamboo, salvaged wood and wood harvested from sustainably managed forests, and revolutionary nonporous surfaces made with recycled paper (they're sturdy, scratchproof, and fire and bacteria resistant). If you are building or remodeling a kitchen or bathroom, step up your surface style by going green.

*When it comes to kitchen and bathroom counters, check out this array of green materials available for eco-savvy form and function.*

## AVONITE SURFACES

Avonite, a member of the USGBC (see "4 Green Standards to Look For in Sustainable Products and Services" on page 312 for details), manufactures composite counters made with recycled materials. You can choose from eight styles, including Crushed Lava, featuring complementary ebony, brown, and pearl tones; Kaleidoscope, which has bold, multihued textures suspended in a translucent matrix; Crater, with its large accents of yellow, gray, red, and brown on a black base; and Palm Desert, an earthy taupe with light accents.

*Available:* at kitchen and bath design centers and online

www.avonitesurfaces.com

## BEDROCK INDUSTRIES BLAZESTONE TILE

Blazestone tiles are crafted entirely from postconsumer and postindustrial recycled glass. They are available in a wide variety of shapes, colors, and finishes, including Glossy Finish Classic in seven colors, Matte Finish Classic in 11 colors, Water Color Series in 10 colors, New Caribbean Colors in six colors, and Stripes and Dots.

*Available:* online at www.bedrockindustries.com

## COVERINGS ETC. ECO-TERR

Coverings Etc., a member of the USGBC, is committed to providing building materials that have environmentally friendly and sustainable attributes. One such product is Eco-Terr, an eco-friendly terrazzo made with recycled content that's available in tiles and slabs.

*Available:* at select design, flooring, and tile stores and online

www.coveringsetc.com

## ELEEK RECYCLED ALUMINUM COUNTERTOPS AND TILES

Eleek specializes in designing and making handcrafted, beautifully durable products, including stylish recycled aluminum counters. The company's signature finishing process smoothes and polishes the metal to give it the look of weathered stone and a feeling of silky softness (without holding fingerprints like stainless steel). Eleek is a very green company; it uses 100 percent green electricity, prints everything on 100 percent recycled paper, recycles materials during manufacture, and sources 80 percent of its supplies from within 50 miles of the shop.

*Available:* at select home and design stores and online

www.eleek.com

## ENVIROGLAS ENVIROSLAB

EnviroSLAB is a terrazzo counter made with 100 percent recycled glass and porcelain that is formed into a counter of standard size. You can choose from more than 100 existing color designs and 22 standard resin colors, or customize your own. EnviroGLAS is a member of the USGBC and use of its products can contribute LEED points toward certification.

*Available:* at select kitchen and bathroom design stores and online

www.enviroglasproducts.com

*(continued)*

## ICESTONE

IceStone is a durable surface made with recycled glass and cement that is as strong as granite, less porous than marble, and heat resistant like stone. IceStone is Cradle to Cradle–certified, and its installation can contribute points toward LEED certification. It's VOC free and available in 27 standard colors that can be mixed to make almost any background color and then combined with glass of various sizes and colors to create a unique surface.

**Available:** at select design stores and online

www.icestone.biz

## KLIP BIOTECHNOLOGIES ECOTOP

EcoTop is a chic, durable biocomposite surface that binds an FSC-certified fifty-fifty blend of bamboo and wood fiber salvaged from demolition sites to a petroleum- and VOC-free water-based resin. Klip BioTechnologies is a member of the USGBC, and the purchase of EcoTop can contribute to LEED certification.

**Available:** at select design stores and online

www.kliptech.com

## OCEANSIDE GLASSTILE

Oceanside Glasstile makes handcrafted glass tiles containing up 87 percent recycled material. The company uses more than 2 million pounds of glass from curbside recycling programs annually. Eight collections are available in a wide range of colors, sizes, and styles.

**Available:** at select design stores and online

www.glasstile.com

## RICHLITE

Richlite is a composite counter surface made with paper pulp from trees harvested from certified managed forests. Some recycled content is used, though the company does not have a set percentage requirement for recycled content. It is available in eight colors and many sizes and with edge treatments ranging from simple rounded and squared to artistic.

**Available:** at select kitchen and design stores and online

www.richlite.com

## SANDHILL INDUSTRIES

Sandhill's 100 percent recycled glass tiles come in 36 colors with a gloss or matte finish and five deco designs. Choose from a spectrum of beautiful designs in borders, field concepts, and mosaic blends, or customize your own.

**Available:** at select design stores and online

www.sandhillind.com

## SHETKAWORKS SHETKASTONE

ShetkaSTONE, a revolutionary surface made with pre- and postconsumer paper, has a 100 percent sustainable life cycle, meaning that all by-products and manufacturing waste can be recycled back into the manufacturing process. It's resistant to scratching, bacteria, stains, and water, and it is fire resistant without the need for added chemicals. Available in seven colors, it is finished to standard sizes but can be customized.

**Available:** at select design stores and online

www.shetkastone.com

## TOTALLY BAMBOO

Counters made by Totally Bamboo are, well, totally bamboo! Light and dark styles are available in three grains: Vertical Grain, with a thin grain stripe; Flat Grain, with wider grain stripes, and Parquet End Grain, with short, rectangular stripes grouped in squares. Nontoxic, food-grade, and formaldehyde-free adhesives are used in fabricating these counters. Ready for contractor installation, the counters are available in standard sizes that can be cut to size.

*Available:* online at www.totallybamboo.com

## TERAGREN

This manufacturer makes formaldehyde-free, food-safe bamboo parquet butcher block panels that can be used to make counters or tabletops. The panels are available in two sizes and in natural and caramelized colors. Custom sizes are also available.

*Available:* at select design stores and online
www.teragren.com

## VETRAZZO

Vetrazzo makes dazzling counter surfaces made with 85 percent glass, all of it recycled, and 15 percent cement and pigments. Most of the glass used by Vetrazzo is collected from curbside recycling, but they also reclaim glass from windows, dinnerware, windshields, stained-glass traffic lights, and buildings. The manufacturing plant even has respectable green attributes, including natural daylight illumination, dust filters to minimize air pollution, and a state-of-the-art system to recycle water used during manufacturing. The counters are available in a rainbow palette of colors such as Alehouse Amber, Bistro Green, Cubist Clear, and Cobalt Skyy.

*Available:* at kitchen, bath, and design stores and online

www.vetrazzo.com

# Cabinets

Going green with cabinets means choosing materials that are nontoxic and sustainable. Cabinets typically are made with unsustainably harvested wood, composite materials, or synthetic materials, all of which are usually processed with formaldehyde and glued with adhesives that contain formaldehyde and emit toxic VOCs. PVC, another unhealthy material often used for edge banding on cabinet boxes and drawers, contains and emits chlorine. But more and more gorgeous green options are now available for constructing cabinetry, including FSC-certified wood; bamboo, a durable, beautiful, rapidly renewable material; and, most important, formaldehyde-free glues, resins, and adhesives. Green cabinetry is better for you, your home, and the planet.

*Go green with cabinets! Take a look at these nontoxic, sustainable products made from classic and innovative materials.*

## BERKELEY MILLS

Berkeley Mills makes custom wood and bamboo furniture and cabinets. Committed to ecologically sound manufacturing and business practices, the company is certified by the FSC for its conscientious use of sustainable, responsibly harvested wood.

*Available:* at the Berkeley Mills Showroom in Berkeley, California, and online

www.berkeleymills.com

## CASE GREEN CONSTRUCTION AND CABINETRY

Case Green uses eco-friendly products, materials, and construction practices for its wide range of cabinets. The company uses wheat board composites (made with wheat straw) and formaldehyde-free resins as substrate materials. You can choose from environmentally friendly wood options like bamboo, lyptus (eucalyptus, a fast-growing tree), and veneers (a thin slice of wood that gives you the look and feel of wood but doesn't use much of it). Reconstituted veneers, which are engineered from sustainably harvested woods to replicate exotic species, are also available. No PVC is used for the edge banding on the cabinet boxes or drawers.

*Available:* at select design and cabinetry stores and online

www.casegreen.com

## COATES WALKER CABINETRY HEALTHE GREEN DESIGN

HealthE Green Design is Coates Walker's proprietary cabinetry design. The company uses eco-friendly manufacturing and processes, including using woods certified by the FSC, materials that don't emit formaldehyde, low- or zero-VOC finishes, no PVC, and products that contribute to LEED certification requirements.

*Available:* at select design stores and online

www.coateswalker.com

## HUMABUILT WHEATCORE CABINETS

Humabuilt Wheatcore Cabinets are made with wheat chaff waste (a rapidly renewable resource that can be grown in one season) and are manufactured without formaldehyde.

*Available:* at select design stores and online

www.humabuilt.com

## NEIL KELLY CABINETS

Neil Kelly Cabinets' Naturals Collection uses FSC-certified woods and bamboo; formaldehyde-free agriboard materials; and low-VOC glues, adhesives, and finishes, the latter including clear, water-based finishes, renewable natural oil and hard wax finishes, and low-VOC-paint finishes. They are available in a variety of beautiful styles.

*Available:* at select design and cabinet stores and online

www.neilkellycabinets.com

# Candles

Candles are a sumptuous way to instill ambience and subtle aroma in any room. Clean, natural candles like those made from soy, palm, or pure beeswax are a great choice to create a soft, diffused atmosphere without dealing with the fumes released by artificially scented, petroleum-based paraffin wax candles. Naturally based candles are the green choice because they're made with renewable resources, burn cleanly, and are biodegradable.

## Paraffin Pollution

Unless otherwise specified, conventional candles are generally made from paraffin, which is a group of petroleum compounds. Paraffin belongs to a group of alkane hydrocarbons. To give you an idea of their characteristics, the lightest and simplest form of paraffin is methane gas (a global-warming bully), and a heavier, liquid paraffin is octane (think of a gas pump). For candles, a solid form of paraffin known as paraffin wax is needed. It is really a waste product of petroleum refining. The jury is out on how harmful paraffin wax fumes are, but it's a good bet that they're not super-good. In Britain, kerosene is commonly called *paraffin oil*, which it's not, but, like kerosene, low-grade paraffin produces a heck of a lot of soot (particulate pollution that is not good to breathe), so maybe that's why it got that name. Since paraffin is a petroleum product, it may contain toxins like benzene and acetone,[50] which, when burned in candles, can pollute indoor air with unhealthy fumes and soot.

So why is paraffin used for candles? Well, it's cheap, it burns readily and melts at the right temperature, and it doesn't much react with other stuff. The fact that it's insoluble in water makes processing easy. It is, however, soluble in petrochemicals like benzene and esters, which are used for processing paraffin candles. So, while it's questionable whether paraffin itself is benign or malignant to breathe, those petrochemical solvents used to make paraffin candles are definitely the latter and then some.

The good news is that if you enjoy both the ambience of candles *and* healthy indoor air, there are a number of lovely green alternatives to paraffin candles.

## Beeswax

Beeswax is one of the longest-used and most highly valued natural materials for candle making. It burns long and clean, and high-quality beeswax is relatively dripless if it is kept out of drafts. Beeswax is the only autonomous, naturally occurring wax on planet Earth, which means that it's a true wax that doesn't require processing to become a wax. It is, after all, wax.

*(continued on page 341)*

*Check out the spectrum of green, clean-burning candles made from pure, renewable materials and natural fragrances for eco-friendly ambience and sumptuous smells.*

## ALOHA BAY PALM CANDLES

I have an affinity for Aloha Bay candles, in part because I am a dozen-year transplant to Hawaii, but also because their 100 percent palm wax candles burn fantastically cleanly and long. Using naturally pressed and distilled cosmetic-grade palm tree oil (and no petroleum solvents) and pure essential oils, Aloha Bay makes candles in a bouquet of scents (and unscented too) and a rainbow of colors. The wicks are braided cotton or cotton with a paper core. The company's scented candles are infused with pure essential oils and available as votives, chakra votives, pillars, Bright Bouquets (two wicked candles with three fragrances in a glass vase), and highly fragranced (made with concentrated essential oils). Its unscented candles come as 9-inch tapers, tea lights, votives, chakra jars, and river rock candles.

*Available:* at large natural markets and natural home stores and online

www.alohabay.com

## ANNA SOVA

These 100 percent soy candles have gorgeous aromatherapy scents that come from pure essential oils. The eco-friendly wicks were recently reformulated for a cleaner burn. Options include poured candles in a heavy glass votive and single candles with scents like vanilla with patchouli and cedarwood with lime. They even come in a 100 percent postconsumer-waste recycled gift box. How cool.

*Available:* online at www.annasova.com

## ARCHIPELAGO BOTANICALS

Archipelago Botanicals' candles fill a room with the rich, delightful smells of the unique and enticing blends the company makes using fine essential oils and natural fragrances. Hand poured into heavy glass votives, the candles are made with a premium wax blend containing more than 50 percent soy wax and clean burning wicks. Six collections of candles are available in a variety of shapes and sizes—votives, pillars, glass jars, and tins—all of which are naturally inviting. Scents include blends like avocado, teakwood, and amber; iris, sweet pea, and violet; chocolate soy; rhubarb vanilla; and linden leaf, white fig, and rose.

*Available:* at select natural markets and home stores and online

www.amazon.com; www.sensia.com

## BLUEWICK

Bluewick was the first to use 100 percent soy wax for candles in the early 1990s. Kudos! The company now has five distinctive collections of hand-poured candles in more than 50 varieties, including fragrances like citrus basil berry, Macintosh pear, spicy chai green tea, and ginger nectarine. Bluewick knows how to infuse good sense and good scents. All of its candles have organic paper-core wicks for clean burning and are available in a great range of sizes in glass tumblers and tins.

*Available:* at select natural markets and online

www.bluewick.com

## CANDLE BEE FARM

Candle Bee Farm produces 100 percent pure beeswax candles with no additives and all-cotton wicks. Handcrafted by beekeepers, these artisan candles burn cleanly and come in a fun variety of shapes, styles, and sizes. They have a subtle, clean honey aroma that comes naturally from the high-quality wax; no fragrances are added. The company uses a solar melt method instead of steam melt machines to purify the wax, with pure, clean results. No additives, hardeners, or toxic release spray is ever used. Instead, the process includes a long setting time, slow cooling, and careful hands.

*Available:* online at www.candlebeefarm.com

## FLORAPATHICS

Florapathics knows all about aromatherapy and delivers an enticing range of pure, delectable fragrances using the highest quality organic essential oils in its luxury soy candles. Made with pure soy wax poured into a heavy-bottomed glass votive, the candles have a double cotton wick to augment the release of pure aromatherapeutic essential oil blends extracted from flowers, stems, seeds, leaves, bark, roots, rinds, and grasses. Scents include blends like bergamot, lime, and petitgrain; Chai Fusion; basil; and blood orange.

*Available:* at select natural markets and online www.florapathics.com

## GREEN TREE CANDLE

Green Tree Candle makes its 100 percent pure beeswax candles with 100 percent cotton wicks by hand at its upstate New York studio. The company has a rich palette of colors and a spread of unique shapes, including tapers, pillars, and woodland molds like twigs and pinecones.

*Available:* online at www.greentreecandleco.com

## LUMINUS AROMATHERAPY BODY CARE AND ENVIRONMENTALLY SOUND CANDLES

Luminus produces a nice spread of aromatherapy and unscented candles in a variety of shapes and sizes. They are made with vegetable oil and have cotton wicks. Luminus tea lights are my favorite because natural tea lights

are hard to find, and they're versatile and useful for refilling glass votives and essential oil diffusers. Available in ivory and colors, they come in boxes of six and bulk packs of 100 for a price that's reasonable considering their fine quality.

*Available:* at natural markets and online www.luminusonline.com

## MRS. MEYER'S CLEAN DAY

These candles from the makers of hardworking, great-smelling ecological cleaning products are made with soy and vegetable wax and offer potent aromas from plant-based fragrances and the essential oils of lavender, lemon verbena, and geranium. Unbleached cotton wicks with a paper core are used for clean burning. They're simply good all around.

*Available:* at natural markets and some home stores and online www.mrsmeyers.com

## N.K.D. NAKED CANDLE

N.K.D. candles are made in the United States with 100 percent pure soy wax and without chemicals, added colors, or paraffin. They have 100 percent cotton wicks and come in a stunning array of scents, such as Mulling Spice, Orchid Rain, and Mint Julep, as well as unscented. You can choose from two sizes, one in tin, the other in glass. The company even uses recycled paper packaging and labels made from corn that are printed with soy-based ink. Fantastic.

*Available:* at select natural markets and online www.nkdpure.com

*(continued)*

## PACIFICA

Pacifica produces a beautiful spread of hand-poured soy wax candles in an incredible spectrum of alluring natural scents, such as Moroccan Chamomile, Egyptian Bergamot Rose, Tuscan Blood Orange, Waikiki Pikake, and Mexican Cocoa, using plant-based fragrances and essential oils. All of the candles have cotton wicks and are available in two sizes—a 3-ounce glass votive and 7-ounce tin. Pacifica also makes a wide selection of round and square pillars and votives that are a mixture of soy wax and food-grade paraffin (which is probably as clean as paraffin gets, but it's still petroleum).

*Available:* at most natural markets and online

www.pacificacandles.com

## RED FLOWER

All Red Flower products, candles included, embody pure, provocative scents by using the highest-grade plant-based ingredients and essential oils. Made with pure vegetable oils, their candles have an aroma profile that is delectably divine, including Thai honeysuckle, Japanese peony, and Icelandic moonflower. Poured into glass votives and given striking colors, the 6-ounce candles are topped with a heap of real flower petals to complement the seductive, complex aromas of the candles. "Little Flower" candles are also available in 1.5-ounce votives without petals.

*Available:* at select spas and home stores and online

www.redflower.com

## SCANDLE

Scandle makes one of the most interesting natural candles out there—a soy candle and massage oil/lotion in one. Specially formulated with a complex blend of soy and all-natural vegetable oils (including palm kernel oil, shea butter, cosmetic-grade soy butter, and vitamin E), Scandle candles are designed to melt at a slightly lower temperature than regular candles, yielding a pure, warm massage lotion. Pretty cool, and just the right temperature for an inviting rub down. Only plant-based fragrances and pure essential oils are used for the company's signature fragrances, which include Oatmeal Milk and Honey, Warm Vanilla Sugar, and Green Tea Aloe. Natural wicks are used. Each candle provides enough lotion for 20 full-body massages, has a burn time of 15 to 120 hours depending on its size, and is available in a glass votive or travel tin.

*Available:* at select natural markets and online

www.abodycandle.com

## SUNBEAM CANDLES

Sunbeam's candles are handmade in small batches using the purest ingredients. The wax, wicks, and oils are all from the earth. Sunbeam is committed to environmentally sound business practices based on sustainable values. Its central New York State candle shop runs on solar energy, and it supports the local economy by buying locally produced beeswax. In addition to a wide variety of triple-filtered, 100 percent beeswax candles in a great spread of shapes, sizes, and styles, the company also pours soy wax candles and scents them with enticing fragrances from pure essential oils. All wicks are made with 100 percent unbleached cotton for clean burning.

*Available:* at some natural markets and home stores and online

www.sunbeamcandles.com

## VOTIVO

Votivo candles have a decadent signature. The complex portfolio of distinct fragrances is inviting and delicious. Each of the eight hand-poured collections is more amazing than the last. Two lines (Kyoto and Nola) are made with soy wax and the rest are naturally based (though they may contain some paraffin). It's hard to say whether all of the fragrances are natural, though Votivo's commitment to quality suggests that the company put thoughtful research into all of its ingredients. My favorites include Fresh Tomato Leaf, Celadon Tea, and Mandarin Teak, though I could easily spend a small fortune buying candles from among the other 50. Most are poured into substantial glass votives and some into terra-cotta vases. Lovely all around.

*Available:* at select home stores and natural markets and online

www.votivo.com

The quality and sourcing of beeswax are both essential parts of the game. To begin with, the quality of beeswax can vary big-time. Toxic chemicals applied to beehives to ward off pests and disease are largely unregulated abroad and even in some states, and they can end up in the beeswax. Some countries ban the importation of bee products because of the possible chemical residues, but no regulatory measures exist for these chemicals in the United States. Most small bee-product producers take pride in the purity of their goods, and those that go to the wall for their bees and make pure products won't be shy about letting you know what they're up to.

Though some products claim to be 100 percent beeswax, many companies put additives and hardeners in the wax to quicken its setting and create a super-smooth finish.

The color of beeswax can vary from cream to honey brown. It all depends on the source and purity of the product. High-quality beeswax is generally golden with hints of yellow and orange pollen, like the sun. Be wary of beeswax that is toward the dark end of the spectrum. Dull brown beeswax is generally of the lowest quality and may contain impurities or chemical residues, or it could be from diseased hives. Creamy white beeswax may be a result of chlorine bleaching or chemical filtering. However, extremely high quality beeswax can be naturally filtered to a creamy color. When bees secrete wax, it is actually creamy white; it turns golden when nectar and pollen are brought into the hive. Careful, repeated filtration can return the wax to its original buttery color without chemicals or bleach. Again, producers who take these painstaking measures to turn out pure products will flaunt it. Look for them! Pure beeswax candles also have a lovely honey smell that just can't be synthesized.

Many people consider supporting small-scale, local beekeeping to be one of the best ways to support local agriculture, because bees are the pollen carriers and keepers. Bees are responsible for pollinating the vast majority of fruits and flowers. Those wild lupines that spring forth in royal purple glory in the early summer? Thank the bees. Those luscious cherries of delectably firm crimson? Bees again. Without bees, most of our food crops could not produce their harvest. Therefore, buying beeswax (and honey!) products from small-scale producers is a noble green move with benefits that go way beyond some romantic candlelight.

## Palm Wax

Palm wax is made from the fruit and berries of palm trees. Doesn't that sound harmlessly inviting? It's obviously derived from a renewable resource, which is a good thing. In addition, 100 percent palm wax candles are clean and long burning.

## Soy Wax

Soy wax is a clean-burning, renewable candle option made with soybeans. It's reputed to burn longer than paraffin, and it emits less soot than paraffin by a good margin. Soy wax doesn't diffuse carcinogenic fumes into the air, either. That's a good thing.

## Green Wicks

Wicks are the essential detail that differentiates a delightful, soft-burning candle from a hunk of wax. What they're made of determines how cleanly or sootily a candle burns and what kind of fumes accompany the illumination. Conventional paraffin candles typically use synthetic wicks that may have a core of metal or zinc, both of which emit toxic stuff. While lead wicks are not permitted for use in US-made candles, they are consistently found in cheap imported candles, especially those from China. One study revealed that burning lead-wicked candles just once a week emits enough lead into the air to contaminate kids' blood beyond federally accepted levels. Yikes! So be very wary of imported candles (the country of manufacture is usually printed on the packaging or on stickers found on the bottom of the candle), period.

Natural candles, on the other hand, opt for cotton- or paper-core wicks for a nice, clean burn. It's a detail that makes a big difference for your lungs.

Why are synthetic wicks with cores of metal or zinc used? Because they're cheap and stiff, so they stay where they were placed in the mold when the wax is poured. That's great, but they can also emit toxic smoke, soot, and lead. If you want to see if a candlewick has a metal core, just peel back the fiber and see if there is metallic stuff underneath. If you want to check for lead, rub the peeled wick on a piece of white paper—if it leaves a gray smudge, it likely contains lead. By all means, don't burn the thing. Instead, look for candles that brag about having paper-core or cotton wicks—they burn brilliantly and cleanly, with no fuss and no muss.

# Endnotes

# Chapter 1:
# Green Living Is Easy

1   Tufts University. "How to Save Energy and Money in Your Home." 2005. www.tufts.edu/tie/tci/excel%20and%20word/SaveEnergy.doc.

2   Agency for Toxic Substances and Disease Registry. "Toxicological Profile for Chlorinated Dibenzo-p-dioxins (CDDs). Chapter 5: Potential for Human Exposure." p. 458. http://www.atsdr.cdc.gov/toxprofiles/tp104-c5.pdf.

3   Ibid.

4   Hamilton, M. "Liquid Assets, Pure and Simple." *Washington Post* September 14, 1996.

5   "Uncapping Consumers' Thirst for Bottled Water." *Bottled Water Reporter* December/January 1994.

6   Natural Resources Defense Council. "Bottled Water: Pure Drink or Pure Hype?" http://www.nrdc.org/water/drinking/bw/exesum.asp.

7   US PIRG. "Polluters Continue to Violate Clean Water Act: 60 Percent Exceeded Pollution Permits in Recent 18-Month Period." March 30, 2004. http://www.uspirg.org/news-releases/our-rivers-lakes-and-streams/our-rivers-lakes-and-streams/polluters-continue-to-violate-clean-water-act-60-percent-exceeded-pollution-permits-in-recent-18-month-period. [press release]

8   Conacher, D. *Troubled Water on Tap: Organic Chemicals in the Public Drinking Water Systems and the Failure of Regulation.* Washington, DC: Center for Study of Responsive Law, 1988.

9   Llanos, M. "Plastic bottles pile up as mountains of waste." MSNBC, March 3, 2005. http://www.msnbc.msn.com/id/5279230.

10  County of Sacramento, Municipal Services Agency, Department of Water Resources. "SCWA Ultra-Low Flow Toilet Rebate Program." http://www.msa.saccounty.net/waterresources/water/ULFT.asp.

11  US Environmental Protection Agency. "Use Your WaterSense." http://www.epa.gov/watersense/water/simple.htm.

12  Ibid.

13  Woods, M. "Shoes often a vehicle for tracking pesticides into house." *Pittsburgh Post-Gazette* June 22, 1999. http://www.post-gazette.com/healthscience/19990622htrackin2.asp.

14  US Environmental Protection Agency. "The Inside Story: A Guide to Indoor Air Quality." http://www.epa.gov/iaq/pubs/insidest.html.

15  Center for Development of Recycling. "Know the Facts." http://recyclestuff.org/JunkMail.asp.

16  Ibid.

17  New American Dream. "Just the Facts: Junk Mail Facts and Figures." http://www.newdream.org/junkmail/facts.php.

18  McAliney, M. "Arguments for Land Conservation: Documentation and Information Sources for Land Resource Protection." Sacramento, CA: Trust for Public Land, 1993.

19  Colorado Tree Coalition. "Benefits of Trees in Urban Areas: Urban Forests Improve Our Air." http://www.coloradotrees.org/benefits.htm.

20  Cotrone, V., compiler. "The Social and Economic Benefits of Trees." Massachusetts Department of Conservation and Recreation. http://www.mass.gov/dcr/stewardship/forestry/urban/previouscitfor.htm#socialEconomic.

21  Coder, R.D. "Identified Benefits of Community Trees and Forests." October 1996. University of Georgia Cooperative Extension Service Forest Resources Unit Publication #FOR96-39. http://www.marshalltrees.com/upload/articles_files/art_31attached_file.pdf.

22  Arbor Day Foundation. "The Value of Trees to a Community." http://www.arborday.org/trees/Benefits.cfm.

23  Scott, K.I., Simpson, J.R., McPherson, E.G. "Effects of Tree Cover on Parking Lot Microclimate and Vehicle Emissions." *Journal of Arboriculture* 1999;25(3):129-142. http://www.fs.fed.us/psw/programs/cufr/products/11/cufr_68.pdf.

24  Schwaab, E.C., Alban, L., Riley, J., Rabaglia, R., Miller, K.E. *Maryland's Forests: A Health Report.* Annapolis, MD: Maryland Department of Natural Resources Forest Service, 1995.

25  US Department of Agriculture Forest Service Southern Region. "The Benefits of Urban Trees: Urban and Community Forestry: Improving Our Quality of Life." Forestry Report R8-FR 71, September 2003. http://www.urbanforestrysouth.org/resources/collections/benefits-of-urban-trees.

26  University of Washington, College of Forest Resources, Center for Urban Horticulture. "Urban Forest Values: Economic Benefits of Trees in Cities." Fact Sheet #29, 1998. http://www.cfr.washington.edu/news_pubs/fact%20sheets/fact_sheets/29-UrbEconBen.pdf.

27  Neely, D. *Valuation of Landscape Trees, Shrubs, and Other Plants: A Guide to the Methods and Procedures for Appraising Amenity Plants.* 7th edition. Urbana, IL: International Society of Arboriculture, 1988.

28  Arzamassova, E., Lerner, J., Peterson, C. "Enhancing Rhode Island's Urban/Suburban Forests: The Economic Benefits of Urban/ Suburban Forestry." Brown University Center for Environmental Studies, February 7, 2004. http://envstudies.brown.edu/oldsite/Web/ special%20reports/Classes/ES201/2003/Forestry/econbene.htm#prop.

29  University of Washington, College of Forest Resources, Center for Urban Horticulture. "Urban Forest Values: Economic Benefits of Trees in Cities." Fact Sheet #29, 1998. http://www.cfr.washington.edu/news_pubs/fact%20sheets/fact_sheets/29-UrbEconBen.pdf.

30  US Environmental Protection Agency. "Municipal Solid Waste in the United States: 2005 Facts and Figures." EPA530-R-06-011, October 2006. http://www.epa.gov/msw/pubs/mswchar05.pdf.

31  Center for Development of Recycling. "Know the Facts." http://recyclestuff.org/JunkMail.asp.

32  Horrigan, L., Lawrence, R.S., Walker, P. "How Sustainable Agriculture Can Address the Environment and Human Health Harms of Industrial Agriculture." *Environmental Health Perspectives* 2002;110(5):445-456. http://www.ehponline.org/members/2002/110p445-456horrigan/EHP110p445PDF.PDF.

33  Natural Resources Defense Council. *Forces for Nature: 50 Ways You Can Help.* Natural Resources Defense Council, 2007.

34  Natural Resources Defense Council. "America's Animal Factories: How States Fail to Prevent Pollution from Livestock Waste." http://www.nrdc.org/water/pollution/factor/cons.asp.

35  Marks, R. "Cesspools of Shame: How Factory Farm Lagoons and Sprayfields Threaten Environmental and Public Health." Natural Resources Defense Council and Clean Water Network, 2001. http://www.nrdc.org/water/pollution/cesspools/cesspools.pdf.

36  Halverson, M.K. "The Price We Pay for Corporate Hogs." Institute for Agriculture and Trade Policy, 2000. http://www.iatp.org/ hogreport/indextoc.html.

37  Wing, S., Wolf, S. "Intensive Livestock Operations, Health, and Quality of Life Among Eastern North Carolina Residents." *Environmental Health Perspectives* 2000;108(3):233-238.

38  Jackson, L.L. "Large-Scale Swine Production and Water Quality." *Pigs, Profits, and Rural Communities.* Thu, K.M., Durrenberger, E.P., editors. Albany, NY: State University of New York Press, 1998. p. 107.

39  Mulla, D.J., Sekely, A., Birr, A., Perry, J., Vondracek, B., Bean, E., Macbeth, E., Goyal, S., Wheeler, B., Alexander, C., Randall, G., Sands, G., Linn, J. "Generic Environmental Impact Statement on Animal Agriculture: A Summary of the Literature Related to the Effects of Animal Agriculture on Water Resources." University of Minnesota College of Agriculture, Food, and Environmental Sciences, 1999. p. G-195.

40  US Environmental Protection Agency. "Methane." http://www.epa.gov/methane.

41  Natural Resources Defense Council. *Forces for Nature: 50 Ways You Can Help.* Natural Resources Defense Council, 2007.

42  Pace Law School Energy Project. "Power Scorecard: Twenty Things You Can Do to Conserve Energy." http://powerscorecard.org/ reduce_energy.cfm.

43  Ibid.

44  Natural Resources Defense Council. "A Dozen Things You Can Do to Keep Yourself—and the Earth—Healthy." http://www.nrdc.org/ cities/living/dozenthings.pdf.

45  Energy Information Administration. *Annual Energy Review 2006.* 2007. http://www.eia.doe.gov/emeu/aer/pdf/pages/sec1_8.pdf

46  Ibid.

47  Halweil, B. "Home Grown: The Case for Local Food in a Global Market." Worldwatch Paper No. 163. Worldwatch Institute, 2002. pp. 16-21. http://www.worldwatch.org/system/files/EWP163.pdf.

48  Heller, M.C., Keoleian, G.A. "Life Cycle-Based Sustainability Indicators for Assessment of the U.S. Food System." Report No. CSS00-04. Center for Sustainable Systems, University of Michigan, 2000. http://css.snre.umich.edu/css_doc/CSS00-04.pdf.

49  Ibid.

50  Pimentel, D., Giampietro, M. " Food, Land, Population and the U.S. Economy." Carrying Capacity Network, 1994. http://dieoff.org/ page55.htm.

51  Ibid.

52  Heller, M.C., Keoleian, G.A. "Life Cycle-Based Sustainability Indicators for Assessment of the U.S. Food System." Report No. CSS00-04. Center for Sustainable Systems, University of Michigan, 2000. http://css.snre.umich.edu/css_doc/CSS00-04.pdf.

53  Halweil, B. "Home Grown: The Case for Local Food in a Global Market." Worldwatch Paper No. 163. Worldwatch Institute, 2002. pp. 16-21. http://www.worldwatch.org/system/files/EWP163.pdf.

54  US Environmental Protection Agency. "Questions About Your Community: Shopping Bags: Paper or Plastic or...?" http://web.archive. org/web/20060426235724/http://www.epa.gov/region1/communities/shopbags.html.

55  US Department of Energy and US Environmental Protection Agency. "Keeping Your Car in Shape." http://www.fueleconomy.gov/feg/ maintain.shtml.

56  Green Car Congress. " Study: Under-Inflated Tires in the EU Waste 8.1 Billion Liters of Fuel Each Year." March 8, 2007. http://www.greencarcongress.com/2007/03/study_underinfl.html.

57  Natural Resources Defense Council. "A Dozen Things You Can Do to Keep Yourself—and the Earth—Healthy." http://www.nrdc.org/ cities/living/dozenthings.pdf.

58  Reed, P., Hudson, M. "We Test the Tips: What Really Saves Gas? And How Much?" http://www.edmunds.com/advice/fueleconomy/ articles/106842/article.html.

59  Natural Resources Defense Council. "A Dozen Things You Can Do to Keep Yourself—and the Earth—Healthy." http://www.nrdc.org/ cities/living/dozenthings.pdf.

60  Ibid.

61  "Ceres Praises National Launch of 'Eco-Friendly' Paper Coffee Cup." July 26, 2006. http://www.ceres.org/news/news_item.php?nid=215. [press release]

62  Ibid.

63  Conservatree. "Trees into Paper." http://www.conservatree.org/learn/EnviroIssues/TreeStats.shtml.

64  US Environmental Protection Agency. "Municipal Solid Waste in the United States: 2005 Facts and Figures." EPA530-R-06-011, October 2006. http://www.epa.gov/msw/pubs/mswchar05.pdf.

65  American Bar Association. "The ABA-EPA Law Office Eco-Challenge." https://www.abanet.org/environ/ecochallenge/overview.shtml.

66  Conservatree. "Trees into Paper." http://www.conservatree.org/learn/EnviroIssues/TreeStats.shtml.

67  Based on figures from US Environmental Protection Agency. "Municipal Solid Waste in the United States: 2005 Facts and Figures." EPA530-R-06-011, October 2006. http://www.epa.gov/msw/pubs/mswchar05.pdf.

68  Based on calculations from Environmental Defense. "Paper Calculator." http://www.environmentaldefense.org/papercalculator/incompat.cfm.

69  US Department of Energy. "When to Turn Off Personal Computers." http://www.eere.energy.gov/consumer/your_home/appliances/index.cfm/mytopic=10070.

70  US Environmental Protection Agency and US Department of Energy. "Summary of Assumptions for EPA Energy Star Savings Estimates: Energy Star Preliminary Draft Computer Specification (Version 4.0)." 2005. http://www.energystar.gov/ia/partners/prod_development/revisions/downloads/computer/Assumptions_Prelim_Draft_Comp_Spec.pdf.

71  Magid, L. "Putting Energy Hogs in the Home on a Strict Low-Power Diet." *New York Times* June 14, 2007. http://www.nytimes.com/2007/06/14/technology/14basics.html.

72  US Environmental Protection Agency and US Department of Energy. "Energy Star @ Home Tips." http://www.energystar.gov/index.cfm?c=products.es_at_home_tips.

73  US Environmental Protection Agency and US Department of Energy. "Heat and Cool Efficiently." http://www.energystar.gov/index.cfm?c=heat_cool.pr_hvac.

74  US Department of Energy. "Air Conditioners." http://www1.eere.energy.gov/consumer/tips/air_conditioners.html.

75  Sacramento Municipal Utility District. " Stay cool, save energy and money." 2007. http://www.smud.org/residential/saving/conservation.html.

76  Prince, D., Butselaar, E. "Fifty Ways to Help Save the Planet." *Vanity Fair* May 2006. http://www.vanityfair.com/politics/features/2006/05/savetheplanet200605.

77  US Environmental Protection Agency, Region 5 Air and Radiation Division. "Ozone." 2007. http://www.epa.gov/ARD-R5/naaqs/ozone.htm.

78  White, M.V. "Air Pollution and Respiratory Health Effects." 2006. http://www.aqpartners.state.pa.us/news/presentations/2006spring_markwhite.pdf.

79  "U.S. Department of Energy Turns to Window Film for Efficiency, Safety." *Building Operating Management* March 2004. http://findarticles.com/p/articles/mi_qa3922/is_200403/ai_n9346675.

80  US Department of Energy. "Water Heating." http://www1.eere.energy.gov/consumer/tips/water_heating.html.

81  US Environmental Protection Agency. "High Efficiency Water Heaters: Provide Hot Water for Less." http://www.energystar.gov/ia/new_homes/features/WaterHtrs_062906.pdf.

82  US Department of Energy. "Radiant Barrier Attic Fact Sheet." http://www.ornl.gov/sci/roofs+walls/radiant/rb_02.html.

83  US Environmental Protection Agency and US Department of Energy. "Energy Star reflective roof products." http://www.energystar.gov/index.cfm?c=roof_prods.pr_roof_products.

84  Arzamassova, E., Lerner, J., Peterson, C. "Enhancing Rhode Island's Urban/Suburban Forests: The Economic Benefits of Urban/Suburban Forestry." Brown University Center for Environmental Studies, February 7, 2004. http://envstudies.brown.edu/oldsite/Web/special%20reports/Classes/ES201/2003/Forestry/econbene.htm#prop.

85  University of Washington, College of Forest Resources, Center for Urban Horticulture. "Urban Forest Values: Economic Benefits of Trees in Cities." Fact Sheet #29, 1998. http://www.cfr.washington.edu/news_pubs/fact%20sheets/fact_sheets/29-UrbEconBen.pdf.

86  Colorado Tree Coalition. "Benefits of Trees in Urban Areas: Urban Forests Save Energy." http://www.coloradotrees.org/benefits.htm.

87  "Down the Drain." *Forest Voice* Summer 2001. p. 15. http://www.forestcouncil.org/pdf/summer01.pdf.

88  Moll, G., Ebenreck, S, editors. *Shading Our Cities: A Resource Guide for Urban and Community Forests.* Washington, DC: Island Press, 1989. p. 50. http://books.google.com/books?id=zX_4mBswpo8C&pg=PA50&lpg=PA50&dq=us+forest+service+houses+with+trees+use+20+to+25+percent+less+energy+than+houses+in+%22wide+open%22+areas&source=web&ots=HZL6fgimFU&sig=_9lWq5NC22GZJu-PhEUomxXZ4F4.

89  US Department of Agriculture Forest Service and Northeastern Area State and Private Forestry. "Urban and Community Forestry Appreciation Tool Kit: Statistics Sheet." NA-IN-02-04. http://www.fs.fed.us/na/morgantown/macucf/toolkit/StatisticsSheet.pdf.

90  US Department of Agriculture. "United States Standards for Livestock and Meat Marketing Claims." *Federal Register* 2002;67(250):79552-79556. http://www.ams.usda.gov/lsg/stand/ls0202.txt.

91  US Department of Agriculture. "United States Standard for Livestock and Meat Marketing Claim, Grass (Forage) Fed Claim." *Federal Register* 2006;71(92):27662-27665. http://a257.g.akamaitech.net/7/257/2422/01jan20061800/edocket.access.gpo.gov/2006/E6-7276.htm.

92  US Department of Agriculture. "United States Standards for Livestock and Meat Marketing Claims." *Federal Register* 2002;67(250):79552-79556. http://www.ams.usda.gov/lsg/stand/ls0202.txt.

93  Federal Trade Commission. "Guides for the Use of Environmental Marketing Claims: 260.7: Environmental Marketing Claims: (b): Degradable/Biodegradable/Photodegradable." http://www.ftc.gov/bcp/grnrule/guides980427.htm.

94  US Environmental Protection Agency. "Organic Gases (Volatile Organic Compounds—VOCs)." 2007. http://www.epa.gov/iaq/voc.html.

95  US Environmental Protection Agency. "Ozone Layer Depletion: Regulatory Programs." http://www.epa.gov/ozone/title6.

96  Co-op America. "Screening Green Businesses." http://www.coopamerica.org/greenbusiness/screening.cfm.

97  Federal Trade Commission. "Guides for the Use of Environmental Marketing Claims." http://www.ftc.gov/bcp/grnrule/guides980427.htm.

98  US Environmental Protection Agency and US Department of Energy. "About Energy Star." http://www.energystar.gov/index.cfm?c=about.ab_index.

99  Rainforest Alliance. "SmartWood: FSC Endorsed versus Rediscovered Wood Certified Products." http://www.ra-smartwood.org.

100 US Environmental Protection Agency. "Municipal Solid Waste Generation, Recycling, and Disposal in the United States: Facts and Figures for 2006." http://www.epa.gov/epaoswer/non-hw/muncpl/pubs/msw06.pdf.

101 Ibid.

102 Center for Sustainable Systems, University of Michigan. "Municipal Solid Waste." CSS04-15E07.
http://css.snre.umich.edu/css_doc/CSS04-15.pdf.

103 US Environmental Protection Agency. "Municipal Solid Waste Generation, Recycling, and Disposal in the United States: Facts and Figures for 2006." http://www.epa.gov/epaoswer/non-hw/muncpl/pubs/msw06.pdf.

104 Ibid.

105 Ibid.

106 Ibid.

107 Ibid.

108 Ibid.

109 Ibid.

110 Ibid.

111 Ibid.

112 Ibid.

113 Ibid.

114 Ibid.

115 Ibid.

116 Ibid.

117 Ibid.

118 Ibid.

119 Ibid.

120 Ibid.

121 Ibid.

122 Ibid.

123 Ibid.

124 Ibid.

125 Ibid.

126 Ibid.

127 Ibid.

128 Ibid.

129 Ibid.

130 Ibid.

131 Paper Industry Association Council. "Recycling: It Starts with You." 2007. http://www.paperrecycles.org/recycling/index.html.

132 Ibid.

133 Bureau of International Recycling. "About Recycling." 2008. http://www.bir.org/aboutrecycling/index.asp.

134 Ibid.

135 Ibid.

136 American Forest and Paper Association. "Pulp and Paper." http://www.afandpa.org/Content/NavigationMenu/Pulp_and_Paper/Fun_Facts/Fun_Facts.htm.

137 US Environmental Protection Agency. "Municipal Solid Waste in the United States: 2006 MSW Characterization Data Tables: Table 4: Paper and Paperboard Products in MSW, 2006." http://www.epa.gov/epaoswer/non-hw/muncpl/pubs/06data.pdf.

138 Based on calculations from US Environmental Protection Agency. "Municipal Solid Waste Generation, Recycling, and Disposal in the United States: Facts and Figures for 2006." http://www.epa.gov/epaoswer/non-hw/muncpl/pubs/msw06.pdf.

139 Ibid.

140 Ibid.

141 US Environmental Protection Agency. "Municipal Solid Waste in the United States: 2006 MSW Characterization Data Tables: Table 7: Plastics in Products in MSW, 2006." http://www.epa.gov/epaoswer/non-hw/muncpl/pubs/06data.pdf.

142 Washington State Department of Ecology, Hazardous Waste and Toxics Reduction Program. "Hazards of Dioxins." Publication #01-04-010. http://www.ecy.wa.gov/pubs/0104010.pdf.

143 Agency for Toxic Substances and Disease Registry. "Toxicological Profile for Chlorinated Dibenzo-p-Dioxins." 1998.
http://www.atsdr.cdc.gov/toxprofiles/tp104.pdf.

144 Mackie, D., Liu, J., Loh, Y.S., Thomas, V. "No Evidence of Dioxin Cancer Threshold." *Environmental Health Perspectives* 2003;111(9):1145-1147.

145 Yoon, B.I., Inoue, T., Kaneko, T. "Teratological effect of 2,3,7,8-tetrachlorodibenzo-*p*-dioxin (TCDD): Induction of cleft palate in the ddY and C57BL/6 mouse." *Journal of Veterinary Science* 2000;1(2):113-119. http://www.ncbi.nlm.nih.gov/entrez/query.fcgi?cmd=Retrieve&db=PubMed&list_uids=14614306&dopt=Abstract.

146 Agency for Toxic Substances and Disease Registry. "Congressional Testimony: Public Health Implications of Dioxins." June 10, 1992. http://www.atsdr.cdc.gov/testimony/testimony-1992-06-10.html.

147 Donnelly, K.C., Brown, K.W., Estiri, M., Jones, D.H., Safe, S. "Mutagenic potential of binary mixtures of nitro-polychlorinated dibenzo-*p*-dioxins and related compounds." *Journal of Toxicology and Environmental Health* 1988;24(3):345-356. http://www.osti.gov/energycitations/product.biblio.jsp?osti_id=6834585.

148 National Institute of Environmental Health Sciences. "TCDD—Dioxin—Is Listed as 'Known Human Carcinogen' in Federal Government's *Ninth Report on Carcinogens*." January 19, 2001. http://www.niehs.nih.gov/oc/news/dioxadd.htm. [press release]

149 Agency for Toxic Substances and Disease Registry. "ToxFAQs: Chemical Agent Briefing Sheet: Dioxins." March 2006. http://www.atsdr.cdc.gov/cabs/dioxins/dioxins_cabs.pdf.

150 Ibid.

151 Ibid.

152 Ibid.

153 Ibid.

154 Ibid.

155 Ibid.

156 Ibid.

157 Ibid.

158 Ibid.

159 Agency for Toxic Substances and Disease Registry. "Congressional Testimony: Public Health Implications of Dioxins." June 10, 1992. http://www.atsdr.cdc.gov/testimony/testimony-1992-06-10.html.

160 National Toxicology Program. "Substance Profiles: 2,3,7,8-Tetrachlorodibenzo-*p*-Dioxin (TCDD); 'Dioxin': CAS No. 1746-01-6." *Report on Carcinogens, Eleventh Edition* 2005. http://ntp.niehs.nih.gov/ntp/roc/eleventh/profiles/s168tcdd.pdf.

161 Agency for Toxic Substances and Disease Registry. "ToxFAQs: Chemical Agent Briefing Sheet: Dioxins." March 2006. http://www.atsdr.cdc.gov/cabs/dioxins/dioxins_cabs.pdf.

162 Ibid.

163 Agency for Toxic Substances and Disease Registry. "ToxFAQs for Chlorinated Dibenzo-p-Dioxins." 1999. http://www.atsdr.cdc.gov/tfacts104.html.

164 Somogyi, A. "Nurturing and Breast-Feeding: Exposure to Chemicals in Breast Milk." *Environmental Health Perspectives* 1993;101(2):45-52.

165 US Environmental Protection Agency. "Non-Regulated Contaminants: Existing and Future Pollutants in Water Supplies, Old Pollutants, New Concern—New Pollutants, Unknown Issues," Daughton, CG, 10/16/03, prepared for the National Academies Institute of Medicine: Roundtable on Environmental Health Sciences, Research, and Medicine (EHSRT), Washington DC, Workshop #5, From Source Water to Drinking Water: Emerging Challenges for Public Health. http://epa.gov/nerlesd1/bios/daughton/EIAR.pdf.

166 Ibid.

167 Ibid.

168 Ibid.

169 Thomsen, C., Becher, G., editors. *26th International Symposium on Halogenated Persistent Organic Pollutants: Plenary Lecture Abstracts and Session Summaries.* http://209.85.165.104/search?q=cache:IUL6difGtHEJ:x-cd.com/dioxin06/Summaries.pdf+"International+Symposium+on+Halogenated+Persistent+Organic+Pollutants"+tomsen&hl=en&ct=clnk&cd=1&gl=us.

170 Ibid.

171 Ibid.

172 Ibid.

173 Norwegian Pollution Control Authority. "Hazardous substance in the Arctic." March 6, 2004. http://www.sft.no/artikkel____33485.aspx.

174 Mazdai, A., Dodder, N.G., Abernathy, M.P., Hites, R.A., Bigsby, R.M. "Polybrominated diphenyl ethers in maternal and fetal blood samples." *Environmental Health Perspectives* 2003;111(9):1249-1252.

175 Guvenius, D.M., Aronsson, A., Ekman-Ordeberg, G., Bergman, A., Noren, K. "Human prenatal and postnatal exposure to polybrominated diphenyl ethers, polychlorinated biphenyls, polychlorobiphenylols, and pentachlorophenol." *Environmental Health Perspectives* 2003;111(9):1235-1241.

176 Choi, J.W., Fujimaki, T.S., Kitamura, K., Hashimoto, S., Ito, H., Suzuki, N., Sakai, S., Morita, M. "Polybrominated dibenzo-*p*-dioxins, dibenzofurans, diphenyl ethers in Japanese human adipose tissue." *Environmental Science and Technology* 2003;37;(5):817-821.

177 She, J., Petreas, M., Winkler, J., Visita, P., McKinney, M., Kopec, D. "PBDEs in San Francisco Bay area: Measurements in harbor seal blubber and human breast adipose tissue." *Chemosphere* 2002;46(5):697-707.

178 Stapleton, H.M., Alaee, M., Letcher, R.J., Baker, J.E. "Debromination of the flame retardant decabromodiphenyl ether by juvenile carp (*Cyprinus carpio*) following dietary exposure." *Environmental Science and Technology* 2004;38(1):112-119.

179 Hites, R.A., Foran, J.A., Schwager, S.J., Knuth, B.A., Hamilton, M.C., Carpenter, D.O. "Global Assessment of Polybrominated Diphenyl Ethers in Farmed and Wild Salmon." *Environmental Science and Technology* 2004;38(19):4945-4959. http://pubs.acs.org/subscribe/journals/esthag-a/38/free/es049548m.html.

180 Landrigan, P.J., Carlson, J.E., Bearer, C.F., Cranmer, J.S., Bullard, R.D., Etzel, R.A., Groopman, J., McLachlan, J.A., Perera, F.P., Reigart, J.R., Robison, L., Schell, L., Suk, W.A. "Children's health and the environment: A new agenda for prevention research." *Environmental Health Perspectives* 1998;106(Suppl 3):787-794.

181 Raloff, J. "New PCBs?" *Science News* 2003;164(17):266.

182 Agency for Toxic Substances and Disease Registry. "Toxicological Profile for Polybrominated Biphenyls and Polybrominated Diphenyl Ethers (PBBs and PBDEs)." 2004. http://www.atsdr.cdc.gov/toxprofiles/tp68.html.

183 Environmental Working Group. "EPA Science Panel Says Teflon Chemical 'Likely' Cause of Cancer." January 30, 2006. http://www.ewg.org/node/21302.

184 Sandy, M. "Petition for Expedited CIC Consideration of Perfluorooctanoic Acid (PFOA)." California Office of Environmental Health Hazard Assessment. http://www.oehha.ca.gov/prop65/public_meetings/pdf/pfoacic%20slides121206.pdf.

185 Environmental Working Group. "EPA Science Panel Says Teflon Chemical 'Likely' Cause of Cancer." January 30, 2006. http://www.ewg.org/node/21302.

186 van de Plassche, E., Schwegler, A. "Polychlorinated naphthalenes." 2002. http://www.unece.org/env/popsxg/2000-2003/pcn.pdf.

187 Houlihan, J., Kropp, T., Wiles, R., Gray, S., Campbell, C. "Cord Blood: Detailed Findings." Environmental Working Group Report, 2005. p. 8. http://www.drgreene.org/body.cfm?xyzpdqabc=0&id=21&action=detail&ref=1985.

188 Bogdal, C., Kohler, M., Schmid, P., Sturm, M., Grieder, E., Scheringer, M., Hungerbühler, K. "Polychlorinated naphthalenes: Congener specific analysis and source identification in a dated sediment core from Lake Thun, Switzerland." *Organohalogen Compounds* 2006; 68:300-303. http://www.nrp50.ch/fileadmin/user_upload/Dokumente/Hall_of_Fame/Bogdal_et_al_OrganohalogenCompounds2006_01.pdf.

189 Environmental Working Group. "Human Toxome Project: Polychlorinated naphthalenes (PCNs)." http://www.ewg.org/sites/humantoxome/chemicals/chemical_classes.php?class=Polychlorinated+naphthalenes+(PCNs).

190 Domingo, J. "Polychlorinated naphthalenes in animal aquatic species and human exposure through the diet: A review." *Journal of Chromatography A* 2004;1054(1-2):327-334.

191 van de Plassche, E., Schwegler, A. "Polychlorinated naphthalenes." 2002. http://www.unece.org/env/popsxg/2000-2003/pcn.pdf.

192 Thomsen, C., Becher, G., editors. *26th International Symposium on Halogenated Persistent Organic Pollutants: Plenary Lecture Abstracts and Session Summaries.* http://209.85.165.104/search?q=cache:IUL6difGtHEJ:x-cd.com/dioxin06/Summaries.pdf+"International+Symposium+on+Halogenated+Persistent+Organic+Pollutants"+tomsen&hl=en&ct=clnk&cd=1&gl=us.

193 Ibid.

194 Ibid.

195 Ibid.

196 World Health Organization. "Polybrominated dibenzo-p-dioxins and dibenzofurans." Environmental Health Criteria No. 205, 1998.

197 US Environmental Protection Agency. "Organic Gases (Volatile Organic Compounds—VOCs)." http://www.epa.gov/iaq/voc.html.

198 Ibid.

199 Ibid.

200 Ibid.

201 State of California, Environmental Protection Agency, Office of Environmental Health Hazard Assessment. "Chemicals Known to the State to Cause Cancer or Reproductive Toxicity." Safe Drinking Water and Toxic Enforcement Act of 1986. 2007. http://www.oehha.ca.gov/prop65/prop65_list/files/060107LST.pdf.

202 US Environmental Protection Agency. "Organic Gases (Volatile Organic Compounds—VOCs)." http://www.epa.gov/iaq/voc.html.

203 Ibid.

204 Ibid.

# Chapter 2:
# Green Cleaning Basics

1 Material Safety Data Sheet. "Quaternary Ammonium 10% Solution." CAS No. 68391-01-5, MSDS No. CFYDS.

2 Physical and Theoretical Chemistry Laboratory, Oxford University. "Safety Data for Ammonium Hydroxide." CAS No. 1336-21-6, Annex I Index No. 007-001-01-2.

3 Ibid.

4 Ibid.

5 Material Safety Data Sheet. "2-Butoxyethanol." CAS No, 111-76-2, MSDS No. CJNRJ, Product ID No. 2138.

6 Ibid.

7 Agency for Toxic Substances and Disease Registry. "Medical Management Guideline for Chlorine." CAS No. 7782-50-5. http://www.atsdr.cdc.gov/MHMI/mmg172.html.

8 Ibid.

9 Ibid.

10   Ibid.

11   Ibid.

12   Ibid.

13   Physical and Theoretical Chemistry Laboratory, Oxford University. "Safety Data for Chlorine." CAS No. 7782-50-5, EC No. 231-959-5.

14   Material Safety Data Sheet. "Diethanolamine." Account No. 00532, CAS No. 111-42-2.

15   Ibid.

16   Ibid.

17   Material Safety Data Sheet. "Dipropylene Glycol, Tech., 99%." Account No. 32455, CAS No. 25265-71-8.

18   Ibid.

19   Physical and Theoretical Chemistry Laboratory, Oxford University. "Safety Data for Ethylene Glycol." CAS No. 107-21-1.

20   Ibid.

21   Ibid.

22   Ibid.

23   Ibid.

24   Material Safety Data Sheet. "Diethylene Glycol." MSDS No. 08764, CAS No. 111-46-6.

25   Material Safety Data Sheet. "Glycolic Acid." MSDS No. G6820, CAS No. 79-14-1.

26   Ibid.

27   Ibid.

28   Ibid.

29   Physical and Theoretical Chemistry Laboratory, Oxford University. '"Safety Data for Naphtha." CAS No. 8030-30-6.

30   Ibid.

31   Ibid.

32   Ibid.

33   Material Safety Data Sheet. "Petroleum Distillate." CAS No. 8030-30-6. http://www.mcgillairseal.com/textDocs/msds/uniFast.htm.

34   Ibid.

35   Ibid.

36   Ibid.

37   Material Safety Data Sheet. "Nonylphenol." CAS No. 84852-15-3.

38   Ibid.

39   Ibid.

40   Ibid.

41   Ibid.

42   Material Safety Data Sheet. "Sodium Hydroxide Solution, 0.5-1.0M (2-4%)." Account No. 02023, CAS No. 1310-73-2.

43   Ibid.

44   Ibid.

45   Ibid.

46   Ibid.

47   Material Safety Data Sheet. "Sodium Hypochlorite Solution, 4-6%." Account No. 40179, CAS No. 7681-52-9.

48   Ibid.

49   Material Safety Data Sheet. "Triethanolamine." Account No. 01071, CAS No. 102-71-6.

50   Ibid.

51   Ibid.

52   Ibid.

53   Seventh Generation. http://www.seventhgen.com/our_products/free_and_clear/free_clear_all_purpose_cleaner.html.

54   Material Safety Data Sheet. "Sodium Dodecylbenzene Sulfate." CAS No. 25155-30-0.

55   Ibid.

56   US Environmental Protection Agency. "Cleaning National Parks: Using Environmentally Preferable Janitorial Products at Yellowstone and Grand Teton National Parks." 2000, Pollution Prevention Program (8P-P3T), EPA/908/R-00-001.

57   Agency for Toxic Substances and Disease Registry. "Medical Management Guideline for Chlorine." CAS No. 7782-50-5 http://www.atsdr.cdc.gov/MHMI/mmg172.html.

58   Ibid.

59   Ibid.

60   Ibid.

61   Kim, J., Marshall, M., Wei, C. "Antibacterial Activity of Some Essential Oil Components Against Five Foodborne Pathogens." *Journal of Agricultural Food Chemistry* 1995;43:2839-2845. http://pubs.acs.org/cgi-bin/abstract.cgi/jafcau/1995/43/i11/f-pdf/ f_jf00059a013.pdf?sessid=6006l3.

62   Ibid.

63   Dorman, H., Deans, S. "Antimicrobial agents from plants: antibacterial activity of plant volatile oils." *Journal of Applied Microbiology* 2000;88(2):308–316.

64   Cavanagh, H., Wilkinson, J. "Biological Activities of Lavender Essential Oil." *Phytotherapy Research* 2002;16(4):301-308.

65  Kim, J., Marshall, M., Wei, C. "Antibacterial Activity of Some Essential Oil Components Against Five Foodborne Pathogens." *Journal of Agricultural Food Chemistry* 1995;43:2839-2845. http://pubs.acs.org/cgi-bin/abstract.cgi/jafcau/1995/43/i11/f-pdf/f_jf00059a013.pdf?sessid=60061 3.

66  Hammer, K., Carson, C., Riley, T. "Antimicrobial activity of essential oils and other plant extracts." *Journal of Applied Microbiology* 1999;86:985-990.

67  Kim, J., Marshall, M., Wei, C. "Antibacterial Activity of Some Essential Oil Components Against Five Foodborne Pathogens." *Journal of Agricultural Food Chemistry* 1995;43:2839-2845. http://pubs.acs.org/cgi-bin/abstract.cgi/jafcau/1995/43/i11/f-pdf/f_jf00059a013.pdf?sessid=60061 3.

68  Dorman, H., Deans, S. "Antimicrobial agents from plants: antibacterial activity of plant volatile oils." *Journal of Applied Microbiology* 2000;88(2):308–316.

69  Hammer, K., Riley, T. "Antimicrobial activity of essential oils and other plant extracts." *Journal of Applied Microbiology* 1999;86:985-990.

70  Burt, S., Reinders, R. "Antibacterial activity of selected plant essential oils." *Letters in Applied Microbiology* 2003;36:162-167.

71  Cavanagh, H., Wilkinson, J. "Biological Activities of Lavender Essential Oil." *Phytotherapy Research* 2002;16(4):301-308.

72  Dorman, H., Deans, S. "Antimicrobial agents from plants: antibacterial activity of plant volatile oils." *Journal of Applied Microbiology* 2000;88(2):308–316.

73  Hammer, K., Riley, T. "Antimicrobial activity of essential oils and other plant extracts." *Journal of Applied Microbiology* 1999;86:985-990.

74  Cosentino, S., Tuberoso, C., Pisano, B., Satta, M., Mascia, V., Arzedi, E., Palmas, F. "In-vitro antimicrobial activity and chemical composition of Sardinian *Thymus* essential oils." *Letters in Applied Microbiology* 1999;29(2):130-135.

75  Sherry, E., Boeck, H., Warnke, P.H. "Percutaneous treatment of chronic MRSA osteomyelitis with a novel plant-derived antiseptic." *BMC Surgery* 2001;1(1). http://www.biomedcentral.com/1471-2482/1/1.

76  Material Safety Data Sheet. "Dipropylene Glycol Methyl Ether." CAS No. 34590-94-8. http://www.sciencelab.com/xMSDS-Dipropylene_Glycol_Methyl_Ether-9923864.

77  Material Safety Data Sheet. "2-Butoxyethanol." CAS No. 111-76-2, MSDS No. B6100. http://www.jtbaker.com/msds/englishhtml/b6100.htm.

78  Material Safety Data Sheet. "Monoethanolamine." CAS No. 141-43-5. http://www.sciencelab.com/xMSDS-Monoethanolamine-9922885.

79  Material Safety Data Sheet. "Ammonium Hydroxide." CAS No. 1336-21-6. http://www.jtbaker.com/msds/englishhtml/a5916.htm

80  Seventh Generation. http://www.seventhgen.com/our_products/free_and_clear/free_clear_glass_surface_cleaner.html.

81  Occupational Safety and Health Administration. "Occupational Safety and Health Guidelines for Dipropylene Glycol Methyl Ether." CAS No. 34590-94-8. http://www.osha.gov/SLTC/healthguidelines/dipropyleneglycolmethylether/recognition.html.

82  US Environmental Protection Agency. "CTSA, Public Comment Draft: Chapter 3: Risk: Dipropylene Glycol Methyl Ether." CAS No. 34590-94-8, 2000. pp. 3-13-3-22. http://www.epa.gov/opptintr/dfe/pubs/flexo/ctsa/draft/ch3-risk.pdf.

83  Ibid.

84  Ibid.

85  Ibid.

86  Agency for Toxic Substances and Disease Registry. "2-Butoxyethanol and 2-Butoxyethanol Acetate: Health Effects." http://www.atsdr.cdc.gov/toxprofiles/tp118-c2.pdf.

87  Ibid.

88  Ibid.

89  Agency for Toxic Substances and Disease Registry. "ToxFAQs: 2-Butoxyethanol and 2-Butoxyethanol Acetate." 1999. http://www.atsdr.cdc.gov/tfacts118.html.

90  Occupational Safety and Health Administration. "Ethanolamine." CAS No. 141-43-5. http://www.osha.gov/SLTC/healthguidelines/ethanolamine/index.html.

91  Material Safety Data Sheet. "PH Adjuster I: 2. Hazardous Ingredients/Identity Information, Monoethanolamine." CAS No. 141-43-5. http://www.weyerhaeuser.com/environment/msds/pdfs/328.pdf.

92  Ibid.

93  Ibid.

94  Ibid.

95  Material Safety Data Sheet. "Monoethanolamine." CAS No. 141-43-5. http://www.hillyard.com/images/msds/MSDSHIL00152.pdf.

96  Agency for Toxic Substances and Disease Registry. "Medical Management Guidelines for Ammonia." CAS No. 7664-41-7. http://www.atsdr.cdc.gov/mhmi/mmg126.html.

97  Scorecard. "Ammonium Hydroxide." CAS No. 1336-21-6. http://www.scorecard.org/chemical-profiles/summary.tcl?edf_substance_id=1336-21-6.

98  Agency for Toxic Substances and Disease Registry. "Medical Management Guidelines for Ammonia." CAS No. 7664-41-7. http://www.atsdr.cdc.gov/mhmi/mmg126.html.

99  Material Safety Data Sheet. "Ammonium Hydroxide Solution." CAS No. 7664-41-7. http://www.genchemcorp.com/pdf/msds/Ammonium%20Hydroxide%20-%208-01.pdf.

100 Environmental Risk Management Authority New Zealand. "Evaluation Sheet, Nonylphenol, Nonylphenol Ethoxylates and Octylphenol Ethoxylates." http://www.ermanz.govt.nz/consultations/ceir/s.pdf.

101 Ibid.

102 Nethercott, J.R., Lawrence, M.J. "Allergic contact dermatitis due to nonylphenol ethoxylate (Nonoxynol-6)." *Contact Dermatitis* 1984;10(4):235-239. http://www.blackwell-synergy.com/doi/abs/10.1111/j.1600-0536.1984.tb00106.x?journalCode=cod.

103 US Department of Agriculture. "Human and Ecological Risk Assessment of Nonylphenol Polyethoxylate-based (NPE) Surfactants." 2003. http://www.fs.fed.us/r6/invasiveplant-eis/Risk-Assessments/NPE-Surfactant_RA_final.pdf.

104 Ibid.

105 Ibid.

106 Wallace, L., Nelson, W., Pellizzari, E., Raymer, J., Thomas, K. "Identification of Polar Volatile Organic Compounds in Consumer Products and Common Microenvironments." US Environmental Protection Agency, Paper No. A312, 1991.

107 Lessenger, J.E. "Occupational Acute Anaphylactic Reaction to Assault by Perfume Spray in the Face." *Journal of the American Board of Family Practice* 2001;14(2):137-140. http://www.jabfm.org/cgi/reprint/14/2/137.pdf.

108 Ibid.

109 Griffiths, D.E. "Psi-screen, an in vitro toxicity test system: applications in the bioassay of perfumes and fragrance chemicals." *Alternatives to Laboratory Animals* 2005;33(5):471-486. http://altweb.jhsph.edu/publications/journals/atla/33_5/Griffiths_33.5.pdf.

110 Report by the Committee on Science and Technology. "Neurotoxins: At Home and the Workplace." US House of Representatives, September 16, 1986. Report 99-827.

111 Ibid.

112 Grandjean, P., Landrigan, P.J. "Developmental neurotoxicity of industrial chemicals." *Lancet* 2006;368(9553):2167-2178.

113 Shea, K.M., and Committee on Environmental Health. " Pediatric Exposure and Potential Toxicity of Phthalate Plasticizers." *Pediatrics* 2003;111(6):1467-1474. http://pediatrics.aappublications.org/cgi/content/full/111/6/1467.

114 National Institute of Environmental Health Services. "Endocrine Disruptors." 2006. http://www.niehs.nih.gov/oc/factsheets/pdf/endocrine.pdf.

115 Center for the Evaluation of Risks to Human Reproduction. "NPT Brief on the Potential Human Reproductive and Developmental Effects of Di(2-ethylhexyl) Phthalate (DEHP)." US Department of Health and Human Services, National Toxicology Program. Draft, May 2006. http://cerhr.niehs.nih.gov/chemicals/dehp/DEHP%20Brief%20Draft1.pdf.

116 Graham, S. "Ubiquitous Chemical Associated with Abnormal Human Reproductive Development." *Scientific American* May 27, 2005. http://scientificamerican.com/article.cfm?chanID=sa003&articleID=000240B8-30B1-1296-B0B183414B7F0000.

117 Foster, P. "Effects of Di(n-butyl)phthalate on Reproductive Development." 2006. http://www.americanchemistry.com/s_acc/docs/LRIAbstracts/LRIAbstract_43.pdf.

118 Kleinsasser, N., Wallner, B.C., Kastenbauer, E.R., Weissacher, H., Harreus, U.A. "Genotoxicity of di-butyl-phthalate and di-iso-butyl-phthalate in human lymphocytes and mucosal cells." *Teratogenesis, Carcinogenesis, and Mutagenesis* 2001;21(3):189-196. http://www3.interscience.wiley.com/cgi-bin/abstract/78505490/ABSTRACT.

119 Shea, K., and Committee on Environmental Health. "Pediatric Exposure and Potential Toxicity of Phthalate Plasticizers." *Pediatrics* 2003;111(6):1467-1474. http://pediatrics.aappublications.org/cgi/content/full/111/6/1467.

120 Hu, X., Wen, B., Shan, X. "Survey of phthalate pollution in arable soils in China." *Journal of Environmental Monitoring* 2003;5:649-653. http://www.rsc.org/publishing/journals/EM/article.asp?doi=b304669a.

121 US Environmental Protection Agency. "The Inside Story: A Guide to Indoor Air Quality." http://www.epa.gov/iaq/pubs/insidest.html.

122 US Environmental Protection Agency. "Introduction to Indoor Air Quality: Organic Gasses (Volatile Organic Compounds)." http://www.epa.gov/iaq/voc.html.

123 Ibid.

124 Ibid.

125 Wolverton, B.C. *How to Grow Fresh Air.* New York: Penguin, 1996.

126 Ibid.

127 Wolverton, B.C., Wolverton, J. "Interior Plants: Their Influence on Airborne Microbes Inside Energy Efficient Buildings." *Journal of the Mississippi Academy of Science* 1996;41(2):99-105.

128 Lohr, V.I., Pearson-Mims, C.H., and Goodwin, G.K. "Interior Plants May Improve Worker Productivity and Reduce Stress in a Windowless Environment." *Journal of Environmental Horticulture* 1996;14(2):97-100.

129 Zuckerman, M. "Development of Situation Specific Trait-State Test for Prediction and Measurement of Affective Responses." *Journal of Clinical Psychology* 1977;45(4):97-100.

130 Fjeld, T., Bonneville, C. "Effects of Plants and Artificial Day-Light on the Well-Being and Health of Office Workers, School Children and Health Care Personnel." Presented at the Plants for People "Reducing Health Complaints at Work" Symposium, June 14, 2002.

131 Mercola, J., Droege, R. "Plants Are Good for Your Health: Four Ways to Use Them to Your Advantage." 2004. http://www.mercola.com/2004/may/8/plants_health.htm.

# Chapter 3:
# 5 Steps to a Green Kitchen

1   Agency for Toxic Substances and Disease Registry. "Benzene." CAS No.: 71-43-2. http://www.atsdr.cdc.gov/tfacts3.html.

2   US Environmental Protection Agency. "1,4-Dioxane (1,4-Diethyleneoxide)." http://www.epa.gov/ttn/atw/hlthef/dioxane.html.

3   Breast Cancer Fund. "Cancer-Causing Chemical Found in Children's Bath Products." 2007. http://www.breastcancerfund.org/site/pp.asp?c=kwKXLdPaE&b=2483603.

4   Black, R.E., Hurley, F.J., Havery, D.C. "Occurrence of 1,4-Dioxane in Cosmetic Raw Materials and Finished Cosmetic Products." *Journal of AOAC International* 2001;84(3):666-670. http://www.atypon-link.com/AOAC/doi/abs/10.5555/jaoi.2001.84.3.666.

5   Coastal Watershed Council. "Water Quality Objectives." http://www.coastal-watershed.org/CWC_Library/Water_Quality/index.htm.

6   Mohr, T.K.G. "Solvent Stabilizers: White Paper, Prepublication Copy." June 14, 2001. http://www.valleywater.org/water/Water_Quality/Protecting_your_water/_Solvents/_PDFs/SolventStabilizers.pdf.

7   Sijm, D., de Bruijn, J., Crommentuijn, T., van Leeuwen, K. "Environmental Quality Standards: Endpoints or Triggers for a Tiered Ecological Effect Assessment Approach?" *Environmental Toxicology and Chemistry* 2001;20(11):2644-2648. http://www.setacjournals.org/perlserv/?request=get-abstract&doi=10.1897%2F1551-5028(2001)020%3C2644:EQSEOT%3E2.0.CO%3B2&ct=1&SESSID=b00af2d5601icd2eb9041c0bd14ad32e.

8   Ibid.

9   Ostroumov, S.A. "Studying effects of some surfactants and detergents on filter-feeding bivalves." *Hydrobiologia* 500(1-3):341-344. http://www.springerlink.com/content/k05884h730t228w4.

10  Pesticide Action Network. "Acute Aquatic Ecotoxicity Summaries for Alcohol Ethoxylate (C9-C11, 6 EO) on Fish." CAS No. 68439-46-3. PAN Pesticides Database: Chemical Toxicity Studies on Aquatic Organisms. http://www.pesticideinfo.org/List_AquireAcuteSum.jsp?Rec_Id=PC109&Taxa_Group=Fish.

11  US Environmental Protection Agency. "1,4-Dioxane (1,4-Diethyleneoxide)." http://www.epa.gov/ttn/atw/hlthef/dioxane.html.

12  Breast Cancer Fund. "Cancer-Causing Chemical Found in Children's Bath Products." 2007. http://www.breastcancerfund.org/site/pp.asp?c=kwKXLdPaE&b=2483603.

13  Georgia Strait Alliance. "ToxicSmart: Glossary of Ingredients." http://www.georgiastrait.org/?q=node/504.

14  National Environmental Trust. "Studies on Bisphenol-A Migration from Polycarbonate Plastic." http://www.net.org/health/products/plasticwrap/migration.vtml.

15  Gibson, R.L. "Toxic Baby Bottles: Scientific study finds leaching chemicals in clear plastic baby bottles." Environment California Research and Policy Center, 2007. http://www.environmentcalifornia.org/uploads/Ve/AQ/VeAQsr6MMu4xA3-2ibnr_g/Toxic-Baby-Bottles.pdf.

16  Ibid.

17  Ibid.

18  Ibid.

19  National Environmental Trust. "Studies on Bisphenol-A Migration from Polycarbonate Plastic." http://www.net.org/health/products/plasticwrap/migration.vtml.

20  Agency for Toxic Substances and Disease Registry. "ToxFAQs: Chemical Agent Briefing Sheet (CABS): Dioxins." March 2006. http://www.atsdr.cdc.gov/cabs/dioxins/dioxins_cabs.pdf.

21  Ibid.

22  Ibid.

23  Mackie, D., Liu, J., Loh, Y.S., Thomas, V. "No Evidence of Dioxin Cancer Threshold." *Environmental Health Perspectives* 2003;111(9):1145-1147.

24  Physical and Theoretical Chemistry Laboratory, Oxford University. "Safety Data for Ethylene Glycol." CAS No. 107-21-1.

25  Ibid.

26  Ibid.

27  Physical and Theoretical Chemistry Laboratory, Oxford University. "2-Butoxyethanol." CAS No. 11-72-2.

28  Ibid.

29  Material Safety Data Sheet. "2-Butoxyethanol." MSDS No. CJNRJ, Product ID No.: 2138.

30  Ibid.

31  Georgia Strait Alliance. "Toxic Smart: Glossary of Ingredients: Butyl Cellosolve." http://www.georgiastrait.org/?q=node/504#B.

32  Material Safety Data Sheet. "Sodium Hydroxide." CAS No. 1310-73-2, MSDS No. S4034.

33  Ibid.

34  Ibid.

35  Physical and Theoretical Chemistry Laboratory, Oxford University. "Safety Data for Naphtha." CAS No. 8030-30-6.

36  Material Safety Data Sheet. "Petroleum Distillate." http://www.mcgillairseal.com/textDocs/msds/uniFast.htm.

37  Physical and Theoretical Chemistry Laboratory, Oxford University. "Safety Data for Naphtha." CAS No. 8030-30-6.

38  Material Safety Data Sheet. "Petroleum Distillate." http://www.mcgillairseal.com/textDocs/msds/uniFast.htm.

39  Physical and Theoretical Chemistry Laboratory, Oxford University. "Safety Data for Naphtha." CAS No. 8030-30-6.

40  Material Safety Data Sheet. "Petroleum Distillate." http://www.mcgillairseal.com/textDocs/msds/uniFast.htm.

41  Physical and Theoretical Chemistry Laboratory, Oxford University. "2-Butoxyethanol." CAS No. 11-72-2.

42  Georgia Strait Alliance. "Toxic Smart: Glossary of Ingredients: Butyl Cellosolve." http://www.georgiastrait.org/?q=node/504#B.

43  Lima, P.D.L., Leite, D.S., Vasconcellos, M.C., Cavalcanti, B.C., Santos, R.A., Costa-Lotufo, L.V., Pessoa, C., Moraes, M.O., Burbano, R.R. "Genotoxic effects of aluminum chloride in cultured human lymphocytes treated in different phases of cell cycle." *Food and Chemical Toxicology* 2007;45(7):1154-1159. http://www.sciencedirect.com/science?_ob=ArticleURL&_udi=B6T6P-4MSXT97-F&_user=10&_coverDate=07%2F31%2F2007&_rdoc=1&_fmt=&_orig=search&_sort=d&view=c&_acct=C000050221&_version=1&_urlVersion=0&_userid=10&md5=d2ae77fe6219f136ae53828453e7bb71.

44  Ibid.

45  Darbre, P.D. "Aluminum, antiperspirants and breast cancer." *Journal of Inorganic Biochemistry* 2005;99(9):1912-1929.

46  Bishop, N.J., Morley, R., Day, J.P., Lucas, A. "Aluminum neurotoxicity in preterm infants receiving intravenous-feeding solutions." *New England Journal of Medicine* 1997;336(22):1557-1562.

47  Center for Food Safety and Applied Nutrition, US Food and Drug Administration. "Bottled water: Proposed rule." *Code of Federal Regulations* 21 CFR Part 165. Docket No.: 95N090203, 1995. http://www.cfsan.fda.gov/~lrd/n095-327.txt.

48  Sedman, A. "Aluminum Toxicity in Childhood." *Pediatric Nephrology* 1992;6(4):383-393. http://www.springerlink.com/content/v5h1446t58x26655.

49  Deloncle, R., Guillard, O., Clanet, F., Courtois, P., Piriou, A. "Aluminum transfer as glutamate complex through blood-brain barrier. Possible implication in dialysis encephalopathy." *Biological Trace Element Research* 1990;25(1):39-45. http://www.ncbi.nlm.nih.gov/sites/entrez?cmd=Retrieve&db=PubMed&list_uids=1696110&dopt=Abstract.

50  Yokel, R. "Blood-brain barrier flux of aluminum, manganese, iron and other metals suspected to contribute to metal-induced neurodegeneration." *Journal of Alzheimer's Disease* 2006;10:223-253. http://www.mc.uky.edu/pharmacy/faculty/files/jad.pdf.

51  Trapp, G.A., Miner, G.D., Zimmerman, R.L., Mastri, A.R., Heston, L.L. "Aluminum levels in brain in Alzheimer's disease." *Biological Psychiatry* 1978;13(6):709-718. http://www.ncbi.nlm.nih.gov/sites/entrez?cmd=Retrieve&db=PubMed&list_uids=737258&dopt=Abstract.

52  Perl, D. "Relationship of Aluminum to Alzheimer's Disease." *Journal of Environmental Health Perspectives* 1985;63:149-153. http://links.jstor.org/sici?sici=0091-6765(198511)63%3C149%3AROATAD%3E2.0.CO%3B2-U.

53  Corrigan, F.M., Reynolds, G.P., Ward, N.I. "Hippocampal tin, aluminum and zinc in Alzheimer's disease." *BioMetals* 2005;6(3):149-154. http://www.springerlink.com/content/758257436878500g.

54  CBS News. "Teflon Chemical a Likely Carcinogen." February 15, 2006. http://www.cbsnews.com/stories/2006/02/15/tech/main1321804.shtml.

55  MSNBC, Nightly News. "EPA: Compound in Teflon May Cause Cancer." June 29, 2005. http://www.msnbc.msn.com/id/8408729.

56  Weise, E. "Panel calls chemical a 'likely carcinogen.'" *USA Today* June 29, 2005. http://www.usatoday.com/news/health/2005-06-29-teflon-usat_x.htm.

57  US Environmental Protection Agency. "Basic Information on PFOA." http://www.epa.gov/opptintr/pfoa/pubs/pfoainfo.htm.

58  US Environmental Protection Agency. "Perfluorooctanoic Acid (PFOA)." http://www.epa.gov/oppt/pfoa.

59  Sandy, M. "Petition for Expedited CIC Consideration of Perfluorooctanoic Acid (PFOA)." California Office of Environmental Health Hazard Assessment. http://www.oehha.ca.gov/prop65/public_meetings/pdf/pfoacic%20slides121206.pdf.

60  Environmental Working Group. "EPA Science Panel Says Teflon Chemical 'Likely' Cause of Cancer." January 30, 2006. http://www.ewg.org/node/21302.

61  Sandy, M. "Petition for Expedited CIC Consideration of Perfluorooctanoic Acid (PFOA)." California Office of Environmental Health Hazard Assessment. http://www.oehha.ca.gov/prop65/public_meetings/pdf/pfoacic%20slides121206.pdf.

62  Environmental Working Group. "EPA Science Panel Says Teflon Chemical 'Likely' Cause of Cancer." January 30, 2006. http://www.ewg.org/node/21302.

63  Sandy, M. "Petition for Expedited CIC Consideration of Perfluorooctanoic Acid (PFOA)." California Office of Environmental Health Hazard Assessment. http://www.oehha.ca.gov/prop65/public_meetings/pdf/pfoacic%20slides121206.pdf.

64  Environmental Working Group. "EPA Science Panel Says Teflon Chemical 'Likely' Cause of Cancer." January 30, 2006. http://www.ewg.org/node/21302.

65  DuPont Teflon. "Safety of Teflon Non-Stick Coatings for Cookware." http://www.teflon.com/Teflon/teflonissafe/cookware_safety.html.

66  3M. "3M Phasing Out Some of Its Specialty Materials." May 16, 2000. http://www.chemicalindustryarchives.org/dirtysecrets/scotchgard/pdfs/226-0641.pdf#page=1. [press release]

67  CBS News. "Teflon Chemical a Likely Carcinogen." February 15, 2006. http://www.cbsnews.com/stories/2006/02/15/tech/main1321804.shtml.

68  MSNBC, Nightly News. "EPA: Compound in Teflon May Cause Cancer." June 29, 2005. http://www.msnbc.msn.com/id/8408729.

69  Weise, E. "Panel calls chemical a 'likely carcinogen.'" *USA Today* June 29, 2005. http://www.usatoday.com/news/health/2005-06-29-teflon-usat_x.htm.

70  US Environmental Protection Agency. "Perfluorooctanoic Acid (PFOA)." http://www.epa.gov/oppt/pfoa.

71  US Environmental Protection Agency. "Basic Information on PFOA." http://www.epa.gov/opptintr/pfoa/pubs/pfoainfo.htm.

72  Ibid.

73  Sandy, M. "Petition for Expedited CIC Consideration of Perfluorooctanoic Acid (PFOA)." California Office of Environmental Health Hazard Assessment. http://www.oehha.ca.gov/prop65/public_meetings/pdf/pfoacic%20slides121206.pdf.

74  Environmental Working Group. "EPA Science Panel Says Teflon Chemical 'Likely' Cause of Cancer." January 30, 2006. http://www.ewg.org/node/21302.

75  Environmental Working Group. "EPA Science Panel Says Teflon Chemical 'Likely' Cause of Cancer." January 30, 2006. http://www.ewg.org/node/21302.

76  Sandy, M. "Petition for Expedited CIC Consideration of Perfluorooctanoic Acid (PFOA)." California Office of Environmental Health Hazard Assessment. http://www.oehha.ca.gov/prop65/public_meetings/pdf/pfoacic%20slides121206.pdf.

77  Environmental Working Group. "EPA Science Panel Says Teflon Chemical 'Likely' Cause of Cancer." January 30, 2006. http://www.ewg.org/node/21302.

78  US Environmental Protection Agency. "Perfluorooctanoic Acid (PFOA)." http://www.epa.gov/oppt/pfoa.

79  Sandy, M. "Petition for Expedited CIC Consideration of Perfluorooctanoic Acid (PFOA)." California Office of Environmental Health Hazard Assessment. http://www.oehha.ca.gov/prop65/public_meetings/pdf/pfoacic%20slides121206.pdf.

80 Environmental Working Group. "EPA Science Panel Says Teflon Chemical 'Likely' Cause of Cancer." January 30, 2006. http://www.ewg.org/node/21302.

81 US Environmental Protection Agency. "Perfluorooctanoic Acid (PFOA)." http://www.epa.gov/oppt/pfoa.

82 Environmental Working Group. "EPA Science Panel Says Teflon Chemical 'Likely' Cause of Cancer." January 30, 2006. http://www.ewg.org/node/21302.

83 Sandy, M. "Petition for Expedited CIC Consideration of Perfluorooctanoic Acid (PFOA)." California Office of Environmental Health Hazard Assessment. http://www.oehha.ca.gov/prop65/public_meetings/pdf/pfoacic%20slides121206.pdf.

84 Environmental Working Group. "EPA Science Panel Says Teflon Chemical 'Likely' Cause of Cancer." January 30, 2006. http://www.ewg.org/node/21302.

85 Sandy, M. "Petition for Expedited CIC Consideration of Perfluorooctanoic Acid (PFOA)." California Office of Environmental Health Hazard Assessment. http://www.oehha.ca.gov/prop65/public_meetings/pdf/pfoacic%20slides121206.pdf.

86 Environmental Working Group. "EPA Science Panel Says Teflon Chemical 'Likely' Cause of Cancer." January 30, 2006. http://www.ewg.org/node/21302.

87 Dominiak, M.F. "Emerging Pollutants: Perfluorinated Compunds." Western Region Pollution Prevention Network Conference, October 17, 2003. http://www.p2pays.org/ref/34/33018.pdf.

88 US Environmental Protection Agency. "Nominates for testing by NTP a class study of perfluorosulfonates, carboxylic acids and telomers." August 7, 2003.

89 Environmental Working Group. "EPA Science Panel Says Teflon Chemical 'Likely' Cause of Cancer." January 30, 2006. http://www.ewg.org/node/21302.

90 Sandy, M. "Petition for Expedited CIC Consideration of Perfluorooctanoic Acid (PFOA)." California Office of Environmental Health Hazard Assessment. http://www.oehha.ca.gov/prop65/public_meetings/pdf/pfoacic%20slides121206.pdf.

91 Environmental Working Group. "EPA Science Panel Says Teflon Chemical 'Likely' Cause of Cancer." January 30, 2006. http://www.ewg.org/node/21302.

92 Sandy, M. "Petition for Expedited CIC Consideration of Perfluorooctanoic Acid (PFOA)." California Office of Environmental Health Hazard Assessment. http://www.oehha.ca.gov/prop65/public_meetings/pdf/pfoacic%20slides121206.pdf.

93 Environmental Working Group. "EPA Science Panel Says Teflon Chemical 'Likely' Cause of Cancer." January 30, 2006. http://www.ewg.org/node/21302.

94 World Wildlife Fund. "Wildlife at Risk: Emerging Chemical Threats." Doc. 08-04/1000, 2004. http://www.worldwildlife.org/toxics/pubs/wildlife_at_risk.pdf.

95 Eilperin, J. "Harmful Teflon Chemical to Be Eliminated by 2015." *Washington Post* January 26, 2006.

96 US Environmental Protection Agency. "Perfluorooctanoic Acid (PFOA)." http://www.epa.gov/oppt/pfoa.

97 Environmental Working Group. "EPA Science Panel Says Teflon Chemical 'Likely' Cause of Cancer." January 30, 2006. http://www.ewg.org/node/21302.

98 DuPont Teflon. "Safety of Teflon Non-Stick Coatings for Cookware." http://www.teflon.com/Teflon/teflonissafe/cookware_safety.html.

99 Cortese, A. "Will Environmental Fear Stick to DuPont's Teflon?" *New York Times* July 24, 2005. http://www.nytimes.com/2005/07/24/business/yourmoney/24teflon.html?ex=1183694400&en=5f941521d711c144&ei=5070.

100 Environmental Working Group. "EPA Science Panel Says Teflon Chemical 'Likely' Cause of Cancer." January 30, 2006. http://www.ewg.org/node/21302.

101 Sandy, M. "Petition for Expedited CIC Consideration of Perfluorooctanoic Acid (PFOA)." California Office of Environmental Health Hazard Assessment. http://www.oehha.ca.gov/prop65/public_meetings/pdf/pfoacic%20slides121206.pdf.

102 Environmental Working Group. "EPA Science Panel Says Teflon Chemical 'Likely' Cause of Cancer." January 30, 2006. http://www.ewg.org/node/21302.

103 DuPont Teflon. "Safety of Teflon Non-Stick Coatings for Cookware." http://www.teflon.com/Teflon/teflonissafe/cookware_safety.html.

104 Environmental Working Group. "EWG finds heated Telfon pans can turn toxic faster than DuPont claims." 2007. http://www.ewg.org/reports/toxicteflon.

105 Ibid.

106 DuPont Teflon. "Safety of Teflon Non-Stick Coatings for Cookware." http://www.teflon.com/Teflon/teflonissafe/cookware_safety.html.

107 US Environmental Protection Agency. "Locating and Estimating Air Emissions from Sources of Dioxins and Furans." May 1997. http://www.epa.gov/ttnchie1/le/dioxin.pdf.

108 Pennsylvania State University. "Resource Recovery: Turning Waste into Energy." Garthe, J. W. http://www.age.psu.edu/extension/factsheets/c/C11.pdf

109 Agency for Toxic Substances and Disease Registry. "ToxFAQs for Vinyl Chloride." CAS No. 75-01-4. July 2006. http://www.atsdr.cdc.gov/tfacts20.html#bookmark01.

110 Public Interest Research Group. "It's Perfectly Clear: The Case Against PVC Packaging. Section 2: The Problem with PVC." April 1988. http://www.masspirg.org/enviro/sw/pvc/page3.htm.

111 Schierow, L., Buck, E. "Endocrine Disruption: An Introduction." *CRS Report for Congress* January 11, 2001. http://www.ncseonline.org/nle/crsreports/pesticides/pest-11.cfm.

112 Institute for Agriculture and Trade Policy, Food and Health Program. "Smart Plastics Guide: Healthier Food Uses of Plastics." October 2005. http://www.healthobservatory.org/library.cfm?refID=77083.

113 Agency for Toxic Substances and Disease Registry. "Toxicological Profile for Styrene." CAS No. 100-42-5. September 1992. http://www.atsdr.cdc.gov/toxprofiles/tp53.html.

114 Agency for Toxic Substances and Disease Registry. "ToxFAQs for Styrene." CAS No. 100-42-5. September 1995. http://www.atsdr.cdc.gov/tfacts53.html.

115 Ibid.

116 Agency for Toxic Substances and Disease Registry. "Toxicological Profile for Styrene." CAS No. 100-42-5. September 1992. http://www.atsdr.cdc.gov/toxprofiles/tp53.html.

117 US Environmental Protection Agency. "Integrated Risk Information System: Styrene (CASRN 100-42-5)." http://www.epa.gov/iris/subst/0104.htm.

118 Hiroi, H., Tsutsumi, O., Takeuchi, T., Momoeda, M., Ikezuki, Y., Okamura, A., Yokota, H., Taketani, Y. "Differences in Serum Bisphenol A Concentrations in Premenopausal Normal Women and Women with Endometrial Hyperplasia." *Endocrine Journal* 2004;51(6):595-600. http://biblioteca.sp.san.gva.es/biblioteca/publicaciones/MATERIAL/METABUSQUEDAS/MUJER/15644579.PDF.

119 Ibid.

120 Vom Saal, F.S., Cooke, P.S., Buchanan, D.L., Palanza, P., Thayer, K.A., Nagel, S.C., Parmigiani, S., Welshons, W.V. "A physiologically based approach to the study of bisphenol A and other estrogenic chemicals on the size of reproductive organs, daily sperm production, and behavior." *Toxicology and Industrial Health* 1998;14:239-260.

121 Ibid.

122 Wetherill, Y.B., Hess-Wilson, J.K., Comstock, C.E.S., Shah, S.A., Buncher, C.R., Sallans, L., Limbach, P.A., Schwemberger, S., Babcock, G.F., Knudsen, K.E. "Bisphenol A facilitates bypass of androgen ablation therapy in prostate cancer." *Molecular Cancer Therapeutics* 2006;5:3181-3190. http://www.environmentalhealthnews.org/newscience/2007/2007-0409wetherilletal.html.

123 "Bisphenol A and Breast Cancer Still Linked." *Cancer/Oncology News* August 29, 2006. http://www.medicalnewstoday.com/medicalnews.php?newsid=50587.

124 Institute for Agriculture and Trade Policy, Food and Health Program. "Smart Plastics Guide: Healthier Food Uses of Plastics." October 2005. http://www.healthobservatory.org/library.cfm?refID=77083.

125 Royte, E. "US: Corn Plastic to the Rescue." *Smithsonian* August 1, 2006. http://www.corpwatch.org/article.php?id=13967.

126 Gibson, R. "Toxic Baby Bottles: Scientific study finds leaching chemicals in clear plastic baby bottles." Environment California Research and Policy Center, 2007. http://www.environmentcalifornia.org/uploads/Ve/AQ/VeAQsr6MMu4xA3-2ibnr_g/Toxic-Baby-Bottles.pdf.

127 Ibid.

128 Ibid.

129 Ibid.

130 Ibid.

131 Ibid.

132 Ibid.

133 Harvard School of Public Health. "Study Shows Association between Phthalates and Human Semen Quality." 2003. http://www.hsph.harvard.edu/news/press-releases/2003-releases/press05202003.html.

134 US Environmental Protection Agency. "Bis(2-ethylhexyl) phthalate (DEHP)." http://www.epa.gov/ttnatw01/hlthef/eth-phth.html.

135 Lovecamp-Swant, T., Davis, B. "Mechanisms of Phthalate Ester Toxicity in the Female Reproductive System." *Environmental Health Perspectives* 2003;111:139-145. http://www.questia.com/googleScholar.qst?docId=5001696615.

136 Barrett, J.R. "Phthalates and Baby Boys: Potential Disruption of Human Genital Development." *Environmental Health Perspectives* 2005;113(8):A542. http://www.ehponline.org/docs/2005/113-8/EHP113pa542PDF.PDF.

137 Environmental Working Group. "Beauty Secrets: Phthalates." http://www.ewg.org/reports/beautysecrets/chap2.html.

138 National Environmental Trust. "Health Effects of DINP Phthalate." October 1998. http://www.net.org/health/products/toxictoys/healtheffects.vtml.

139 Deloncle, R., Guillard, O., Clanet, F., Courtois, P., Piriou, A. "Aluminum transfer as glutamate complex through blood-brain barrier: Possible implication in dialysis encephalopathy." *Biological Trace Element Research* 1990;25(1):39-45. http://www.ncbi.nlm.nih.gov/sites/entrez?cmd=Retrieve&db=PubMed&list_uids=1696110&dopt=Abstract.

140 Yokel, R.A. "Blood-brain barrier flux of aluminum, manganese, iron and other metals suspected to contribute to metal-induced neurodegeneration." *Journal of Alzheimer's Disease* 2006;10:223-253. http://www.mc.uky.edu/pharmacy/faculty/files/jad.pdf.

141 Bishop, N.J., Morley, R., Day, J.P., Lucas, A. "Aluminum neurotoxicity in preterm infants receiving intravenous-feeding solutions." *New England Journal of Medicine* 1997;336(22):1557-1561.

142 US Food and Drug Administration. "Beverages: Bottled Water." *Code of Federal Regulations* 21 CFR Part 165. November 3, 1995. http://www.cfsan.fda.gov/~lrd/n095-327.txt.

143 Sedman, A. "Aluminum toxicity in childhood." *Pediatric Nephrology* 1992;6(4):383-393. http://hdl.handle.net/2027.42/47831.

144 Darbre, P.D. "Aluminum, antiperspirants and breast cancer." *Journal of Inorganic Biochemistry* 2005;99(9):1912-1929.

145 Trapp, G.A., Miner, G.D., Zimmerman, R.L., Mastri, A.R., Heston, L.L. "Aluminum levels in brain in Alzheimer's disease." *Biological Psychiatry* 1978;13(6):709-718. http://www.ncbi.nlm.nih.gov/sites/entrez?cmd=Retrieve&db=PubMed&list_uids=737258&dopt=Abstract.

146 Perl, D. "Relationship of aluminum to Alzheimer's disease." *Journal of Environmental Health Perspectives* 1985;63:149-153. http://links.jstor.org/sici?sici=0091-6765(198511)63%3C149%3AROATAD%3E2.0.CO%3B2-U.

147 Corrigan, F.M., Reynolds, G.P., Ward, N.I. "Hippocampal tin, aluminum and zinc in Alzheimer's disease." *BioMetals* 2005;6(3):149-154. http://www.springerlink.com/content/758257436878500g.

148 National Environmental Trust. "Studies on Bisphenol-A Migration from Polycarbonate Plastic." http://www.net.org/health/products/plasticwrap/migration.vtml.

149 Environment California. "Recommendations for Parents." http://www.environmentcalifornia.org/environmental-health/ stop-toxic-toys/toxics-fact-sheet.

150 Gibson, R.L. "Toxic Baby Bottles: Scientific study finds leaching chemicals in clear plastic baby bottles." Environment California Research and Policy Center, 2007. http://www.environmentcalifornia.org/uploads/Ve/AQ/VeAQsr6MMu4xA3-2ibnr_g/Toxic-Baby-Bottles.pdf.

151 Avant, B. "Paper or Plastic? A Simple Question, Right? Wrong!" http://www.state.tn.us/environment/tn_consv/archive/paperplastic.pdf.

152 West, L. "Paper, Plastic, or Something Better?" http://environment.about.com/od/recycling/a/reusablebags.htm.

153 Herrick, T. "Plastic Bag Fight Pits U.S. Makers v. U.S. Importers." *Wall Street Journal* October 10, 2003. http://www.global-trade-law.com/ Article.WSJ%20Series,Battling%20Imports%20(WSJ%20Oct.%202003).htm.

154 Institute for Lifecycle Environmental Assessment. "Paper vs. Plastic Bags." 1990. http://www.ilea.org/lcas/franklin1990.html.

155 Ibid.

156 Ibid.

157 Ibid.

158 Herrick, T. "Plastic Bag Fight Pits U.S. Makers v. U.S. Importers." *Wall Street Journal* October 10, 2003. http://www.global-trade-law.com/ Article.WSJ%20Series,Battling%20Imports%20(WSJ%20Oct.%202003).htm.

159 Institute for Lifecycle Environmental Assessment. "Paper vs. Plastic Bags." 1990. http://www.ilea.org/lcas/franklin1990.html.

160 US Environmental Protection Agency. "Municipal Solid Waste in the United States: Facts and Figures 2005." http://www.epa.gov/msw/ pubs/mswchar05.pdf.

161 Seventh Generation. "Our Products." http://www.seventhgeneration.com/our_products/supplies.php.

162 CBS News. "San Francisco Moves to Ban Plastic Bags." March 28, 2007. http://www.cbsnews.com/stories/2007/03/28/tech/ main2618372.shtml.

163 Goodyear, C. "S.F. First City to Ban Plastic Shopping Bags." *San Francisco Chronicle* March 28, 2007. http://www.sfgate.com/cgi-bin/ article.cgi?file=/c/a/2007/03/28/MNGDROT5QN1.DTL.

164 Ibid.

165 NatureWorks. "Life Cycle Assessment." http://www.natureworksllc.com/our-values-and-views/life-cycle-assessment.aspx.

166 Reusablebags.com. "The Numbers . . . Believe It or Not." http://www.reusablebags.com/facts.php?id=4.

167 BBC News. "Irish Bag Tax Hailed Success." August 20, 2002. http://news.bbc.co.uk/1/hi/world/europe/2205419.stm.

168 American Society for Testing Materials. "Active Standard: ASTM D6400-04 Standard Specification for Compostable Plastics." ICS Number Code 83.080.01. 2007. http://www.astm.org/cgi-bin/SoftCart.exe/database.cart/redline_pages/ d6400.htm?L+mystore+khgg2000+1202374008

169 Ibid.

170 Ibid.

171 Ibid.

172 World Centric. "Compostable, Biodegradable BioPlastics." http://www.worldcentric.org/bio/bioplastics.htm.

173 Based on figures from Seventh Generation. http://www.seventhgen.com/our_products/supplies/trash_bags.html and http://www.seventhgen.com/our_products/supplies/tall_kitchen_bags.html.

174 Ibid.

175 US Environmental Protection Agency. "Municipal Solid Waste in the United States: Facts and Figures 2005." http://www.epa.gov/msw/ pubs/mswchar05.pdf.

176 Ibid.

177 National Institute of Environmental Health Sciences, National Toxicology Program. "Substance Profiles: 2,3,7,8-Tetrachlorodibenzo-*p*-Dioxin (TCDD): Dioxin: CAS No.: 1746-01-6." http://ntp.niehs.nih.gov/ntp/roc/eleventh/profiles/s168tcdd.pdf.

178 Agency for Toxic Substances and Disease Registry. "ToxFAQs: Chemical Agent Briefing Sheet (CABS): Dioxins." March 2006. http://www.atsdr.cdc.gov/cabs/dioxins/dioxins_cabs.pdf.

179 Ibid.

180 Ibid.

181 Ibid.

182 Based on figures from Seventh Generation. http://www.seventhgeneration.com.

183 Ibid.

# Chapter 4:
# 4 Steps to a Spic-and-Span Green Bathroom

1    Huang, C.-M., Wang, C.-C., Kawai, M., Barnes, S., Elmets, C.A. "Surfactant Sodium Lauryl Sulfate Enhances Skin Vaccination: Molecular Characterization via a Novel Technique Using Ultrafiltration Capillaries and Mass Spectrometric Proteomics." *Molecular and Cellular Proteomics* 2006; 5(3):523-532. http://www.mcponline.org/cgi/reprint/M500259-MCP200v1.pdf.

2　Shea, K., and Committee on Environmental Health. "Pediatric Exposure and Potential Toxicity of Phthalate Plasticizers." *Pediatrics* 2003;111(6):1467-1474. http://pediatrics.aappublications.org/cgi/content/full/111/6/1467.

3　National Institute of Environmental Health Services. "Endocrine Disruptors." 2006. http://www.niehs.nih.gov/health/topics/agents/endocrine.

4　Center for the Evaluation of Risks to Human Reproduction, National Toxicology Program, US Department of Health and Human Services. "NTP Brief on the Potential Human Reproductive and Developmental Effects of Di(2-Ethylhexyl) Phthalate (DEHP)." May 2006. http://cerhr.niehs.nih.gov/chemicals/dehp/DEHP%20Brief%20Draft1.pdf.

5　Kleinsasser, N., Wallner, B.C., Kastenbauer, E.R., Weissacher, H., Harréus, U.A. "Genotoxicity of di-butyl-phthalate and di-iso-butyl-phthalate in human lymphocytes and mucosal cells." *Teratogenesis, Carcinogenesis, and Mutagenesis* 2001;21(3):189-196. http://www3.interscience.wiley.com/cgi-bin/abstract/78505490/ABSTRACT.

6　Shea, K., and Committee on Environmental Health. "Pediatric Exposure and Potential Toxicity of Phthalate Plasticizers." *Pediatrics* 2003;111(6):1467-1474. http://pediatrics.aappublications.org/cgi/content/full/111/6/1467.

7　Graham, S. "Ubiquitous Chemical Associated with Abnormal Human Reproductive Development." *Scientific American* May 27, 2005.

8　Foster, P. "Effects of Di(n-butyl)phthalate on Reproductive Development." Long-Range Research Initiative Project Abstract, 2006. http://www.americanchemistry.com/s_acc/docs/LRIAbstracts/LRIAbstract_43.pdf.

9　Black, R.E., Hurley, F.J., Havery, D.C. "Occurrence of 1,4-Dioxane in Cosmetic Raw Materials and Finished Cosmetic Products." *Journal of AOAC International* 2001;84(3):666-670. http://www.atypon-link.com/AOAC/doi/abs/10.5555/jaoi.2001.84.3.666.

10　US Environmental Protection Agency. "1,4-Dioxane (1,4-Diethyleneoxide)." http://www.epa.gov/ttn/atw/hlthef/dioxane.html.

11　Coleman, H.M., Vimonses, V., Leslie, G., Amal, R. "Degradation of 1,4-dioxane in water using $TiO_2$ based photocatalytic and $H_2O_2$/UV processes." *Journal of Hazardous Materials* 146(3):496-501. http://www.sciencedirect.com/science?_ob=ArticleURL&_udi=B6TGF-4NJ20K2-H&_user=10&_rdoc=1&_fmt=&_orig=search&_sort=d&view=c&_acct=C000050221&_version=1&_urlVersion=0&_userid=10&md5=f5723fb06243ecacc9f32b4b9a368f45.

12　Ibid.

13　National Institute of Environmental Health Sciences. "Substance Profiles: *N*-Nitrosodiethanolamine: CAS No. 1116-54-7." http://ntp.niehs.nih.gov/ntp/roc/eleventh/profiles/s126nitr.pdf.

14　Ibid.

15　Levy, S.B. "Antibacterial Household Products: Cause for Concern." *Emerging Infectious Diseases* 2001;7(3 Suppl):512-515. http://www.cdc.gov/ncidod/eid/vol7no3_supp/levy.htm.

16　Ibid.

17　"Study: Soap and water work best in ridding hands of disease viruses." March 10, 2005. http://www.eurekalert.org/pub_releases/2005-03/uonc-ssa031005.php. [press release]

18　Levy, S.B. "Antibacterial Household Products: Cause for Concern." *Emerging Infectious Diseases* 2001;7(3 Suppl):512-515. http://www.cdc.gov/ncidod/eid/vol7no3_supp/levy.htm.

19　Braun-Fahrländer, C., Gassner, M., Grize, L., Neu, U., et al. "Prevalence of hay fever and allergic sensitization in farmer's children and their peers living in the same rural community." *Clinical and Experimental Allergy* 1999;29(1):28-34. http://www.ncbi.nlm.nih.gov/sites/entrez?cmd=Retrieve&db=PubMed&list_uids=10051699&dopt=AbstractPlus.

20　Rook, G.A., Stanford, J.L. "Give us this day our daily germs." *Immunology Today* 1999;20(6):289-290. http://www.ncbi.nlm.nih.gov/sites/entrez?cmd=Retrieve&db=PubMed&list_uids=9540269&dopt=AbstractPlus.

21　Oehme, M. "Ambient Levels and Trends 1+ 2." 26th International Symposium on Halogenated Persistent Organic Pollutants, Dioxin 2006 Session Summary. pp. 43-45. http://72.14.253.104/search?q=cache:4ZrYHDN3PN4J:www.x-cd.com/dioxin06/Summaries.pdf+EPA+triclosan+persistent+organic+pollutant&hl=en&ct=clnk&cd=3&gl=us.

22　Tatarazako, N., Ishibashi, H., Teshima, K., Kishi, K., Arizono, K. "Effects of triclosan on various aquatic organisms." *Environmental Science* 2004;11(2):133-140. http://www.ncbi.nlm.nih.gov/sites/entrez?cmd=Retrieve&db=PubMed&list_uids=15746894&dopt=Abstract.

23　Rule, K.L., Ebbett, V.R., Vikesland, P.J. "Formation of chloroform and chlorinated organics by free-chlorine-mediated oxidation of triclosan." *Environmental Science Technology* 2005;39(9):3176-3185. http://www.ncbi.nlm.nih.gov/sites/entrez?cmd=Retrieve&db=PubMed&list_uids=15926568&dopt=Citation.

24　Latch, D.E., Packer, J.L., Arnold, W.A., McNeill, K. "Photochemical conversion of triclosan to 2,8-dichlorodibenzo-p-dioxin in aqueous solution." *Journal of Photochemistry and Photobiology A: Chemistry* 2000;158(1):63-66.

25　Rule, K.L., Ebbett, V.R., Vikesland, P.J. "Formation of Chloroform and Chlorinated Organics by Free-Chlorine-Mediated Oxidation of Triclosan." *Environmental Science and Technology* 2005;39(9):3176-3185.

26　Cavanagh, H.M., Wilkinson. J.M. "Biological activities of lavender essential oil." *Phytotherapy Research* 2002;16(4):301-8.

27　Allen Woodburn Associates Ltd./Managing Resources Ltd. "Cotton: The Crop and Its Agrochemicals Market." 1995.

28　Team Treehugger. "How to Green Your Wardrobe." November 13, 2006. http://www.treehugger.com/files/2006/11/how_to_green_yo_12.php#top.

29　Material Safety Data Sheet. "2-Butoxyethanol." CAS No. 111-76-2.

30　Material Safety Data Sheet. "2-Butoxyethanol." MSDS No. CJNRJ, Product ID No. 2138.

31　Ibid.

32　Material Safety Data Sheet. "Sodium Hypochlorite Solution A.R." CAS No. 7681-52-9.

33　Material Safety Data Sheet. "Sodium Hypochlorite Solution, 4-6%." Account No. 40179, Case No. 7681-52-9.

34　Ibid.

35　Ibid.

36  Physical and Theoretical Chemistry Laboratory, Oxford University. "Safety data for ammonium hydroxide." CAS No. 1336-21-6.

37  Material Safety Data Sheet. "Ammonia Solution." MSDS No. A5472.

38  Ibid.

39  Ibid.

40  Ibid.

41  Ibid.

42  Ibid.

43  Material Safety Data Sheet. "Diethylene glycol monobutyl ether." Account No. 07330, Case No. 112-34-5.

44  Ibid.

45  Ibid.

46  Ibid.

47  Ibid.

48  International Chemical Safety Cards. "Nitrilotriacetic acid trisodium salt." ICSC No. 1240, Case No. 5064-31-3.

49  Ibid.

50  Ibid.

51  Ibid.

52  Material Safety Data Sheet. "Benzalkonium chloride." CAS No. 8001-54-5.

53  Material Safety Data Sheet. "Quaternary Ammonium 10% Solution." MSDS No. CFYDS.

54  Material Safety Data Sheet. "Sodium Hydroxide." CAS No. 1310-73-2.

55  Ibid.

56  Material Safety Data Sheet. "Sodium Hydroxide 10%." Account No. 88811, Case No. 1310-73-2.

57  Ibid.

58  Ibid.

59  Ibid.

60  Seventh Generation. http://www.seventhgeneration.com/our_products/household/natural_citrus_shower_cleaner.html.

61  Center for Health, Environment and Justice. "About PVC." http://www.besafenet.com/pvc/about.htm.

62  US Environmental Protection Agency. "Basic Information on PFOA." http://www.epa.gov/opptintr/pfoa/pubs/pfoainfo.htm.

63  Environmental Working Group. "EPA Science Panel Says Teflon Chemical 'Likely' Cause of Cancer." January 30, 2006. http://www.ewg.org/node/21302.

64  Anderson, I. *New Scientist* September 1996. http://www.triangularwave.com/f9.htm.

65  Deinzer, H., Schaumburg, F., Klein, E. "Environmental Health Sciences Center Task Force Review on Halogenated Organics in Drinking Water." *Environmental Health Perspectives* 1978;24:209-239. http://www.pubmedcentral.nih.gov/pagerender.fcgi?artid=1637223&pageindex=1.

66  County of Sacramento, Municipal Services Agency, Department of Water Resources. "Flush with Efficiency." http://www.msa.saccounty.net/waterresources/water/ULFT.asp.

67  Seventh Generation. http://www.seventhgeneration.com/our_products/paper/multi_pack_bathroom_tissue.html.

68  Based on figures from Seventh Generation. http://www.seventhgeneration.com/our_products/paper/facial_tissues.html.

# Chapter 5:
# Natural Beauty: The Simple 7

1  US Food and Drug Administration. "Federal Food, Drug, and Cosmetic Act: Chapter II: Definitions." Sec. 201 [21 USC 321]. http://www.fda.gov/opacom/laws/fdcact/fdcact1.htm.

2  Environmental Working Group. Skin Deep Cosmetic Safety Database. http://www.cosmeticdatabase.com.

3  US Food and Drug Administration. "Food and Cosmetics: International Activities." http://www.fda.gov/oia/foodcosm.htm.

4  Ford, R.A., Hawkins, D.R., Mayo, B.C., Api, A.M. "The in vivo dermal absorption and metabolism of [4-$^{14}$C]coumarin by rats and human volunteers under simulated conditions of use in fragrances." *Food and Chemical Toxicology* 2001;39(2):153-162. http://www.sciencedirect.com/science?_ob=ArticleURL&_udi=B6T6P-42M1CN5-8&_user=10&_rdoc=1&_fmt=&_orig=search&_sort=d&view=c&_acct=C000050221&_version=1&_urlVersion=0&_userid=10&md5=327ffb3f820160bd0a68ae0f5a8ed3d4.

5  Brounaugh, R.L., Collier, S.W., Macpherson, S. E., Kraeling, M.E.K. "Influence of Metabolism in Skin on Dosimetry after Topical Exposure." *Environmental Health Perspectives* 1994;102(Suppl 11):71-74. http://www.ehponline.org/members/1994/Suppl-11/bronaugh-full.html.

6  Kao, J., Hall, J. "Skin absorption and cutaneous first pass metabolism of topical steroids: In vitro studies with mouse skin in organ culture." *Journal of Pharmacology and Experimental Therapeutics* 1987;241(2):482-487. http://jpet.aspetjournals.org/cgi/content/abstract/241/2/482.

7  National Toxicology Program. "Butylparaben: Final Review of Toxicological Literature." CAS No. 94-26-8. http://ntp.niehs.nih.gov/files/Butylparaben.pdf.

8  Ibid.

9   Oishi, S. "Effects of butyl paraben on the male reproductive system in mice." *Archives of Toxicology* 2002;76(7):423-429. http://www.ncbi.nlm.nih.gov/entrez/query.fcgi?db=PubMed&cmd=Retrieve&list_uids=12111007.

10  National Toxicology Program. "Butylparaben: Final Review of Toxicological Literature." CAS No. 94-26-8. http://ntp.niehs.nih.gov/files/Butylparaben.pdf.

11  Ibid.

12  Ibid.

13  Darbre, P.D., Aljarrah, A., Miller, W.R., Coldham, N.G., Sauer, M.J., Pope, G.S. "Concentrations of Parabens in Human Breast Tumors." *Journal of Applied Toxicology* 2004;24:5-13.

14  Harvey, P., Everett, D. "Significance of the detection of esters of *p*-hydroxybenzoic acid (parabens) in human breast tumours." *Journal of Applied Toxicology* 2004;24:1-4.

15  Fisher, J.S., Turner, K.J., Brown, D., Sharpe, R.M. "Effect of neonatal exposure to estrogenic compounds on development of the excurrent ducts of the rat testis through puberty to adulthood." *Environmental Health Perspectives* 1999:107:397-405.

16  Routledge, E.J., Parker, J., Odum, J., Ashby, J., Sumpter, J.P. "Some alkyl hydroxy benzoate preservatives (parabens) are estrogenic." *Toxicology and Applied Pharmacology* 1998;153(1):12-19.

17  Elder, R. "Final report on the safety assessment of methylparaben, ethylparaben, propylparaben and butylparaben." *Journal of the American College of Toxicology* 1984;3:147-209.

18  Nagel, J.E., Fuscaldo, J.T., Fireman, P. "Paraben Allergy." *Journal of the American Medical Association* 1977;237(15):1594-1595. http://jama.ama-assn.org/cgi/content/abstract/237/15/1594.

19  Harvell, J., Bason, M., Maibach, H. "Contact Urticaria and Its Mechanisms." *Food and Chemical Toxicology* 1994;32(2):103-112.

20  Darbre, P.D., Aljarrah, A., Miller, W.R., Coldham, N.G., Sauer, M.J., Pope, G.S. "Concentrations of parabens in human breast tumors." *Journal of Applied Toxicology* 2004;24:5-13.

21  Harvey, P., Everett, D. "Significance of the detection of esters of *p*-hydroxybenzoic acid (parabens) in human breast tumours." *Journal of Applied Toxicology* 2004;24:1-4.

22  Routledge, E.J., Parker, J., Odum, J., Ashby, J., Sumpter, J.P. "Some alkyl hydroxy benzoate preservatives (parabens) are estrogenic." *Toxicology and Applied Pharmacology* 1998;153(1):12-19.

23  Elder, R. "Final report on the safety assessment of methylparaben, ethylparaben, propylparaben and butylparaben." *Journal of the American College of Toxicology* 1984;3:147-209.

24  Ibid.

25  Nagel, J.E., Fuscaldo, J.T., Fireman, P. "Paraben Allergy." *Journal of the American Medical Association* 1977;237(15):1594-1595. http://jama.ama-assn.org/cgi/content/abstract/237/15/1594.

26  Oishi, S. "Effects of propyl paraben on the male reproductive system." *Food and Chemical Toxicology* 2002;40(12):1807-1813.

27  Routledge, E.J., Parker, J., Odum, J., Ashby, J., Sumpter, J.P. "Some alkyl hydroxy benzoate preservatives (parabens) are estrogenic." *Toxicology and Applied Pharmacology* 1998;153(1):12-19.

28  Elder, R. "Final report on the safety assessment of methylparaben, ethylparaben, propylparaben and butylparaben." *Journal of the American College of Toxicology* 1984;3:147-209.

29  Ibid.

30  Houlihan, J., Brody, C., Schwan, B. "Not Too Pretty: Phthalates, Beauty Products and the FDA." 2002. http://www.safecosmetics.org/docUploads/NotTooPretty_r51.pdf.

31  DiGangi, J., Schettler, T., Cobbing, M., Rossi, M. "Aggregate Exposures to Phthalates in Humans." Health Care Without Harm, 2002. http://www.noharm.org/library/docs/Phthalate_Report_Europe.pdf.

32  Ibid.

33  Shea, K., and Committee on Environmental Health. "Pediatric Exposure and Potential Toxicity of Phthalate Plasticizers." *Pediatrics* 2003;111(6):1467-1474. http://pediatrics.aappublications.org/cgi/content/full/111/6/1467.

34  Kleinsasser, N.H., Wallner, B.C., Kastenbauer, E.R., Weissacker, H., Harréus, U.A. "Genotoxicity of di-butyl-phthalate and di-iso-butyl-phthalate in human lymphocytes and mucosal cells." *Teratogenesis, Carcinogenesis, and Mutagenesis* 2001;21(3):189-196. http://www3.interscience.wiley.com/cgi-bin/abstract/78505490/ABSTRACT.

35  Shea, K., and Committee on Environmental Health. "Pediatric Exposure and Potential Toxicity of Phthalate Plasticizers." *Pediatrics* 2003;111(6):1467-1474. http://pediatrics.aappublications.org/cgi/content/full/111/6/1467.

36  Graham, S. "Ubiquitous Chemical Associated with Abnormal Human Reproductive Development." *Scientific American* May 27, 2005.

37  Foster, P. "Effects of Di(n-butyl)phthalate on Reproductive Development." 2006. http://www.americanchemistry.com/s_acc/docs/LRIAbstracts/LRIAbstract_43.pdf

38  National Institute of Environmental Health Sciences. "Endocrine Disruptors." 2007. http://www.niehs.nih.gov/health/topics/agents/endocrine.

39  Center for the Evaluation of Risks to Human Reproduction, National Toxicology Program. "NPT Brief on the Potential Human Reproductive and Developmental Effects of Di(2-ethylhexyl) Phthalate (DEHP)." May 2006. http://cerhr.niehs.nih.gov/chemicals/dehp/DEHP%20Brief%20Draft1.pdf.

40  Grandjean, P., Landrigan, P.J. "Developmental neurotoxicity of industrial chemicals." *Lancet* 2006;368(9553):2167-2178. http://www.kevinleitch.co.uk/wp/wp-content/uploads/2006/11/chemicallist.pdf.

41  National Toxicology Program. "Chemical Information Profile for Diethyl Phthalate." CAS No. 84-66-2. 2006. http://ntp.niehs.nih.gov/ntp/htdocs/Chem_Background/ExSumPdf/Diethyl_phthalate.pdf.

42  DiGangi, J., Schettler, T., Cobbing, M., Rossi, M. "Aggregate Exposures to Phthalates in Humans." Health Care Without Harm, 2002. http://www.noharm.org/library/docs/Phthalate_Report_Europe.pdf.

43  Tickner, J.A., Schettler, T., Guidotti, T., McCally, M., Rossi, M. "Health risks posed by use of di-2-ethylhexyl phthalate (DEHP) in PVC medical devices: A critical review." *American Journal of Industrial Medicine* 2001;39(1):100-111.

44  Lampen, A., Zimnik, S., Nau, H. "Teratogenic phthalate esters and metabolites activate the nuclear receptors PPARs and induce differentiation of F9 cells." *Toxicology and Applied Pharmacology* 2003;188(1):14-23.

45  Hu, X., Wen, B., Shan, X. "Survey of phthalate pollution in arable soils in China." *Journal of Environmental Monitoring* 2003;5:649-653. http://www.rsc.org/publishing/journals/EM/article.asp?doi=b304669a.

46  Centers for Disease Control and Prevention. "National Report on Human Exposure to Environmental Chemicals." 2001.

47  National Industrial Chemicals Notification and Assessment Scheme, Department of Health and Ageing, Australia. "Sodium Lauryl Sulfate: CAS No: 151-21-3." 2007 http://www.nicnas.gov.au/Publications/Information_Sheets/Existing_Chemical_Information_Sheets/ecis_SLS_PDF.pdf.

48  Huang, C.M., Wang, C.C., Kawai, M., Barnes, S., Elmets, C.A. "Surfactant Sodium Lauryl Sulfate Enhances Skin Vaccination: Molecular Characterization via a Novel Technique Using Ultrafiltration Capillaries and Mass Spectrometric Proteomics." *Molecular and Cellular Proteomics* 2006;5:523-532. http://www.mcponline.org/cgi/content/abstract/5/3/523.

49  Ibid.

50  Ibid.

51  Ibid.

52  Ibid.

53  Ibid.

54  Black, R.E., Hurley, F.J., Havery, D.C. "Occurrence of 1,4-Dioxane in Cosmetic Raw Materials and Finished Cosmetic Products." *Journal of AOAC International* 2001;84(3):666-670. http://www.atypon-link.com/AOAC/doi/abs/10.5555/jaoi.2001.84.3.666.

55  Ibid.

56  Ibid.

57  Ibid.

58  Ibid.

59  US Food and Drug Administration, Center for Food Safety and Applied Nutrition. "1,4-Dioxane." 2007. http://www.cfsan.fda.gov/~dms/cosdiox.html.

60  US Environmental Protection Agency. "1,4-Dioxane (1,4-Diethyleneoxide): Hazard Summary." http://www.epa.gov/ttn/atw/hlthef/dioxane.html.

61  Breast Cancer Fund. "Cancer-Causing Chemical Found in Children's Bath Products." February 8, 2007. http://www.breastcancerfund.org/site/pp.asp?c=kwKXLdPaE&b=2483603. [press release]

62  Coleman, H.M., Hon, H., Amal, R., Leslie, G., Wehner, M., Fitzsimmons, S. "Removal of oestrogenic and carcinogenic substances from water using alternative water treatments." Australian Water Association Specialty Conference II in Public Health, Contaminants of Concern: Chemicals, Pathogens, Toxins. Canberra, Australia. June 22-23, 2005.

63  Ibid.

64  National Toxicology Program. "*N*-Nitrosodiethanolamine: CAS No. 1116-54-7." *Report on Carcinogens, Eleventh Edition*, 2005. http://ntp.niehs.nih.gov/ntp/roc/eleventh/profiles/s126nitr.pdf.

65  Ibid.

66  Chapman, D.V., editor. "Water Quality Assessments: A Guide to the Use of Biota, Sediments and Water in Environmental Monitoring." 2nd edition. New York: E&FN Spon, 1996.

67  Barber, L.B. II, Leenheer, J.A., Pereira, W.E., Noyes, T.I., Brown, G.K., Tabor, C.F., Writer, J.H. "Organic Contamination of the Mississippi River from Municipal and Industrial Wastewater." US Geological Survey Circular 1133, 1995. http://pubs.usgs.gov/circ/circ1133/organic.html.

68  Kimura, M., Kawada, A. "Contact dermatitis due to trisodium ethylenediaminetetra-acetic acid (EDTA) in a cosmetic lotion." *Contact Dermatitis* 1999;41(6):341.

69  Ibid.

70  Material Safety Data Sheet. "Ethylenediamine Tetraacetic Acid." CAS No. 60-00-4. https://fscimage.fishersci.com/msds/09570.htm.

71  Ibid.

72  Ibid.

73  International Agency for Research on Cancer. "IARC Classifies Formaldehyde as Carcinogenic to Humans." Press release no. 153, June 15, 2004. http://www.iarc.fr/ENG/Press_Releases/archives/pr153a.html. [press release]

74  Epstein, S.S. "Losing the Cancer War." *The Stop Cancer Before It Starts Campaign: How to Win the Losing War Against Cancer.* Chicago: Cancer Prevention Coalition, 2003. http://www.preventcancer.com/losing/nci/experimental.htm.

75  Ibid.

76  National Toxicology Program. "Imidazolidinyl Urea: 39236-46-9." http://ntp.niehs.nih.gov/ntp/htdocs/Chem_Background/ExSumPdf/ImidazolidinylUrea.pdf.

77  Environmental Working Group. "Diazolidinyl Urea." http://www.cosmeticsdatabase.com/ingredient.php?ingred06=701923&refurl=%2Fwordsearch.php%3Fquery%3Durea%26.

78  de Groot, A.C., Bruynzeel, D.P., Jagtman, B.A., Weyland, J.W. "Contact allergy to diazolidinyl urea (Germall II)." *Contact Dermatitis* 1998;18(4):202-205.

79 Material Safety Data Sheet. "Diazolidinyl Urea." CAS No. 78491-02-8.

80 Environmental Working Group. "Diazolidinyl Urea." http://www.cosmeticsdatabase.com/ingredient.php?ingred06=701923&refurl=%2F wordsearch.php%3Fquery%3Durea%26.

81 Saripalli, Y.V. "The Detection of Clinically Relevant Contact Allergens Using a Standard Screening Tray of Twenty-Three Allergens." *Journal of the American Academy of Dermatology* 2003;49(1):65-69.

82 National Toxicology Program. "Imidazolidinyl Urea: 39236-46-9." http://ntp.niehs.nih.gov/ntp/htdocs/Chem_Background/ExSumPdf/ImidazolidinylUrea.pdf.

83 Ibid.

84 Ibid.

85 de Groot, A.C., Bos, J.D., Jagtman, B.A., Bruynzeel, D.P., Van Joost, T., Weyland, J.W. "Contact allergy to preservatives—II." *Contact Dermatitis* 1986;15(4):218-222. http://www.blackwell-synergy.com/doi/abs/10.1111/j.1600-0536.1986.tb01340.x?journalCode=cod.

86 Environmental Working Group. "DMDM Hydantoin." http://www.cosmeticdatabase.com/ingredient.php?ingred06=702196&refurl=%2F wordsearch.php%3Fquery%3Ddimethyl+dimethyl+hydantoin%26.

87 Ibid.

88 Brown, J.A. "Quaternium-15." CAS No. 4080-31-3. Haz-Map: Information on Hazardous Chemicals and Occupational Diseases. http://hazmap.nlm.nih.gov/cgi-bin/hazmap_generic?tbl=TblAgents&id=843.

89 Cahill, J., Nixon, R. "Allergic contact dermatitis to quaternium 15 in a moisturizing lotion." *Australian Journal of Dermatology* 2005;46(4): 284-285. http://pt.wkhealth.com/pt/re/aujd/abstract.00000936-200511000-00017. htm;jsessionid=HFcQl81vLpdDqT5pQ1NPnZXrvvhQ5J5lX4KnCJpdvgBV9rSwbk4c!-1297386286!181195629!8091!-1.

90 Mathur, A.K., Khanna, S.K. "Dermal Toxicity Due to Industrial Chemicals." *Skin Pharmacology and Applied Skin Physiology* 2002;15(3):147-153. http://content.karger.com/ProdukteDB/produkte.asp?Aktion=ShowPDF&ProduktNr=224194&Ausgabe=228459&ArtikelNr=63543.

91 Cahill, J., Nixon, R. "Allergic contact dermatitis to quaternium 15 in a moisturizing lotion." *Australian Journal of Dermatology* 2005;46(4): 284-285. http://pt.wkhealth.com/pt/re/aujd/abstract.00000936-200511000-00017. htm;jsessionid=HFcQl81vLpdDqT5pQ1NPnZXrvvhQ5J5lX4KnCJpdvgBV9rSwbk4c!-1297386286!181195629!8091!-1.

92 Mathur, A.K., Khanna, S.K. "Dermal Toxicity Due to Industrial Chemicals." *Skin Pharmacology and Applied Skin Physiology* 2002;15(3):147-153. http://content.karger.com/ProdukteDB/produkte.asp?Aktion=ShowPDF&ProduktNr=224194&Ausgabe=228459&ArtikelNr=63543.

93 Cahill, J., Nixon, R. "Allergic contact dermatitis to quaternium 15 in a moisturizing lotion." *Australian Journal of Dermatology* 2005;46(4): 284-285. http://pt.wkhealth.com/pt/re/aujd/abstract.00000936-200511000-00017. htm;jsessionid=HFcQl81vLpdDqT5pQ1NPnZXrvvhQ5J5lX4KnCJpdvgBV9rSwbk4c!-1297386286!181195629!8091!-1.

94 Mathur, A.K., Khanna, S.K. "Dermal Toxicity Due to Industrial Chemicals." *Skin Pharmacology and Applied Skin Physiology* 2002;15(3):147-153. http://content.karger.com/ProdukteDB/produkte.asp?Aktion=ShowPDF&ProduktNr=224194&Ausgabe=228459&ArtikelNr=63543.

95 Peters, M.S., Connolly, S.M., Schroder, A.L. "Bronopol allergic contact dermatitis." *Contact Dermatitis* 1983;9(5):397-401. http://www.blackwell-synergy.com/doi/abs/10.1111/j.1600-0536.1983.tb04436.x.

96 Brown, J.A. " Bronopol." CAS No. 52-51-7. Haz-Map: Information on Hazardous Chemicals and Occupational Diseases. http://hazmap.nlm.nih.gov/cgi-bin/hazmap_generic?tbl=TblAgents&id=1010.

97 US Environmental Protection Agency. "Addition of Certain Chemicals; Toxic Chemical Release Reporting; Community Right-to-Know." *Federal Register* 40 CFR Part 372, November 30, 1994. http://www.epa.gov/EPA-TRI/1996/October/Day-18/pr-61DIR/Other/ tri5396.txt.html.

98 US Environmental Protection Agency. "R.E.D. Facts: Bronopol." EPA-738-F-95-029, October 1995. http://www.epa.gov/oppsrrd1/ REDs/factsheets/2770fact.pdf.

99 US Environmental Protection Agency. "Bronopol; Notice of Filing a Pesticide Petition to Establish a Tolerance for a Certain Pesticide Chemical in or on Food." *Federal Register* 2002;67(247):78459-78467. http://www.epa.gov/EPA-PEST/2002/December/Day-24/ p32400.htm.

100 Humane Society of the United States. "Protocols for Embalming Donated Animals." Tufts University, 2001. http://www.educationalmemorial.org/resource_embalming.html.

101 Agency for Toxic Substances and Disease Registry. "ToxFAQs for Ethylene Glycol." CAS No. 107-21-1. 2007. http://www.atsdr.cdc.gov/ tfacts96.html.

102 Ibid.

103 Ibid.

104 Ibid.

105 Material Safety Data Sheet. "Propylene Glycol MSDS." CAS No. 57-55-6. 2005. http://www.sciencelab.com/ xMSDS-Propylene_glycol-9927239.

106 Material Safety Data Sheet. "Propylene Glycol." CAS No. 57-55-6, MSDS No. P6928. 2005. http://environmentalchemistry. com/yogi/periodic/Al.html.

107 Gonzalo, M.A., de Argila, D., Garcia, J.M., Alvarado, M.I. "Allergic Contact Dermatitis to Propylene Glycol." *Allergy* 1999;54(1):82-83.

108 Agency for Toxic Substances and Disease Registry. "Toxicological Profile for Ethylene Glycol." CAS No. 107-21-1. 2007. http://www.atsdr.cdc.gov/toxprofiles/tp96.html.

109 Morshed, K.M., Jain, S.K., McMartin, K.E. "Propylene Glycol-Mediated Cell Injury in a Primary Culture of Human Proximal Tubule Cells." *Toxicological Sciences* 1998;46:410-417. http://toxsci.oxfordjournals.org/cgi/reprint/46/2/410.pdf.

110 Ibid.

111 Ibid.

112 Ibid.

113 Agency for Toxic Substances and Disease Registry. "Toxicological Profile for Toluene." CAS No. 108-88-3. September 2000. http://www.atsdr.cdc.gov/toxprofiles/tp56.html.

114 Ibid.

115 Ibid.

116 Ibid.

117 Ibid.

118 Agency for Toxic Substances and Disease Registry. "Asbestos Toxicity: How Are People Exposed to Asbestos?" http://www.atsdr.cdc.gov/HEC/CSEM/asbestos/exposure_pathways.html.

119 Agency for Toxic Substances and Disease Registry. "Asbestos Toxicity: What Respiratory Conditions Are Associated with Asbestos?" http://www.atsdr.cdc.gov/HEC/CSEM/asbestos/physiologic_effects.html#other.

120 Material Safety Data Sheet. "Talc." CAS No. 014807-96-6, MSDS No. T0026. 2005.

121 Ibid.

122 Harlow, B.L., Cramer, D.W., Bell, D.A., Welch, W.R. "Perineal exposure to talc and ovarian cancer risk." *Obstetrics and Gynecology* 1992;80:19-26.

123 Kabacoff, B.L., Douglass, M.L., Rosenberg, I.E., Levan, L.W., Punwar, J.K., Vielhuber, S.F., Lechner, R.J. "Formation of nitrosamines in non-ionic and anionic emulsions in the presence and absence of inhibitors." *IARC Scientific Publications* 1984;57:347-352.

124 Spiegelhalder, B., Preussmann, R. "Contamination of toiletries and cosmetic products with volatile and nonvolatile *N*-nitroso carcinogens." *Journal of Cancer Research and Clinical Oncology* 1984;108(1):160-163. http://www.springerlink.com/content/v2w0914827332645.

125 Ibid.

126 Dow Chemical. "Product Safety Assessment: Monoethanolamine." CAS No. 141-43-5. http://www.dow.com/productsafety/finder/mea.htm.

127 Material Safety Data Sheet. "Diethanolamine." Account No. 00532, Case No. 111-42-2.

128 Ibid.

129 Dow Chemical. "Product Safety Assessment: Monoethanolamine." CAS No. 141-43-5. http://www.dow.com/productsafety/finder/mea.htm.

130 Ibid.

131 Ibid.

132 York, R.G., Barnwell, P.L., Pierrera, M., Schuler, R.L., Hardin, B.D. "Evaluation of 12 chemicals in a preliminary developmental toxicity test." *Teratology* 1988;37:503-504.

133 Mankes, R.F., "Studies on the embryopathic effects of ethanolamine in Long-Evans rats: Preferential embryopathy in pups contiguous with male siblings in utero." *Teratogenesis, Carcinogenesis, and Mutagenesis* 1986;6:403-417.

134 Material Safety Data Sheet. "Triethanolamine." CAS No. 102-71-6, EC No. 203-049-8. http://ptcl.chem.ox.ac.uk/MSDS/TR/triethanolamine.html.

135 Ibid.

136 Dow Chemical. "Product Safety Assessment: Triethanolamine." CAS No. 102-71-6. http://www.dow.com/productsafety/finder/tea.htm.

137 Material Safety Data Sheet. "Triethanolamine." CAS No. 102-71-6, EC No. 203-049-8. http://ptcl.chem.ox.ac.uk/MSDS/TR/triethanolamine.html.

138 Material Safety Data Sheet. "Triethanolamine." Account No. 01071, Case No. 102-71-6.

139 US Food and Drug Administration. "Federal Food, Drug, and Cosmetic Act: Chapter II: Definitions." Sec. 201 [21 USC 321]. http://www.fda.gov/opacom/laws/fdcact/fdcact1.htm.

140 National Industrial Chemicals Notification and Assessment Scheme, Department of Health and Ageing, Australia. "Sodium Lauryl Sulfate: CAS No: 151-21-3." 2007 http://www.nicnas.gov.au/Publications/Information_Sheets/Existing_Chemical_Information_Sheets/ecis_SLS_PDF.pdf.

141 Nagel, J.E., Fuscaldo, J.T., Fireman, P. "Paraben Allergy." *Journal of the American Medical Association* 1977;237(15):1594-1595. http://jama.ama-assn.org/cgi/content/abstract/237/15/1594.

142 Routledge, E.J., Parker, J., Odum, J., Ashby, J., Sumpter, J.P. "Some alkyl hydroxy benzoate preservatives (parabens) are estrogenic." *Toxicology and Applied Pharmacology* 1998;153(1):12-19.

143 National Institute of Environmental Health Sciences. "Endocrine Disruptors." 2007. http://www.niehs.nih.gov/oc/factsheets/pdf/endocrine.pdf.

144 Oishi, S. "Effects of propyl paraben on the male reproductive system." *Food and Chemical Toxicology* 2002;40(12):1807-1813.

145 Graham, S. "Ubiquitous Chemical Associated with Abnormal Human Reproductive Development." *Scientific American* May 27, 2005.

146 National Toxicology Program. "Butylparaben: Final Review of Toxicological Literature." CAS No. 94-26-8. http://ntp.niehs.nih.gov/files/Butylparaben.pdf.

147 Harvell, J., Bason, M., Maibach, H. "Contact Urticaria and Its Mechanisms." *Food and Chemical Toxicology* 1994;32(2):103-112.

148 Darbre, P.D., Aljarrah, A., Miller, W.R., Coldham, N.G., Sauer, M.J., Pope, G.S. "Concentrations of Parabens in Human Breast Tumors." *Journal of Applied Toxicology* 2004;24:5-13.

149 Harvey, P., Everett, D. "Significance of the detection of esters of *p*-hydroxybenzoic acid (parabens) in human breast tumours." *Journal of Applied Toxicology* 2004;24:1-4.

150 "In Chocolate, More Cocoa Means Higher Antioxidant Capacity." *ScienceDaily* April 23, 2005. http://www.sciencedaily.com/releases/2005/04/050421234416.htm.

151 "Red Wine's Health Benefits May Be Due in Part to 'Estrogen' in Grape Skin." *ScienceDaily* December 19, 1997. http://www.sciencedaily.com/releases/1997/12/971219062019.htm.

152 Lu, C.Y., Lee, H.C., Fahn, H.J., Wei, Y.H. "Oxidative damage elicited by imbalance of free radical scavenging enzymes is associated with large-scale mtDNA deletions in aging human skin." *Mutation Research* 1999;423(1-2):11-21.

153 National Cancer Institute. "Tea and Cancer Prevention: Fact Sheet." 2002. http://www.cancer.gov/newscenter/pressreleases/tea.

154 Nagao, T. "Ingestion of a tea rich in catechins leads to a reduction in body fat and malondialdehyde-modified LDL in men." *American Journal of Clinical Nutrition* 2005;81(1):122-129. http://www.ajcn.org/cgi/content/abstract/81/1/122.

155 Kuriyama, S., Hozawa, A., Ohmori, K., Shimazu, T., Matsui, T., Ebihara, S., Awata, S., Nagatomi, R., Arai, H., Tsuji, I. "Green tea consumption and cognitive function: a cross-sectional study from the Tsurugaya Project." *American Journal of Clinical Nutrition* 2006;83(2): 355-361. http://www.ajcn.org/cgi/content/full/83/2/355.

156 Baltimore Washington Medical Center. "Skin Wrinkles and Blemishes." 2006. http://health.bwmc.umms.org/patiented/articles/what_causes_wrinkles_000021_1.htm.

157 Ibid.

158 Afaq, F., Malik, A., Syed, D., Maes, D., Matsui, M.S., Mukhtar, H. "Pomegranate Fruit Extract Modulates UV-B–Mediated Phosphorylation of Mitogen-Activated Protein Kinases and Activation of Nuclear Factor Kappa B in Normal Human Epidermal Keratinocytes." *Photochemistry and Photobiology* 2005;81(1):38-45. http://www.bioone.org/perlserv/?request=get-abstract&doi=10.1562%2F2004-08-06-RA-264.1.

159 Ibid.

160 Zhang, Y., Kensler, T.W., Cho, C.G., Posner, G.H., Talalay, P. "Anticarcinogenic activities of sulforaphane and structurally related synthetic norbornyl isothiocyanates." *Proceedings of the National Academy of Sciences of the United States of America* 1994;91(8):3147-3150. http://www.pubmedcentral.nih.gov/articlerender.fcgi?artid=43532.

161 Ibid.

162 Aggarwal, B.B., Bhardwaj, A., Aggarwal, R.S., Seeram, N.P., Shishodia, S., Takada, Y. "Role of Resveratrol in Prevention and Therapy of Cancer: Preclinical and Clinical Studies." *Anticancer Research* 2004;24(5A):2783-2840. http://www.chiroonline.net/_fileCabinet/resveratrol_medicalreview.pdf.

163 Adhami, V.M., Afaq, F., Ahmad, N. "Suppression of Ultraviolet B Exposure-Mediated Activation of NF-χB in Normal Human Keratinocytes by Resveratrol." *Neoplasia* 2003;5(1):74-82. http://www.pubmedcentral.nih.gov/articlerender.fcgi?artid=1502124.

164 "In Chocolate, More Cocoa Means Higher Antioxidant Capacity." *ScienceDaily* April 23, 2005. http://www.sciencedaily.com/releases/2005/04/050421234416.htm.

165 Biello, D. "Forget Resveratrol, Tannins Key to Heart Health from Wine." *Scientific American* November 29, 2006. http://www.sciam.com/article.cfm?articleID=356161C7-E7F2-99DF-3CD9171A34A9BC3F.

166 Schroeter, H., Heiss, C., Balzer, J., Kleinbongard, P., Keen, C.L., Hollenberg, N.K., Sies, H., Kwik-Uribe, C., Schmitz, H.H., Kelm, M. "(-)-Epicatechin mediates beneficial effects of flavanol-rich cocoa on vascular function in humans." *Proceedings of the National Academy of Sciences of the United States of America* 2006;103(4):1024-1029. http://www.pnas.org/cgi/content/abstract/103/4/1024.

167 Allan Woodburn Associates Ltd. "Cotton: The Crop and Its Agrochemicals Market." 1995.

168 United States Department of Agriculture. "Agriculture Chemical Usage: 2003 Field Crop Summary."

169 Organic Consumers Association. "Clothes for a Change: Background Info." http://www.organicconsumers.org/clothes/background.cfm.

170 Swedish Society for Nature Conservation. "The invesitgation of zinc pyrithione in dandruff shampoo: A presentation of the facts." 2004. http://www.snf.se/pdf/rap-hmv-dandruffeng.pdf.

171 Material Safety Data Sheet. "Zinc Pyrithione, 48% Aqueous Dispersion." http://www.sciencelab.com/xMSDS-Zinc_Pyrithione_48_Aqueous_Dispersion-9925493.

172 Ibid.

173 Ibid.

174 US Environmental Protection Agency. "Selenium Sulfide (CASRN 7446-34-6)." http://www.epa.gov/iris/subst/0458.htm.

175 Ibid.

176 US Food and Drug Administration. "Hair Dye Products." 1997. http://www.cfsan.fda.gov/~dms/cos-hdye.html.

177 Ibid.

178 Physical and Theoretical Chemistry Laboratory, Oxford University. "Safety Data for Ammonium Hydroxide," CAS No. 1336-21-6, Annex I Index No. 007-001-01-2.

179 Agency for Toxic Substances and Disease Registry. "Toxicological Profile for Ammonia." CAS No. 766-41-7. 2004. http://www.atsdr.cdc.gov/toxprofiles/tp126.html.

180 Agency for Toxic Substances and Disease Registry. *Interaction Profile for Benzene, Toluene, Ethylbenzene, and Xylenes: Appendix A: Background Information for Benzene.* Atlanta: US Department of Health and Human Services, Public Health Service, 2004. http://www.atsdr.cdc.gov/interactionprofiles/IP-btex/ip05-a.pdf.

181 Ibid.

182 Ibid.

183 Ibid.

184 Ibid.

185 Ibid.

186 Ibid.

187 US Environmental Protection Agency. "Consumer Factsheet on: Benzene." 2006. http://www.epa.gov/OGWDW/dwh/c-voc/benzene.html.

188 US Food and Drug Administration. "Hair Dye Products." 1997. http://www.cfsan.fda.gov/~dms/cos-hdye.html.

189 Agency for Toxic Substances and Disease Registry. "Creosote." CAS No. 8021-39-4, 8001-58-9, 8007-45-2. 2002. 2002. http://www.atsdr.cdc.gov/tfacts85.pdf.

190 US Environmental Protection Agency. "Lead and compounds (inorganic) (CASRN 7439-92-1)." 2007. http://www.epa.gov/iris/subst/0277.htm.

191 Ibid.

192 Ibid.

193 Agency for Toxic Substances and Disease Registry. "Public Health Statement for Lead." CAS No. 7439-92-1. 2007. http://www.atsdr.cdc.gov/toxprofiles/phs13.html.

194 Farley, D. "Dangers of Lead Still Linger." *FDA Consumer* January-February 1998. http://www.cfsan.fda.gov/~dms/fdalead.html.

195 Agency for Toxic Substances and Disease Registry. "Public Health Statement for Lead." CAS No. 7439-92-1. 2007. http://www.atsdr.cdc.gov/toxprofiles/phs13.html.

196 Ibid.

197 Ibid.

198 International Chemical Safety Cards. "P-Phenylenediamine." CAS No. 106-50-3, ICSC No. 0805.

199 Epstein, S.S. "Losing the Cancer War." *The Stop Cancer Before It Starts Campaign: How to Win the Losing War Against Cancer.* Chicago: Cancer Prevention Coalition, 2003. http://www.preventcancer.com/losing/nci/experimental.htm.

200 Kirkland, D.J. "The mutagenicity and carcinogenicity of hair dyes." *International Journal of Cosmetic Science* 1983;5(2):51-71. http://www.blackwell-synergy.com/doi/abs/10.1111/j.1467-2494.1983.tb00326.x?journalCode=ics.

201 Ibid.

202 International Chemical Safety Cards. "P-Phenylenediamine." CAS No. 106-50-3, ICSC No. 0805.

203 Ibid.

204 International Agency for Research on Cancer. "Toluene (Group 3): 5. Summary of Data Reported and Evaluation." CAS No. 108-88-3. 1999. http://www.inchem.org/documents/iarc/vol71/030-toluene.html.

205 National Toxicology Program. "NTP Toxicology and Carcinogenesis Studies of Toluene (CAS No.108-88-3) in F344/N Rats and B6C3F1 Mice (Inhalation Studies)." *National Toxicology Program Technical Report Series* 1990;371:1-253. http://www.ncbi.nlm.nih.gov/sites/entrez?cmd=Retrieve&db=PubMed&list_uids=12692650&dopt=Abstract.

206 Ames, B.N., Kammen, H.O., Yamasaki, E. "Hair Dyes Are Mutagenic: Identification of a Variety of Mutagenic Ingredients." *Proceedings of the National Academy of Sciences of the United States of America* 1975;72(6):2423-2427.

207 Ibid.

208 US Environmental Protection Agency. "Consumer Factsheet on: Toluene." 2006 http://www.epa.gov/OGWDW/dwh/c-voc/toluene.html.

209 Almas, K., Al-Sanawi, E., Al-Shahrani, B. "The effect of tongue scraper on mutans streptococci and lactobacilli in patients with caries and periodontal disease." *Odonto-stomatologie tropicale* 2005;28(109):5-10. http://www.ncbi.nlm.nih.gov/sites/entrez?cmd=Retrieve&db=PubMed&list_uids=16032940&dopt=Abstract.

210 Agency for Toxic Substances and Disease Registry. "Toxicological Profile for Fluorides, Hydrogen Fluoride, and Fluorine." April 1993. http://www.fluoridealert.org/ATSDR-Fluoride.pdf.

211 Hutchings, H.E.P. "Improvements in or relating to rat and other vermin poisons." British Patent GB 187,424, filed September 15, 1921, and issued October 26, 1922.

212 Roark, R.C. "Insecticide." US Patent 1,524,884, filed August 6, 1923, and issued February 3, 1925.

213 US Food and Drug Administration. "Anticaries Drug Products for Over-the-Counter Human Use; Final Monograph; Technical Amendment; Partial Delay of Effective Date." *Federal Register* 61(195):52285-52287. http://www.fda.gov/ohrms/dockets/98fr/96-25599.pdf.

214 Diesendorf, M. "Sustainable development and toxic chemicals: The case of fluoride." *Chemistry in Australia* 2005;January/February:14-16. http://www.raci.org.au/chemaust/docs/pdf/2005/CiAJan-Feb2005p14.pdf.

215 Online Legal Marketing Limited. "Fluoride: To Rinse or Not to Rinse?" 2006. http://www.lawyersandsettlements.com/case/fluoride.html.

216 Centers for Disease Control and Prevention. "Community Water Fluoridation Now Reaches Nearly Two-Thirds of U.S. Population." February 21, 2006. http://www.fluoridationcenter.org/papers/pdf/2002fluoridationcensus.pdf. [press release]

217 National Primary Drinking Water Regulations. "Fluoride." 50 *Code of Federal Regulations* 47, pp. 142-155.

218 Cohn, P.D. "A Brief Report on the Association of Drinking Water Fluoridation and the Incidence of Osteosarcoma Among Young Males."1992. http://www.slweb.org/cohn-1992.html.

219 Agency for Toxic Substances and Disease Registry. "ToxFAQs for Fluorine, Hydrogen Fluoride, and Fluorides." CAS No. 7782-41-4, 7664-39-3, 7681-49-4. 2007. http://www.atsdr.cdc.gov/tfacts11.html.

220 Ibid.

221 Huang, C.M., Wang, C.C., Kawai, M., Barnes, S., Elmets, C.A. "Surfactant Sodium Lauryl Sulfate Enhances Skin Vaccination: Molecular Characterization via a Novel Technique Using Ultrafiltration Capillaries and Mass Spectrometric Proteomics." *Molecular and Cellular Proteomics* 2006;5:523-532. http://www.mcponline.org/cgi/content/abstract/5/3/523.

222 Ibid.

223 Reuber, M.D. "Carcinogenicity of saccharin." *Environmental Health Perspectives* 1978;25:173-200. http://www.pubmedcentral.nih.gov/articlerender.fcgi?artid=1637197.

224 Black, R.E., Hurley, F.J., Havery, D.C. "Occurrence of 1,4-Dioxane in Cosmetic Raw Materials and Finished Cosmetic Products." *Journal of AOAC International* 2001;84(3):666-670. http://www.atypon-link.com/AOAC/doi/abs/10.5555/jaoi.2001.84.3.666.

225 Ibid.

226 US Environmental Protection Agency. "1,4-Dioxane (1,4-Diethyleneoxide)." Hazard Summary. http://www.epa.gov/ttn/atw/hlthef/dioxane.html.

227 National Toxicology Program. "*N*-Nitrosodiethanolamine: CAS No. 1116-54-7." *Report on Carcinogens, Eleventh Edition.* 2005. http://ntp.niehs.nih.gov/ntp/roc/eleventh/profiles/s126nitr.pdf.

228 Breast Cancer Fund. "Cancer-Causing Chemical Found in Children's Bath Products." http://www.breastcancerfund.org/site/pp.asp?c=kwKXLdPaE&b=2483603.

229 National Toxicology Program. "*N*-Nitrosodiethanolamine: CAS No. 1116-54-7." *Report on Carcinogens, Eleventh Edition.* 2005. http://ntp.niehs.nih.gov/ntp/roc/eleventh/profiles/s126nitr.pdf.

230 Reuber, M.D. "Carcinogenicity of saccharin." *Environmental Health Perspectives* 1978;25:173-200. http://www.pubmedcentral.nih.gov/articlerender.fcgi?artid=1637197.

231 Fukushima, S., Uwagawa, S., Shirai, T., Hasegawa, R., Ogawa, K. "Synergism by sodium L-ascorbate but inhibition by L-ascorbic acid for sodium saccharin promotion of rat two-stage bladder carcinogenesis." *Cancer Research* 50(14):4195-4198. http://www.ncbi.nlm.nih.gov/pubmed/2364375?ordinalpos=1887&itool=EntrezSystem2.PEntrez.Pubmed.Pubmed_ResultsPanel.Pubmed_RVDocSum.

232 Bidwell, J., Regan, B. "Saccharin: Regulatory History of Saccharin." 2005. http://enhs.umn.edu/saccharin/reghistory.html,

233 Reisch, M.S. "From Coal Tar to Crafting a Wealth of Diversity." *Chemical and Engineering News* January 12, 1998. http://pubs.acs.org/hotartcl/cenear/980112/coal.html.

234 Tonne, P., Jaedicke, H. "Preparation of Saccharine." US Patent 4464537, filed November 12, 1981, and issued August 7, 1984. http://www.freepatentsonline.com/4464537.html.

235 US Food and Drug Administration. "Food Color Facts." 1993. http://www.cfsan.fda.gov/~lrd/colorfac.html.

236 US Food and Drug Administration. "FDA Public Health Advisory: Reports of Blue Discoloration and Death in Patients Receiving Enteral Feeding Tinted with the Dye FD&C Blue No. 1." September 29, 2003. http://www.cfsan.fda.gov/%7Edms/col-ltr2.html.

237 US Food and Drug Administration, Center for Food Safety and Applied Nutrition. "Summary of Color Additives Listed for Use in the United States in Food, Drugs, Cosmetics, and Medical Devices." 2007. http://www.cfsan.fda.gov/~dms/opa-col2.html#ftnote6.

238 "Artificial food colouring warning." BBC News, May 8, 2007. http://news.bbc.co.uk/2/hi/health/6634071.stm.

239 Lawrence, F. "New fears over additives in children's food." *The Guardian* May 8, 2007. http://www.guardian.co.uk/food/Story/0,,2074346,00.html.

240 US Food and Drug Administration, Center for Food Safety and Applied Nutrition. "Summary of Color Additives Listed for Use in the United States in Food, Drugs, Cosmetics, and Medical Devices." 2007. http://www.cfsan.fda.gov/~dms/opa-col2.html#ftnote6.

241 UK Food Guide. "E129: Allura Red AC, FD&C Red 40." http://www.ukfoodguide.net/e129.htm.

242 Macioszek, V.K., Kononowicz, A.K. "The evaluation of the genotoxicity of two commonly used food colors: Quinoline Yellow (E 104) and Brilliant Black BN (E 151)." *Cellular and Molecular Biology Letters* 2004;9(1):107-122. http://www.ncbi.nlm.nih.gov/sites/entrez?Db=pubmed&Cmd=ShowDetailView&TermToSearch=15048155&ordinalpos=1&itool=EntrezSystem2.PEntrez.Pubmed.Pubmed_ResultsPanel.Pubmed_RVDocSum.

243 "Artificial food colouring warning." BBC News, May 8, 2007. http://news.bbc.co.uk/2/hi/health/6634071.stm.

244 Landa, A.S., Makin, S.A., McKay, V.A. "Anti-microbial antiperspirant products." US Patent 6,893,630, filed January 17, 2001, and issued May 17, 2005.

245 Ibid.

246 Ibid.

247 Barbalace, K. "Periodic Table of Elements: Aluminum." EnvironmentalChemistry.com. 1995-2008. http://environmentalchemistry.com/yogi/periodic/Al.html.

248 Exley, C. "Aluminum in antiperspirants: More than just skin deep." *American Journal of Medicine* 2004;117(12):969-970.

249 Ibid.

250 National Breast Cancer Coalition. "No Proven Link Between Antiperspirant Use and Breast Cancer." 2005. http://www.stopbreastcancer.org/index.php?option=com_content&task=view&id=351&Itemid=170.

251 Pitman, S. "Years on and the debate over aluminum deodorants goes on." CosmeticsDesign.com, March 6, 2006. http://www.cosmeticsdesign.com/news/ng.asp?id=66222-dedorant-aluminum-salts-ctfa.

252 Darbre, P.D. "Metalloestrogens: An emerging class of inorganic xenoestrogens with potential to add to the oestrogenic burden of the human breast." *Journal of Applied Toxicology* 2006;26(3):191-197. http://www.ncbi.nlm.nih.gov/pubmed/16489580.

253 "Potential Link Between Aluminum Salts in Deodorants and Breast Cancer Warrants Further Research." *Medical News Today* March 2, 2006. http://www.medicalnewstoday.com/articles/38619.php.

254 Lima, P.D.L., Leite, D.S., Vasconcellos, M.C., Cavalcanti, B.C., Santos, R.A., Costa-Lotufo, L.V., Pessoa, C., Moraes, M.O., Burbano, R.R. "Genotoxic effects of aluminum chloride in cultured human lymphocytes treated in different phases of cell cycle." *Food and Chemical Toxicology* 2007;45(7):1154-1159. http://www.sciencedirect.com/science?_ob=ArticleURL&_udi=B6T6P-4MSXT97-F&_user=10&_coverDate=07%2F31%2F2007&_rdoc=1&_fmt=&_orig=search&_sort=d&view=c&_acct=C000050221&_version=1&_urlVersion=0&_userid=10&md5=d2ae77fe6219f136ae53828453e7bb71.

255 Ibid.

256 Darbre, P.D. "Aluminum, antiperspirants and breast cancer." *Journal of Inorganic Biochemistry* 2005;99(9):1912-1929.

257 Ibid.

258 Bishop, N.J., Morley, R., Day, J.P., Lucas, A. "Aluminum neurotoxicity in preterm infants receiving intravenous-feeding solution." *New England Journal of Medicine* 1997;336(22):1557-1562.

259 US Food and Drug Administration. "Beverages: Bottled Water." *Code of Federal Regulations* 21 CFR Part 165. November 3, 1995. http://www.cfsan.fda.gov/~lrd/n095-327.txt.

260 Sedman, A. "Aluminum toxicity in childhood." *Pediatric Nephrology* 1992;6(4):383-393. http://hdl.handle.net/2027.42/47831.

261 Deloncle, R., Guillard, O., Clanet, F., Courtois, P., Piriou, A. "Aluminum transfer as glutamate complex through blood-brain barrier: Possible implication in dialysis encephalopathy." *Biological Trace Element Research* 1990;25(1):39-45. http://www.ncbi.nlm.nih.gov/sites/entrez?cmd=Retrieve&db=PubMed&list_uids=1696110&dopt=Abstract.

262 Yokel, R.A. "Blood-brain barrier flux of aluminum, manganese, iron and other metals suspected to contribute to metal-induced neurodegeneration." *Journal of Alzheimer's Disease* 2006;10:223-253. http://www.mc.uky.edu/pharmacy/faculty/files/jad.pdf.

263 Ibid.

264 Perl, D. "Relationship of aluminum to Alzheimer's disease." *Journal of Environmental Health Perspectives* 1985;63:149-153. http://links.jstor.org/sici?sici=0091-6765(198511)63%3C149%3AROATAD%3E2.0.CO%3B2-U.

265 Corrigan, F.M., Reynolds, G.P., Ward, N.I. "Hippocampal tin, aluminum and zinc in Alzheimer's disease." *BioMetals* 2005;6(3):149-154. http://www.springerlink.com/content/758257436878500g.

266 Tatarazako, N., Ishibashi, H., Teshima, K., Kishi, K., Arizono, K. "Effects of triclosan on various aquatic organisms." *Environmental Sciences* 2004;11(2):133-140. http://www.ncbi.nlm.nih.gov/sites/entrez?cmd=Retrieve&db=PubMed&list_uids=15746894&dopt=Abstract.

267 Jones, K.C., de Voogt, P. "Persistent organic pollutants (POPs): State of the science." *Environmental Pollution* 1999;100(1-3): 209-221. http://www.sciencedirect.com/science?_ob=ArticleURL&_udi=B6V5B-3X3BXS6-F&_user=10&_rdoc=1&_fmt=&_orig=search&_sort=d&view=c&_acct=C000050221&_version=1&_urlVersion=0&_userid=10&md5=d52a75f9b64873 1cd94d117bc9a5bcf9.

268 Allmyr, M., Adolfsson-Erici, M., McLachlan, M.S., Sandborgh-Englund, G. "Triclosan in plasma and milk from Swedish nursing mothers and their exposure via personal care products." *Science of the Total Environment* 2006;372(1):87-93. http://www.sciencedirect.com/science?_ob=ArticleURL&_udi=B6V78-4M04J06-1&_user=10&_coverDate=12%2F15%2F2006&_rdoc=1&_fmt=&_orig=search&_sort=d&view=c&_acct=C000050221&_version=1&_urlVersion=0&_userid=10&md5=01c3b6186a2e73608c5cd8236b119bce.

269 Rule, K.L., Ebbett, V.R., Vikesland, P.J. "Formation of chloroform and chlorinated organics by free-chlorine-mediated oxidation of triclosan." *Environmental Science and Technology* 2005;39(9):188A-189A. http://www.ncbi.nlm.nih.gov/sites/entrez?cmd=Retrieve&db=PubMed&list_uids=15926568&dopt=Citation.

270 Latch, D.E., Packer, J.L., Arnold, W.A., McNeill, K. "Photochemical conversion of triclosan to 2,8-dichlorodibenzo-*p*-dioxin in aqueous solution." *Journal of Photochemistry and Photobiology, A: Chemistry* 2003;158(1):63-66.

271 Rule, K.L., Ebbett, V.R., Vikesland, P.J. "Formation of Chloroform and Chlorinated Organics by Free-Chlorine-Mediated Oxidation of Triclosan." *Environmental Science and Technology* 2005;39(9):188A-189A.

272 National Institute of Environmental Health Sciences. "TCDD—Dioxin—Is Listed as 'Known Human Carcinogen' in Federal Government's *Ninth Report on Carcinogens*." January 19, 2001. http://www.niehs.nih.gov/oc/news/dioxadd.htm.

273 Agency for Toxic Substances and Disease Registry. "Toxicological Profile for Chloroform." CAS No. 67-66-3. 1997. http://www.atsdr.cdc.gov/toxprofiles/tp6.html.

274 Latch, D.E., Packer, J.L., Arnold, W.A., McNeill, K. "Photochemical conversion of triclosan to 2,8-dichlorodibenzo-*p*-dioxin in aqueous solution." *Journal of Photochemistry and Photobiology, A: Chemistry* 2003;158(1):63-66.

275 US Environmental Protection Agency. "Dioxin and Related Compounds." 2007. http://cfpub.epa.gov/ncea/cfm/recordisplay.cfm?deid=55264.

276 US Environmental Protection Agency. "Exposure and Human Health Reassessment of 2,3,7,8-Tetrachlorodibenzo-*p*-Dioxin (TCDD) and Related Compounds, National Academy of Sciences (NAS) Review Draft: Part I: Estimating Exposure to Dioxin-Like Compounds. Volume 2: Properties, Environmental Levels, and Background Exposures." 2007. pp. 3-54.

277 Material Safety Data Sheet. "Ethyl Alcohol, 70%." CAS No. 64-17-5. 2001. http://www.nafaa.org/ethanol.pdf.

278 Ibid.

279 Ibid.

280 Ophanswongse, O., Maibach, H. "Alcohol dermatitis: Allergic contact dermatitis and contact urticaria syndrome." *Contact Dermatitis* 1994;30(1):1-6.

281 Ibid.

282 Ibid.

283 Ibid.

284 Material Safety Data Sheet. "Ethyl Alcohol, 70%." CAS No. 64-17-5. 2001. http://www.nafaa.org/ethanol.pdf.

285 Ibid.

286 Ibid.

287 Material Safety Data Sheet. "Talc." CAS No. 014807-96-6, MSDS No. T0026. 2005.

288 Agency for Toxic Substances and Disease Registry. "Asbestos Toxicity: How Are People Exposed to Asbestos?" http://www.atsdr.cdc.gov/HEC/CSEM/asbestos/exposure_pathways.html.

289 Agency for Toxic Substances and Disease Registry. "Asbestos Toxicity: What Respiratory Conditions Are Associated with Asbestos?" http://www.atsdr.cdc.gov/HEC/CSEM/asbestos/physiologic_effects.html#other.

290 Material Safety Data Sheet. "Talc." CAS No. 014807-96-6, MSDS No. T0026. 2005.

291 Ibid.

292 Harlow, B.L., Hartge, P.A. "A Review of Perineal Talc Exposure and Risk of Ovarian Cancer." *Regulatory Toxicology and Pharmacology* 1995;21(2):254-260.

293 Harlow, B.L., Cramer, D.W., Bell, D.A., Welch, W.R. "Perineal exposure to talc and ovarian cancer risk." *Obstetrics and Gynecology* 1992;80:19-26.

294 Agency for Toxic Substances and Disease Registry. "ToxFAQs for Ethylene Glycol." CAS No. 107-21-1. 2007. http://www.atsdr.cdc.gov/tfacts96.html.

295 Ibid.

296 Humane Society of the United States. "Protocols for Embalming Donated Animals." Tufts University, 2001. http://www.educationalmemorial.org/resource_embalming.html.

297 Morshed, K.M., Jain, S.K., McMartin, K.E. "Propylene Glycol-Mediated Cell Injury in a Primary Culture of Human Proximal Tubule Cells." *Toxicological Sciences* 1998;46:410-417. http://toxsci.oxfordjournals.org/cgi/reprint/46/2/410.pdf.

298 Material Safety Data Sheet. "Propylene Glycol MSDS." CAS No.: 57-55-6. 2005. http://www.sciencelab.com/xMSDS-Propylene_glycol-9927239.

299 Perlingieri, I.S. "The Trouble with Tampons." *E/The Environmental Magazine* 2004;15(5). http://www.emagazine.com/view/?2022.

300 Tierno, P.M. *The Secret Life of Germs: Observations and Lessons from a Microbe Hunter.* New York: Pocket Books, 2001.

301 US Environmental Protection Agency. "List of Chemicals Evaluated for Carcinogenic Potential."

302 Organic Consumers Association. "Clothes for a Change: Background Info." http://www.organicconsumers.org/clothes/background.cfm.

303 US Food and Drug Administration. "Office of Science and Technology Annual Report Fiscal Year 1999: Risk Assessment of Dioxin in Tampons." May 2000. http://www.fda.gov/cdrh/ost/reports/fy99/OSTfy99.html#risk_assessment_of_dioxin.

304 Endometriosis Association. "Education Support Research." 2005. http://www.ivf.com/endoassn.html

305 Perloe, M., Christie, L.G. "Endometriosis: Conquering the Silent Invader." *Miracle Babies and Other Happy Endings for Couples with Fertility Problems.* New York: Rawson, 1986. http://www.ivf.com/ch17mb.html.

306 Endometriosis Association. "Toxic Link to Endo." http://www.endometriosisassn.org/environment.html.

307 Rier, S.E., Martin, D.C., Bowman, R.E., Dmowski, W.P., Becker, J.L. "Endometriosis in Rhesus Monkeys (*Macaca mulatta*) Following Chronic Exposure to 2,3,7,8-Tetrachlorodibenzo-*p*-dioxin." *Fundamental and Applied Toxicology* 1993;21:433-441.

308 Endometriosis Association. "Toxic Link to Endo." http://www.endometriosisassn.org/environment.html.

309 Ibid.

310 US Food and Drug Administration. "Tampons and Asbestos, Dioxin, and Toxic Shock Syndrome." 1999. http://www.fda.gov/cdrh/consumer/tamponsabs.html.

311 Ibid.

312 US Food and Drug Administration. "Tampons and Asbestos, Dioxin, and Toxic Shock Syndrome." 1999. http://www.fda.gov/cdrh/consumer/tamponsabs.html.

313 Ibid.

314 National Institute of Environmental Health Sciences. "TCDD—Dioxin—Is Listed as 'Known Human Carcinogen' in Federal Government's *Ninth Report on Carcinogens.*" January 19, 2001. http://www.niehs.nih.gov/oc/news/dioxadd.htm.

315 Agency for Toxic Substances and Disease Registry. "ToxFAQs: Chemical Agent Briefing Sheet (CABS), Dioxins." 2006. http://www.atsdr.cdc.gov/cabs/dioxins/dioxinscabs_route.html.

316 US Food and Drug Administration. "Tampons and Asbestos, Dioxin, and Toxic Shock Syndrome." 1999. http://www.fda.gov/cdrh/consumer/tamponsabs.html.

317 Ibid.

318 Ibid.

319 Mackie, D., Liu, J., Loh, Y.S., Thomas, V. "No Evidence of Dioxin Cancer Threshold." *Environmental Health Perspectives* 2003;111(9):1145-1147.

320 US Environmental Protection Agency. "Dioxin Reassessment: NAS Review Draft 2004." http://cfpub.epa.gov/ncea/cfm/recordisplay.cfm?deid=87843.

321 Perlingieri, I.S. "The Trouble with Tampons." *E/The Environmental Magazine* 2004;15(5). http://www.emagazine.com/view/?2022.

322 Saripalli, Y.V. "The Detection of Clinically Relevant Contact Allergens Using a Standard Screening Tray of Twenty-Three Allergens." *Journal of the American Academy of Dermatology* 2003;49(1):65-69.

323 National Toxicology Program. "Imidazolidinyl Urea: 39236-46-9." http://ntp.niehs.nih.gov/ntp/htdocs/Chem_Background/ExSumPdf/ImidazolidinylUrea.pdf.

324 Ibid.

325 National Toxicology Program. "NTP toxicology and carcinogenesis studies of talc (CAS No. 14807-96-6) (non-asbestiform) in F344/N rats and B6C3F1 mice (inhalation studies)." *National Toxicology Program Technical Report Series* 1993;421:1-287.

326 Hartge P., Hoover R., Lesher L.P., McGowan L. "Talc and ovarian cancer." *Journal of the American Medical Association* 1983;250(14):1844.

327 Rosenblatt, K.A., Szklo, M., Rosenshein, N.B. "Mineral fiber exposure and the development of ovarian cancer." *Gynecologic Oncology* 1992;45:20-25.

328 Harlow, B.L., Cramer, D.W., Bell, D.A., Welch, W.R. "Perineal exposure to talc and ovarian cancer risk." *Obstetrics and Gynecology* 1992;80:19-26.

329 Kabacoff, B.L., Douglass, M.L., Rosenberg, I.E., Levan, L.W., Punwar, J.K., Vielhuber, S.F., Lechner, R.J. "Formation of nitrosamines in non-ionic and anionic emulsions in the presence and absence of inhibitors." *IARC Scientific Publications* 1984;57:347-352.

330 US Food and Drug Administration, Center for Food Safety and Applied Nutrition. "Cosmetic Handbook: 3: Cosmetic Product-Related Regulatory Requirements and Health Hazard Issues: Ingredient Labeling." 1992. http://www.cfsan.fda.gov/~dms/cos-hdb3.html.

331 Material Safety Data Sheet. "Triethanolamine." CAS No. 102-71-6, EC No. 203-049-8. http://ptcl.chem.ox.ac.uk/MSDS/TR/triethanolamine.html.

332 Material Safety Data Sheet. "Triethanolamine." Account No. 01071, CAS No. 102-71-6.

333 Material Safety Data Sheet. "Triethanolamine." CAS No. 102-71-6, EC No. 203-049-8. http://ptcl.chem.ox.ac.uk/MSDS/TR/triethanolamine.html.

334 National Toxicology Program. "Imidazolidinyl Urea: 39236-46-9." http://ntp.niehs.nih.gov/ntp/htdocs/Chem_Background/ExSumPdf/ImidazolidinylUrea.pdf.

335 Ibid.

336 Ibid.

337 Ibid.

# Chapter 6:
# 6 Steps to Eco-Fresh Laundry

1 Seventh Generation. http://www.seventhgeneration.com/our_products/laundry/lavender_laundry.html; http://www.seventhgeneration.com/our_products/laundry/laundry_powder.html.

2 Soto, A.M., Justicia, H., Wray, J.W., Sonnenschein, C. "p-Nonyl-Phenol: An Estrogenic Xenobiotic Released from 'Modified' Polystyrene." *Environmental Health Perspectives* 1991;92:167-173.

3 Ibid.

4 Janitorial Products Pollution Prevention Project. http://www.westp2net.org/janitorial/tools/haz2.htm.

5 Ibid.

6 Ibid.

7 Material Safety Data Sheet. "Sodium Silicate Solution." CAS No. 1344-09-8, MSDS No. S4982.

8 Ibid.

9 Material Safety Data Sheet. "Sodium Silicate Na$_2$O/SiO2." CAS No. 1344-09-8.

10 Material Safety Data Sheet. "Sodium sulfate anhydrous." CAS No. 7757-82-6, ACC No. 21630.

11 Ibid.

12 Ibid.

13 Material Safety Data Sheet. "Sodium Hypochlorite Solution." CAS No. 7681-52-9, MSDS No. S4106.

14 Ibid.

15 Ibid.

16 Main, E. "Cleaner and Greener Laundry." *National Geographic* No. 119, March/April 2007. http://www.thegreenguide.com/doc/119/laundry.

17 US Environmental Protection Agency. "Sodium and Calcium Hypochlorite Salts." EPA 738-F-91-108, September 1991. http://www.epa.gov/oppsrrd1/REDs/factsheets/0029fact.pdf.

18 Ibid.

19 Material Safety Data Sheet. "Decylbenzene sodium sulfonate." CAS No. 68081-81-2.

20 Ibid.

21 Ibid.

22 Material Safety Data Sheet. "Triethylene Glycol (All Grades)." CAS No. 112-27-6.

23 Material Safety Data Sheet. "Triethylene Glycol." CAS No. 112-27-6, MSDS No. T5382.

24 Konishi, N., Donovan, P., Ward, J. "Differential effects of renal carcinogens and tumor promoters on growth promotion and inhibition of gap junctional communication in two rat epithelial cell lines." *Carcinogenesis* 1990;11(6):903-908.

25 Material Safety Data Sheet. "Trisodium Nitrilotriacetate." CAS No. 5064-31-3. http://www.kochmembrane.com/pdf/msds/KOCHKLEEN%20230.pdf.

26 International Programme on Chemical Safety. "Nitrilotriacetic Acid Trisodium Salt (1240)." CAS No. 5064-31-3, RTECS No. MB8400000. May 2003. http://www.ilo.org/public/english/protection/safework/cis/products/icsc/dtasht/_icsc12/icsc1240.pdf.

27 Ibid.

28 Ibid.

29 Seventh Generation. "Optical brighteners." http://www.seventhgeneration.com/household_hazards/glossary.php#O.

30 Tufts University. "How to Save Energy and Money in Your Home." 2005. www.tufts.edu/tie/tci/excel%20and%20word/SaveEnergy.doc.

31 Van Hoof, G., Schowanek, D., Feijtel, T.C.J. "Comparative Life-Cycle Assessment of Laundry Detergent Formulations in the UK. Part I: Environmental Fingerprint of Five Detergent Formulations in 2001." *Tenside Surfactants Detergents* 2003;40(5):266-275. http://www.scienceinthebox.com/en_UK/pdf/TS_20035PartI.PDF.

32  Shea, K., and Committee on Environmental Health. "Pediatric Exposure and Potential Toxicity of Phthalate Plasticizers." *Pediatrics* 2003;111(6):1467-1474.

33  Hu, X.Y., Wen, B., Shan, X.Q. "Survey of phthalate pollution in arable soils in China." *Journal of Environmental Monitoring* 2003;5(4): 649-653.

34  Pace Law School Energy Project. "Power Scorecard." 2000. http://www.powerscorecard.org/reduce_energy.cfm.

35  Centers for Disease Control and Prevention, US Department of Health and Human Services. "Facts about chlorine." March 25, 2005. http://www.bt.cdc.gov/agent/chlorine/basics/facts.asp.

36  US Environmental Protection Agency, Technology Transfer Network, Air Toxics Web Site. "Chlorine." January 2000. http://www.epa.gov/ttn/uatw/hlthef/chlorine.html.

37  International Joint Commission for the Great Lakes. *Global Pesticide Campaigner* 7(4).

38  Occupational Safety and Health Administration. "Occupational Safety and Health Guidelines for Dipropylene Glycol Methyl Ether." CAS No. 34590-94-8. http://www.osha.gov/SLTC/healthguidelines/dipropyleneglycolmethylether/recognition.html.

39  US Environmental Protection Agency. "Flexographic Ink Options: A Cleaner Technologies Substitutes Assessment (Draft): Chapter 3: Risk: Dipropylene Glycol Methyl Ether." CAS No. 34590-94-8. 2000. http://www.epa.gov/opptintr/dfe/pubs/flexo/ctsa/draft/ch3-risk.pdf.

40  Ibid.

41  Ibid.

42  Ibid.

43  Material Safety Data Sheet. "Linear primary alcohol ethoxylate." CAS No. 6839-46-3

44  Ibid.

45  National Institute of Environmental Health Sciences. "1,4-Dioxane CAS No. 123-91-1." Report on Carcinogens, Eleventh Edition. First Listed in the *Second Annual Report on Carcinogens* (1981). http://ntp.niehs.nih.gov/ntp/roc/eleventh/profiles/s080diox.pdf

46  Ibid.

47  Material Safety Data Sheet. "Sodium Dodecylbenzene Sulfonate." CAS No. 25155-30-0.

48  Ibid.

49  Ibid.

50  US Environmental Protection Agency. "Cleaning National Parks: Using Environmentally Preferable Janitorial Products at Yellowstone and Grand Teton National Parks." 2000. EPA/908/R-00-001. http://www.epa.gov/epp/pubs/cleaning.pdf.

51  Physical and Theoretical Chemistry Laboratory, Oxford University. "Safety Data for Ethylene Glycol." CAS No. 107-21-1.

52  Ibid.

53  Ibid.

54  Ibid.

55  Ibid.

56  Material Safety Data Sheet. "Nonoxynol-9 MSDS." CAS No. 26027-38-3 or 127087-87-0. http://www.sciencelab.com/xMSDS-Nonoxynol_9-9926291

57  Ibid.

58  Ibid.

59  Ibid.

60  Material Safety Data Sheet. "Petroleum Distillate." http://www.mcgillairseal.com/textDocs/msds/uniFast.htm.

61  Ibid.

62  Ibid.

63  Ibid.

64  Material Safety Data Sheet. "Sodium Hydroxide." CAS No. 1310-73-2, MSDS No. S4034.

65  Ibid.

66  Ibid.

67  Ibid.

68  US Environmental Protection Agency. "Design for the Environment: Garment and Textile Care Partnership." http://www.epa.gov/opptintr/dfe/pubs/about/index.htm.

69  Environmental Health and Safety Online. "Drycleaning." http://www.ehso.com/ehshome/drycleaningdangers.php.

70  Environmental Health and Safety Online. "Frequently Asked Questions about Drycleaning." http://www.ehso.com/ehsohome/drycleaningfaqs.htm.

71  Proctor, N., Hughes, G. *Chemical Hazards of the Workplace.* Hoboken, NJ: John Wiley, 2004, pp. 564-566.

72  Occupational Safety and Health Administration. "Tetrachloroethylene." CAS No. 127-18-4. http://www.osha.gov/dts/chemicalsampling/data/CH_270620.html.

73  US Environmental Protection Agency. "Chemicals in the Environment: Perchloroethylene (CAS No. 127-18-4)." EPA 749-F-94-020, 1994. http://www.epa.gov/chemfact/f_perchl.txt.

74  Seventh Generation. *Non-Toxic Times* 2(10)

75  Barrows, M.E., Petrocelli, S.R., Macek, K.J., Carroll, J.J. "Bioconcentration and elimination of selected water pollutants by bluegill sunfish (*Lepomis macrochirus*)." *Dynamics, Exposure and Hazard Assessment of Toxic Chemicals.* Ann Arbor, MI: Ann Arbor Science, 1980. pp. 379-392.

76  International Programme on Chemical Safety. "Environmental Health Criteria 31: Tetrachloroethylene." http://www.inchem.org/documents/ehc/ehc/ehc31.htm.

77  Ibid.

78  Correia, Y., Martens, G., Van Mensch, F., Whim, B. "The occurrence of trichloroethylene, tetrachloroethylenes and 1,1,1-trichloroethane in Western Europe in air and water." *Atmospheric Environment* 1977;11:1113-1116.

79  Murray, A., Riley, J. "Occurrence of some chlorinated aliphatic hydrocarbons in the environment." *Nature* 1973;242:37-38.

80  "Dressed to Kill: The Dangers of Dry Cleaning and the Case for Chlorine-Free Alternatives: 3.2: Environmental Fate." http://archive.greenpeace.org/toxics/reports/dtk/dtk.html#Fate.

81  US Environmental Protection Agency, Office of Pollution Prevention and Toxics. "Chemicals in the Environment: Perchloroethylene (CAS No. 127-18-4)." EPA 749-F-94-020, 1994. http://www.epa.gov/chemfact/f_perchl.txt.

82  Ibid.

83  US Environmental Protection Agency. "Frequently Asked Questions about Drycleaning." http://epa.gov/dfe/pubs/garment/ctsa/factsheet/ctsafaq.htm#10.%20November%2010.%20Accessed%20January%2025,%202006.

84  Committee on Source Removal of Contaminants in the Subsurface, National Research Council. *Contaminants in the Subsurface: Source Zone Assessment and Remediation.* Washington, DC: National Academies Press, 2004. http://books.nap.edu/openbook.php?record_id=11146&page=16.

85  Material Safety Data Sheet. "Alpha-Terpineol." Account No. 00855, CAS No. 98-55-5.

86  International Agency for Research on Cancer. "Summaries and Evaluations—Benzyl Acetate (Group 3)." CAS No. 140-11-4. 1999. Vol. 71, p. 1255.

87  National Institute for Occupational Safety and Health. "International Chemical Safety Cards: Benzyl Acetate." ICSC: 1331. http://www.cdc.gov/niosh/ipcsneng/neng1331.html.

88  National Institutes of Health, National Library of Medicine. "Household Products Database: Benzyl Alcohol." CAS No. 100-51-6. http://householdproducts.nlm.nih.gov/cgi-bin/household/brands?tbl=chem&id=142.

89  Ibid.

90  Material Safety Data Sheet. "Chloroform." Account No. 04770. CAS No. 67-66-3.

91  Ibid.

92  Ibid.

93  Ibid.

94  Material Safety Data Sheet. "Dimethyl sulfate." Account No. 41252, CAS No. 77-78-1.

95  Ibid.

96  Ibid.

97  Ibid.

98  Ibid.

99  Kendall, J. "The Health Risks of Twenty Most Common Chemicals Found in Thirty-One Fragrance Products." http://www.herc.org/news/perfume/risks.htm.

100 Material Safety Data Sheet. "Isopropyl alcohol 70% in water." Account No. 89530, CAS No. 67-63-0.

101 Ibid.

102 Ibid.

103 Material Safety Data Sheet. "(-)-Limonene, 92%." Account No. 50173, CAS No. 5989-54-8.

104 Material Safety Data Sheet. "Quaternary Ammonium 10% Solution." MSDS No. CFYDS.

105 Hatcher, M. "Save energy, save money." *Miami Herald* October 3, 2006.

# Chapter 7;
# 4 Corners of a Green Bedroom

1  Kooistra, K.J., Pyburn, R., Termorshuizen, A.J. "The Sustainability of Cotton: Consequences for Man and the Environment." Report 223, 2006, Science Shop Wageningen University and Research Centre. http://www.wur.nl/wewi.

2  Organic Consumers Association. "Clothes for a Change: Background Info." http://www.organicconsumers.org/clothes/background.cfm.

3  Allan Woodburn Associates Ltd. "Cotton: The Crop and Its Agrochemicals Market." 1995.

4  US Environmental Protection Agency. "List of Chemicals Evaluated for Carcinogenic Potential." http://www.epa.gov/pesticides/health/cancerfs.htm.

5  Sustainable Cotton Project. "Cleaner Cotton Campaign Tool Kit." Oroville, CA.

6  Organic Consumers Association. "Clothes for a Change: Background Info." http://www.organicconsumers.org/clothes/background.cfm.

7  Ibid.

8  Physical and Theoretical Chemistry Laboratory, Oxford University. "Safety Information: Formaldehyde Solution." http://ptcl.chem.ox.ac.uk/MSDS/FO/formaldehyde.html.

9  Ibid.

10  Ibid.

11  Ibid.

12  Organic Consumers Association. "Clothes for a Change: Background Info." http://www.organicconsumers.org/clothes/background.cfm.

13  Ibid.

14  Kooistra, K.J., Pyburn, R., Termorshuizen, A.J. "The Sustainability of Cotton: Consequences for Man and the Environment." Report 223, 2006, Science Shop Wageningen University and Research Centre. http://www.wur.nl/wewi.

15  National Institute for Occupational Safety and Health. "A Summary of Health Hazard Evaluations: Issues Related to Occupational Exposure to Isocyanates, 1989 to 2002." U.S Department of Health and Human Services, Centers for Disease Control and Prevention, January 2004. http://www.cdc.gov/niosh/docs/2004-116/pdfs/2004-116.pdf.

16  Ibid.

17  Schecter, A., Papke, O., Staskal, D., Tung, K.C., Rosen, R., Birnbaum, L.S. "PBDE Contamination of U.S. Food and Human Milk, and PBDE, PCDD/F, PCB, and levels in U.S. Human Blood (1973 and 2003)." http://oaspub.epa.gov/eims/xmlreport.display?deid=81527&z_chk=4671&format=print.

18  Environment Canada, Canadian Environmental Protection Act Environmental Registry. "Substances Lists." http://www.ec.gc.ca/CEPARegistry/documents/subs_list/PBDE_draft/PBDE_P3.cfm.

19  Schecter, A., Papke, O., Staskal, D., Tung, K.C., Rosen, R., Birnbaum, L.S. "PBDE Contamination of U.S. Food and Human Milk, and PBDE, PCDD/F, PCB, and levels in U.S. Human Blood (1973 and 2003)." http://oaspub.epa.gov/eims/xmlreport.display?deid=81527&z_chk=4671&format=print.

20  Ibid.

21  Ibid.

22  Cone, M. "Levels of Common Fire Retardants in Humans Are Rising Rapidly." *Los Angeles Times* April 20, 2003.

23  Eriksson, P., Viberg, H., Jakobsson, E., Orn, U., Fredriksson, A. "A Brominated Flame Retardant, 2,2',4,4',5-Pentabromodiphenyl Ether: Uptake, Retention, and Induction of Neurobehavioral Alterations in Mice During a Critical Phase of Neonatal Brain Development." *Toxicology Science* 2002;67(1):98-103. http://toxsci.oxfordjournals.org/cgi/content/abstract/67/1/98.

24  Eriksson, P., Jakobsson, E., Fredriksson, A. "Brominated flame retardants: A novel class of developmental neurotoxicants in our environment?" *Environmental Health Perspectives* 2001;109(9):903-908.

25  Viberg, H., Fredriksson, A., Eriksson, P. "Neonatal exposure to the brominated flame retardant 2,2',4,4',5-pentabromodiphenyl ether causes altered susceptibility in the cholinergic transmitter system in the adult mouse." *Toxicology Science* 2002;67(1):104-107.

26  Kuriyama, S., Chahoud, I. Maternal exposure to low dose 2,2',4,4',5 pentabromo diphenyl ether (PBDE 99) impairs male reproductive performance in adult male offspring. *Organohalogen Compounds* 2003;(61):92-95.

27  Jianzhong, X., Xiaolong, Z., Hongqiang, Q. "Study on the Thermal Stability of Flame Retardant Wools." *Chemistry Magazine* 2004;6(10):74. www.chemistrymag.org/cji/2004/06a074ne.htm.

28  Zhao, D., Little, J.C., Cox, S.S. "Characterizing Polyurethane Foam as a Sink for or Source of Volatile Organic Compounds in Indoor Air." *Journal of Environmental Engineering* 2004;130(9):983-989.

# Chapter 8:
# Energy-Efficient Lightbulbs

1   Natural Resources Defense Council. "Global Warming Basics." http://www.nrdc.org/globalWarming/f101.asp.

2   Energy Star. "Traffic Signals." http://www.energystar.gov/index.cfm?c=traffic.pr_traffic_signals.

3   US Environmental Protection Agency. "Change a Light and Help Change the World." October 26, 2005. http://www.epa.gov/NE/ra/gb/archives/2005/20051026.html.

4   Natural Resources Defense Council. "Global Warming Basics." http://www.nrdc.org/globalWarming/f101.asp.

5   Energy Star. "Light Bulbs and Fixtures." http://www.energystar.gov/index.cfm?c=lighting.pr_lighting.

6   Wald, M.L. "A U.S. Alliance to Update the Light Bulb." *New York Times* March 14, 2007.

7   BBC News. "Bulbs Must Be Efficient by 2009," November 2, 2006. http://news.bbc.co.uk/2/hi/uk_news/politics/6110448.stm.

8   Canadian Press. "Ontario May Ban Old Light Bulbs." February 21, 2007. http://www.ctv.ca/servlet/ArticleNews/story/CTVNews/20070221/ontario_lightbulbs_070221/20070221.

9   CBC News. "Nova Scotia Ponders Light Bulbs Switch." February 28, 2007. http://www.cbc.ca/canada/nova-scotia/story/2007/02/28/ns-lightbulb.html?ref=rss.

10  Ansley, G. "Standard Light Bulbs to Be Switched Off." *New Zealand Herald* February 21, 2007. http://www.nzherald.co.nz/section/1/story.cfm?c_id=1&objectid=10425018.

11  "Levine Legislation to Make California First State in the Nation to Ban Incandescent Light Bulbs." http://democrats.assembly.ca.gov/members/a40.

12  State of Connecticut General Assembly. "Proposed H.B. No. 6550—An Act Concerning Inefficient Incandescent Lamps." http://www.cga.ct.gov/asp/CGABillStatus/CGAbillstatus.asp?selBillType=Bill&bill_num=HB6550.

13  Environmental Defense. "Make the Switch." http://www.environmentaldefense.org/page.cfm?tagid=630&campaign=480.

14  US Environmental Protection Agency. "Save Money While Staying Cool This Summer." May 22, 2006. http://yosemite.epa.gov/opa/admpress.nsf/a8f952395381d3968525701c005e65b5/ed8901928e947a058525717600638d95!OpenDocument.

15  US Environmental Protection Agency. "EPA and Department of Energy Kick-Off Campaign to Save Energy." October 5, 2005. http://yosemite.epa.gov/opa/admpress.nsf/d9bf8d9315e942578525701c005e573c/85cc5d0227b1863685257091004435b7!OpenDocument.

16  Editors of *E/The Environmental Magazine*. *Green Living*. New York: Plume Publishing, 2005.

# Chapter 9:
# Sustainable, Ecological Home Furnishings and Materials

1   National Institute of Environmental Health Sciences. "Endocrine Disrupters." 2007. http://www.niehs.nih.gov/health/topics/agents/endocrine/index.cfm

2   Sakaue, M.S., et al. "Bisphenol-A Affects Spermatogenesis in the Adult Rat Even at Low Dose." *Journal of Occupational Health*. 2001. Vol. 43:185–190.

3   Material Safety Data Sheet. "Petroleum Distillate." http://www.mcgillairseal.com/textDocs/msds/uniFast.htm.

4   Ibid.

5   Ibid.

6   Material Safety Data Sheet. "N-Butyl Acetate." CAS No. 123-86-4. MSDS No. B6184. http://www.jtbaker.com/msds/englishhtml/b6184.htm.

7   Ibid.

8   Ibid.

9   Ibid.

10  Consumer Products Safety Commission. "What You Should Know About Using Paint Strippers." CPSC Document #423. http://www.cpsc.gov/cpscpub/pubs/423.html.

11  Material Safety Data Sheet. "N-Butyl Acetate." CAS No. 123-86-4. MSDS No. B6184. http://www.jtbaker.com/msds/englishhtml/b6184.htm.

12  Material Safety Data Sheet. "Methyl Ethyl Ketone." CAS No. 78-93-3, MSDS No. M4628. http://www.jtbaker.com/msds/englishhtml/m4628.htm.

13  US Environmental Protection Agency. "Methyl Ethyl Ketone (2-Butanone)." Hazard Summary No.: 78-93-9. 1992. http://www.epa.gov/ttn/atw/hlthef/methylet.html.

14  US Environmental Protection Agency, Environmental Criteria and Assessment Office. "Updated Health Effects Assessment for Methyl Ethyl Ketone." EPA/600/8-89/093. 1990.

15  Ibid.

16  Ibid.

17  Agency for Toxic Substances and Disease Registry. "ToxFAQs for 2-butanone." CAS No. 78-93-9, 1995. http://www.atsdr.cdc.gov/tfacts29.html.

18  Physical and Theoretical Chemistry Laboratory, Oxford University. "Safety Data for Ethylene Glycol." CAS No. 107-21-1.

19  Ibid.

20  Ibid.

21  Ibid.

22  US Environmental Protection Agency. "Indoor Air Quality (IAQ): Organic Gases (Volatile Organic Compounds—VOCs)." http://www.epa.gov/iaq/voc.html.

23  Ibid.

24  Ibid.

25  Ibid.

26  Ibid.

27  Ibid.

28  Ibid.

29  Ibid.

30  Cornish Lime Company. "Aglaia Natural Paints and the Environment." http://www.cornishlime.co.uk/html/technical/aglaia_natural_paints.php

31  Material Safety Data Sheet. "Methylene Chloride." CAS No. 75-09-2, MSDS No. M4420. http://www.jtbaker.com/msds/englishhtml/M4420.htm.

32  Material Safety Data Sheet. "N,N-Dimethylformamide." CAS No. 68-12-2, MSDS No. D6408. http://www.jtbaker.com/msds/englishhtml/d6408.htm.

33  Material Safety Data Sheet. "Methylene Chloride." CAS No. 75-09-2, MSDS No. M4420. http://www.jtbaker.com/msds/englishhtml/M4420.htm.

34  Material Safety Data Sheet. "N,N-Dimethylformamide." CAS No. 68-12-2, MSDS No. D6408. http://www.jtbaker.com/msds/englishhtml/d6408.htm.

35  Material Safety Data Sheet. "Methylene Chloride." CAS No. 75-09-2, MSDS No. M4420. http://www.jtbaker.com/msds/englishhtml/M4420.htm.

36  Ibid.

37  Material Safety Data Sheet. "N,N-Dimethylformamide." CAS No. 68-12-2, MSDS No. D6408. http://www.jtbaker.com/msds/englishhtml/d6408.htm.

38  Ibid.

39  Material Safety Data Sheet. "Methylene Chloride." CAS No. 75-09-2, MSDS No. M4420. http://www.jtbaker.com/msds/englishhtml/M4420.htm.

40  Material Safety Data Sheet. "N,N-Dimethylformamide." CAS No. 68-12-2, MSDS No. D6408. http://www.jtbaker.com/msds/englishhtml/d6408.htm.

41  Material Safety Data Sheet. "Methylene Chloride." CAS No. 75-09-2, MSDS No. M4420. http://www.jtbaker.com/msds/englishhtml/M4420.htm.

42  Material Safety Data Sheet. "Methyl Ethyl Ketone." CAS No. 78-93-3, MSDS No. M4628. http://www.jtbaker.com/msds/englishhtml/m4628.htm.

43  Material Safety Data Sheet. "Phenol Reagent A.C.S., Crystal." CAS No. 108-95-2.

44  US Environmental Protection Agency. "Methyl Ethyl Ketone (2-Butanone)." Hazard Summary No. 78-93-9, 1992. http://www.epa.gov/ttn/atw/hlthef/methylet.html.

45  US Environmental Protection Agency, Environmental Criteria and Assessment Office. "Updated Health Effects Assessment for Methyl Ethyl Ketone." EPA/600/8-89/093, 1990.

46  Material Safety Data Sheet. "Phenol Reagent A.C.S., Crystal." CAS No. 108-95-2.

47  US Environmental Protection Agency, Environmental Criteria and Assessment Office. "Updated Health Effects Assessment for Methyl Ethyl Ketone." EPA/600/8-89/093, 1990.

48  Ibid.

49  Material Safety Data Sheet. "Phenol Reagent A.C.S., Crystal." CAS No. 108-95-2.

50  Nemirovskaya, G.B., Emel'yanova, A.S., Ashmyaan, K.D. "Methods of Analysis of High-Wax Crude Oils: Resins, Asphaltenes, Paraffin Waxes." *Chemistry and Technology of Fuels and Oils* 2005;41(3):236-240.

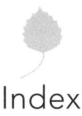

# Index

Underscored page references indicate tables or boxed text.